Strange Allure

Also by Susan Lewis

A Class Apart
Dance While You Can
Stolen Beginnings
Darkest Longings
Obsession
Vengeance
Summer Madness
Last Resort
Wildfire
Chasing Dreams
Taking Chances
Cruel Venus

STRANGE ALLURE

Susan Lewis

WILLIAM HEINEMANN : LONDON

First published in the United Kingdom in 2000 by
William Heinemann

1 3 5 7 9 10 8 6 4 2

Copyright © Susan Lewis 2000

The right of Susan Lewis to be identified as the author of this work has
been asserted by her in accordance with the Copyright, Designs and
Patents Act, 1988

William Heinemann
The Random House Group Limited
20 Vauxhall Bridge Road, London SW1V 2SA

Random House Australia (Pty) Limited
20 Alfred Street, Milsons Point, Sydney,
New South Wales 2061, Australia

Random House New Zealand Limited
18 Poland Road, Glenfield
Auckland 10, New Zealand

Random House (Pty) Limited
Endulini, 5a Jubilee Road, Parktown, 2193, South Africa

The Random House Group Limited Reg. No. 954009
www.randomhouse.co.uk

A CIP catalogue record for this book is available from the British Library

ISBN 0 434 00973 3

Papers used by Random House are natural, recyclable products made from
wood grown in sustainable forests. The manufacturing processes conform to
the environmental regulations of the country of origin

Typeset by SX Composing DTP, Rayleigh, Essex
Printed and bound in Great Britain by Clays Ltd, St Ives plc

For Gary and Jill

Acknowledgements

My gratitude goes to all those who helped with the research on the island of Zanzibar: Raymond Chemah, the management and staff of Fisherman's Resort and of the Mapenzi Beach Hotel.

Most of all my thanks go to Paola Sibilia of the Sultan's Palace Hotel, 00255 811 335828) which is truly exquisite and where the service and exclusivity is second to none. I highly recommend it for a honeymoon, romantic getaway, or pure relaxation after that gruelling safari.

Chapter 1

She sat very still in the aftermath of shock. Seconds passed.
Then, like silvery needles of rain descending on a street lamp,
adrenalin came rushing in, so fast it made her dizzy. Her
heart was thudding in thick, powerful beats of excitement,
then outrage, then relief, then fury. *Thank you God. Oh, thank
you, thank you, God.*

Was she insane? There was nothing to be thankful for here.

So many emotions, it was hard to know how she was
feeling, as they all seemed to shout the truth, and they all *were*
the truth.

Shock returned, rescuing her from the chaos.

She stared at the computer screen for a moment longer.

Then she shouted, 'Sonya! *Sonya!*'

Eddie, the dog, leapt out of a dream, stumbled into the
wall, then came bundling across the room in a flurry of toast-
coloured fur. He was in charge around here, so he needed to
find out what all the fuss was about.

'Are you on fire?' Sonya asked, coming in the door.

'Look at this.' Carla pushed her chair back from the desk,
allowing her sister-in-law room to read the email that was
emblazoned in all its stupefying glory across the screen.

Eddie, from his less advantageous viewpoint, awaited
Sonya's response. As the email consisted of a mere four lines,
it wasn't long in coming.

'Oh my God!' she murmured. 'I don't believe it! *Shit!* Of all
the . . .'

Detecting anger, Eddie growled and moved in closer to
Carla.

Carla looked at Sonya.

1

Sonya looked at Carla, whose normally glowing complexion was, at that moment, starkly white. Her warm, verdant eyes had become vivid lights of confusion; her wide, generous lips were moist, and trembling on the brink of laughter – and horror. The only thing that hadn't changed about her, since Sonya had last seen her, three minutes ago, was her shiny, mahogany hair that waved and curled in its own vain way, refusing ever to look anything but gorgeous, even when tumbling out of a tartan scrunchy as it was now. She even seemed to have lost weight, though Sonya had to concede that probably hadn't happened in the last three minutes.

'What are you going to do?' Sonya asked.

Carla looked at the screen again, and stroked Eddie's ears.

'You're not going to do it?' Sonya cried. 'That man . . .'

'No. *No!* What, do you think I'm insane? Why would I do it?'

Sonya's answer to that was that people did strange things at times, and when confronted by an invitation like this . . .! Well, Sonya knew exactly what she, personally, would do with it, but to her astonishment, and dismay, it seemed that Carla was still making up her mind.

The situation called for a cup of tea.

Ten minutes later Sonya was back with two large glasses of wine. She'd had to run down to the Spar to get it, which was at the other end of the village, and this revolting vintage was all they'd had in the fridge. Teddy Best, who owned the shop, made regular trips across the Channel to get his supplies, and was frequently heard to boast that he'd never yet paid more than eighteen francs a bottle, and Sonya believed him.

When she carried the drinks into the cluttered front room that was Carla's office, it was to find Eddie in his usual position, flat on his back, legs in the air as he honked and snuffled through an apparently erotic dream, while Carla spoke earnestly and rapidly into the phone.

Business as usual.

Putting Carla's wine down on the desk, Sonya sneaked a quick peek at the computer screen. The astounding email had been replaced by a sea of figures – figures that Sonya knew had about as much chance of balancing as a tightrope-walker

2

with no rope. But Carla was known for her optimism, or she had been, once. She'd been known for her easy laughter too, and a quickness of mind that left others reeling. Everyone had loved being around Carla, and those who still knew her, like her family, still did, though she was different now . . .

The other line rang.

'Hello, Carla Craig's office,' Sonya said, taking first the call, then a generous slug of wine. 'Oh, yuk! It's you,' she said, meaning the wine, then her husband. 'Did you pick the kids up from school OK?'

'What?'

Sonya's glass hit the desk. '*Mark!*' she cried, looking at her watch. 'Don't tell me you forgot. My God, you should have been there an hour ago. They've probably been taken into care by now . . .'

'Calm down!' he said, laughing. 'We're all here at home and wanting to know what time to expect you.'

Sonya looked at her watch again, then debated whether or not to tell Mark about the email, and that because of it she would be late back. She glanced over at Carla. Would Carla want her brother to know about the email? Maybe not. Of course, Sonya would tell him anyway, they never had secrets, but she might have to make him swear he didn't know, in the event Carla ended up telling him herself.

'Sonya?'

Remembering the question, she said, 'We're a bit busy here, so I might work on . . .'

Carla was hanging up her call. 'You don't need to do that,' she interrupted. 'There's nothing that can't wait.'

'But what about . . . ?' Sonya nodded towards the computer.

Carla smiled. 'Go home, your family needs you,' she said, in a darkly dramatic voice.

Sonya started to protest again, until she remembered Mark could hear every word. But what about the email? Surely Carla wanted to discuss it. Sonya definitely did.

In the event, Sonya didn't even get to finish her wine – which was no great hardship – for Carla insisted she had to drive over to Trowbridge to see the accountant, and then she was taking Eddie to the vet for his annual injections.

Carla and Eddie stood on the doorstep of their two-up,

two-down cottage watching Sonya drive away, inching reluctantly along the village high street whose cobbles ran raggedly between the dozen or so cottages, all of which had been built in the mid- to late nineteenth century, and created a perfect picture postcard of rural England. Most of the houses were bigger than Carla's, because, over the years, two had been knocked into one, which had inevitably extended the gardens too, and now there were some extremely desirable residences in Cannock Martin, of which hers was not one. Not that she'd have sold, no matter how dire the straits, but nor could she buy either, which was a shame when the cottage attached to hers was for sale. Gilbert Marne, who'd lived there ever since Carla could remember, was now in a nice spick and span nursing home that his daughter had found in Frome, and Carla didn't really expect to get such a gentle and unassuming neighbour again. However, the estate agent wasn't predicting a sale any time soon, for the place was too small, and no-one wanted properties that size any more, no matter how quaint, or great the potential. And Gilbert's didn't have much of that, not with Carla on one side and Maudie Taylor's precious rose garden on the other. And the horse chestnuts at the back were protected, so there was no building out that way either. Of course there was the other reason the house wouldn't sell, but as far as Carla was concerned that was all a lot of superstitious nonsense, for she lived right next door and she'd never heard anyone wailing or singing, nor had she ever spotted anyone coming or going in the dead of night. Eddie hadn't either, because being the alert and sensitive chap he was, he'd have been sure to let the world know if he had.

When Sonya reached the Coach and Horses, which was no more than a stone's throw from Carla's, on the other side of the road, she slowed to wave to Sylvia, the landlady, whose artfully piled curls, and single colour right up to the roots, suggested she'd just got back from Kate's in Radstock, where she went every month to get her hair done.

Sonya's red Fiesta pressed on, around the jutting edge of the duck pond where a fine weeping ash drooped its thin leaves into the weeds; past Teddy's shop, then the smartly clipped privet hedges of the seventeenth-century rectory where Graham Foster the crime writer lived, until she finally disappeared from view behind the old Norman church where the locals claimed King Charles the Second had secretly married Nell Gwyn. Carla didn't know about that, but it was certainly where her grandparents, and her parents had married, and where she and both her brothers had been christened.

Suddenly, the email was right there, at the front of her mind, blocking everything else, and causing her heart to contract with fear. It was drawing her back to a place she just couldn't go, yet there was nowhere else in the world she wanted to be. *Oh dear God, what was this really about? What did it mean?*

She looked up at the sky. It was the colour of stone, seeming to have no depth, or movement, just a stark empty expanse that stretched on and on for ever in a neutral, impenetrable swathe of nothing. Was there actually anything beyond it? The heaven she'd believed in as a child? The place where everyone went, in the end? Fairy tales maybe, but she wanted to know if the dead were there, somewhere, and could see you. What kind of entity were they, after they'd gone? Did they feel anything? Did they know things? Who did they become?

She inhaled sharply, then looked down as a ball bounced softly at her feet. Eddie was gazing up at her. Stooping, she embraced him hard, loving the smell of his shiny coat, and the irregular buttery patches around his chocolatey eyes. His devotion, and curious understanding of her moods, were as soothing as any human embrace and much easier to trust.

She watched him sail over the wall onto the patch of land next to the cottage, in pursuit of the ball. Dumbbell, the cocker spaniel who lived four doors along, suddenly skimmed past the gate and hurtled after Eddie, landing on him as he grabbed the ball, rolling them both over in a riot of leaves and coquettish growls. Dumbbell had a big crush on Eddie, and Eddie, being the male he was, knew it and abused it.

Leaving them to their peculiarly human-style courtship, Carla returned to her desk. One of the windows in the office, that had once been her gran's best room, overlooked the patch of land, so she could keep an eye on Eddie; the other was partly obscured by a lilac bush, the pride of the small garden that separated the cottage from the street.

Putting on the answering machine in case Sonya checked up on her, she returned to the project she'd been working on for the past several months. She couldn't look at the email again yet. It was too demanding of emotions she was unable to control. For now, she needed to reconnect with the reality of her life, to carry on as though nothing was about to change. She pressed a hand to her mouth. Did that mean she was already accepting that change was inevitable?

She picked up the wine Sonya had poured and took a mouthful. It was foul beyond words, but as it was all there was, she braced herself and tried again.

After a while Eddie came trotting back inside and slumped at her feet. She went on with her work, sometimes stopping to feed information into the computer, occasionally checking the reference books she kept at her side. The light faded. She reached out for the desk lamp, which pooled over her papers, and cast the rest of the room, with all its books and files, and the other small desk which Sonya used, into darkness.

Around seven thirty she and Eddie walked over to the pub, where Graham Foster, the writer, already had a lager and black lined up for Carla, and a packet of salt and vinegar for Eddie. There were a few strangers in tonight, tourists as Graham called them, who'd probably driven over from Bath or Bristol. Jack and Sylvia, who ran the pub, were both behind the bar, gossiping with Teddy Best, and occasionally glancing at the TV where someone from *EastEnders* was either working herself up to suicide, or marriage, it was hard to tell.

Though Carla had very few secrets from Graham, whose ruddy, bearded face and steel grey hair had become as dear to her over the years as the features of any member of her family, tonight she didn't trouble his ready paternal concern and patient ear with news of the email. Though there was very little that fazed Graham, there was a good chance this would, and she didn't want his reaction to influence the decision she had to make. Maybe she'd tell him tomorrow, after she'd read it again; by then, if she hadn't already come to a conclusion, she might welcome some advice.

At twenty past eight Graham left to go home, where his

wife was cooking dinner. Betty never came to the pub, nor did she ever speak to any of her neighbours. She was painfully shy, and not at all the kind of wife one would imagine for Graham, considering the quiet flamboyance of his character, and the rather dismaying introversion of hers. Even their physical appearances were a surprising contrast, for he was a tall and handsome man, whereas she was small, plump and unyieldingly plain. However, they'd been together for over two decades, and Carla had never once heard Graham utter a word of criticism or disaffection. If he spoke of her at all, it was always with fondness, and the profoundest respect for her ability to bring out the best in him as a writer. That he had been deeply in love with another woman for several years was well known by all, including Betty, though he had never even suggested leaving his wife, nor had the other woman wanted him to. It was an arrangement that had always worked well, until one day the world had started turning the other way, and everything that was right had suddenly become horribly and frighteningly wrong . . .

Carla was home in time to catch the late news. She and Eddie curled up on the sofa in the cosy little sitting room at the back of the cottage, the only light coming from the flickering images on the TV screen. Another devastating earthquake; another small war; another political scandal; another round of peace-talks. Life went on. Locations changed, languages differed, but the tragedies and stories all stayed the same. So did those who reported them.

Her thumb pressed sharply down on the remote, killing the TV. The room was plunged into darkness. She remained where she was, thinking and trying not to. Feeling and trying not to. Remembering and wishing she couldn't.

Her eyes began adjusting to the darkness, until she could see the old armchair next to the fireplace; the clock on the mantelpiece; the old-fashioned brass-wire fireguard.

She wasn't sure she could stand this. She looked out of the window at the moonlit trees. There was no breeze. Nothing moved. Everything was still. *Mother, where are you?*

She didn't want to go back. If she did, it would mean going through it all again. She'd worked so hard to put it all behind her; to forget and move on. But it seemed the pull of the past

7

was too strong, there was nothing she could do to stop her mind slipping back through time.

She turned to look over her shoulder. Her dark eyes were soft and curious, her breath was shallow. She was no longer at the cottage. She was at home, in London, on a dark, wintry night – one of those nights that made home seem as warm and safe as a womb. A key was going into the front door lock, telling her he was here. She imagined the faint creak of the hinges, then the familiar click of the latch as the door closed. She knew his footsteps. They were coming down the hall of the flat, across the sitting room, towards the bedroom . . .

She waited, her heart heavy with emotion, her skin burning with a very special kind of fear. All around her candles flickered and glowed in the darkness. Her limbs were sensuously oiled, her skin shimmered through the transparent folds that draped them. Scented oils burned in small Eastern pots; her nipples were reddened with henna, her eyes were darkly rimmed in kohl. The crimson satin sheets on which she lay seemed to flow like a river in the sunset; the music touched her senses, desire enfolded her – then engulfed her as the bedroom door opened and his eyes moved through the drifting haze of incense and found her.

For a long time neither of them spoke, as he took her in his arms and kissed her, and stroked her through the chiffon, and looked at her with immeasurable love and desire.

'Welcome home,' she finally whispered.

'If I'd known this was waiting for me I'd have come sooner,' he said. His eyes seemed to drink in every part of her face. 'You're beautiful,' he told her.

'So are you.' To her he was. His wavy, sand-coloured hair, pale blue eyes and harshly weathered skin were as precious to her as the tenderness behind his rough masculinity, as inflaming as the sensitivity that drove his ruthless passion for love. His mind was a constant challenge and stimulation, a questing force for knowledge, an infinite source of intellect and insight. The world, in his presence, was a different place.

He'd been gone for two months – two achingly long months, during which he'd called as often as he could, but it was never often enough. In the three years they'd been together their partings had been frequent, but they never got

8

any easier, they seemed only to get worse.

'Richard,' she said softly.

He lifted his eyes from her breasts, back to her face.

She smiled. Then his lips came crushing down on hers, and she knew that this time there would be no holding back. She helped him take off his clothes, feasting her eyes on the maleness of his body, touching his hardness and wanting him beyond endurance. As he lay down with her she felt that special fear again, the one she always felt when her emotions ran so deep and her need became so strong. It was as though the beauty of what they shared encircled them with a mystery and power that transcended understanding, moving them beyond mere love to a place of such total surrender that there was no longer any knowing where they ended or began.

After they made love they went into the kitchen, cooked a risotto, then opened a bottle of Chianti and returned to bed. The flat they shared was in a quiet side street of Barons Court, West London, with noisy plumbing and lively neighbours. But they were moving in five weeks, over to a smart, leafy square in Chelsea.

As they ate they talked and kissed, and she saw the terrible tiredness in his eyes. He'd just returned from Kosovo, an assignment he'd taken for an American news channel, filing reports from outlying areas as well as the capital. His speciality was danger zones; he'd covered all the major wars, political uprisings and military coups of the past ten years, was very nearly killed in East Timor, and was arrested, tortured and sentenced to death in Baghdad during the crisis in the Gulf. The British government had managed to get him out, but he'd been warned by one of his contacts in Saddam's close circle that there was a fatwa on his head. It didn't stop him living his life the way he always had, though Carla – and British Intelligence – knew about the automatic pistol he carried.

'Now, tell me about you, and what you've been doing,' he said, lifting his fork to her lips and watching her eat. They were sitting cross-legged on the bed, facing each other and wearing nothing but the trays that were balanced on their knees. 'Is the final programme in the can yet?'

'Almost,' she answered. 'We finish editing on Friday. They still haven't given us a transmission date though.'

9

'Why?'

'I don't know. They just keep stalling. It's a travel show, and the economy's not picking up as fast as we thought. People might not be able to afford to travel to quite such exotic places.'

'Is that what they're telling you?'

'It's one excuse. Another is, it's too different. They're not sure where to put it in the schedules. It makes no sense, we didn't have these problems when we were out there raising the money. Everyone seemed to love it then – a travel show that dramatized a country's history, or culture. Actors playing the parts of intrepid explorers, or pilgrim fathers; re-enacting ancient rituals and legends; restaging key battles, pirate attacks, old love stories, classic tragedies, even prehistoric pastimes. We've got it all – and it's cost an absolute fortune, so how the heck they think they're going to get their money back if they don't put the programmes out . . .' She sighed and looked anxiously into his eyes. 'Actually, it's not the BBC that bothers me,' she said, 'it's the private investors who we've approached for a new series of six. If we don't get a transmission date soon, they'll never back us for a second series.'

'Have you thought of going to another company and asking them to buy the BBC out?' he suggested.

She smiled. 'I've got a meeting with Sky on Wednesday. Chrissie's going to speak to someone she knows at Channel Four. If nothing else, it might shake the Beeb up to know we're exploring other avenues. Oh Richard, you're exhausted,' she said as he stifled a yawn. 'Why don't I give you a bath and let you sleep?'

As he lay in the hot, steamy water and she sponged his tired limbs he told her about the informer in Milosevic's inner circle, who'd been tortured and hanged after being followed to a secret rendezvous with Richard. Richard had only just managed to escape, with the help of some fellow journalists. 'But I have to go back there,' he told her. 'The chap had a father, a wife and two daughters. I've got to get them out.'

'Can't someone else do it?' she protested. 'It's too dangerous for you to go back, at least straight away.'

'If I wait it'll be too late. And they're my responsibility. It was me the guy was giving information to, I was the one who was paying him.'

'But what about the intelligence agencies? They've got people who're trained to do that kind of thing.'

'They backed right off the minute the guy was picked up. The family are no use to them, they've already moved on.'

She looked at his handsome face, so ravaged with guilt, and knowing better than to argue any further, she simply said, 'When are you planning to go?'

His eyes moved away from hers. 'I'm not sure,' he answered. 'Soon.'

She pulled him round to face her.

'Bruce Godfrey's still there, he's keeping in touch,' he said.

She gazed deeply into his eyes, all her fears and misgivings gathering such strength inside her they might burst free in a panic. 'One day you're going to go and never come back,' she told him.

'Not true,' he said, stroking her face.

'I just can't bear . . .' She stopped and tried to disguise the dread with a smile. Her mouth made a funny kind of twist, and, laughing, he pulled her into the bath with him.

'We're so much a part of each other, Richard,' she said, lying in his arms. 'If anything happened to you . . .'

'It won't,' he assured her.

She wasn't convinced.

'I promise.'

'Not yours to give,' she reminded him. 'You don't have a say. If death wants you . . .'

'It doesn't. Trust me.'

'But you keep taunting it . . .'

'Stop,' he said, putting a finger over her lips. 'Let's change the subject. What have you been reading while I was away?'

He had a first-class literary mind, with a special love of the French classics – though lately he'd developed an interest in Byzantine verse. Despite her own university education she'd never even heard of these epics until he'd introduced them to her, and she had to confess it was still a struggle trying to remember them now – understanding them was another kind of feat altogether. So should she come clean and tell him she hadn't managed to get very far with *Digenis Akritas*? After all,

11

it was a bit of a stretch believing the chap was already an outstanding warrior by the age of three. But that wasn't the point, and she knew it. It was all allegory and metaphor, and right now she wanted something much more exact, like an assurance that he felt the specialness of the bond between them as keenly, even as painfully sometimes, as she did.

'Don't worry,' he said, 'nothing's going to break us apart,' and she laughed, because in reading her mind he'd just shown her that the power of their love was still working its magic in ways that were much harder to grasp even than the meanings of *Digenis Akritas*.

The next morning Chrissie Fields, Carla's partner and closest friend, was already at her desk in the office they shared in a sunny studio loft over an exotic dance-club in Soho. The club's owner had rented them the space at an exorbitant price, but the location was so perfect, and the enormous room, plus bathroom and kitchen, so unexpectedly bright and welcoming in the midst of Soho's Victorian darkness, that they hadn't even hesitated. The artist who'd occupied the loft before them had painted the walls with huge pastel-coloured waves, creating a rainbow ocean that almost seemed to swell and swirl in the changing light that shone down through the enormous skylight.

In keeping with the airy feel they'd furnished the place with bleached-oak desks, light-coloured filing cabinets and white-painted bookshelves. Posters promoting the six travel programmes they'd made hung from beige linen screens, while dozens of video cassettes, stills photographs, special props and strange location memorabilia were stacked up on the metal-framed shelves that occupied the entire west wall of the room. Carla's and Chrissie's desks were facing each other, just off-centre of the room, with the half-dozen other desks, for the production team's use, spaced evenly round the walls. Currently none of those desks was occupied, and wouldn't be until the second series got under way and a new team was hired. The fear of the moment was that the second series might never get under way.

'You're going to love this,' Chrissie declared, as Carla shrugged off her coat and hooked it on the wrought-iron stand they'd found in Camden market. Because of the weather the loft seemed slightly gloomy this morning, with the rain on the skylight casting eerie blobs of grey shadow over the walls.

'If that was sarcasm leading up to bad news I don't want to hear it,' Carla responded, going to drop her umbrella in the kitchen sink.

Chrissie waited for her to come back, her face almost as beautiful in repose as it was in laughter. At forty she looked closer to thirty, and at five foot eleven she stood closer to God – or she'd certainly been nearby when he was giving out glossy blonde curls, seductively blue eyes, sensuously pouted lips and flawless peachy skin. And she definitely hadn't wandered far afield when he was allocating pert, curvy breasts, superb long legs and tight little bottoms. By the age of twenty Chrissie had already strutted the catwalks of Paris, Milan, Tokyo and New York, and by thirty she was a household name for the various parts she'd played in several TV dramas and two semi-hit movies. However, from there it had gone sharply downhill, when it was revealed that her husband, now ex, had gambled away all their assets, putting them both in the bankruptcy court, then had got himself arrested, and convicted, for raping a seventeen-year-old girl. To cap that, from his prison cell he'd sold the story of Chrissie's drug habit to a Sunday tabloid, claiming she was on everything from blue acid to amyl nitrate to smack. It was all true, she was a mess, and so were most of those she supplied, whom he'd also named. So, with her life and reputation in ruins Chrissie's work had dried up overnight, along with her self-esteem, belief in the world and hope for the future. She had no-one. Her parents were both dead, her husband evidently despised her, and what friends she'd once had rapidly deserted her. Eventually, after a second, and damn near successful, attempt at suicide, a caring female doctor had persuaded her to go into rehab, and three long and difficult years later she had returned to the world, nervous, but eager to make a comeback. It wasn't easy, with no money and nowhere to live, and she might well have been sucked right back into the depths, had a director she'd once known not appeared out of the blue with the offer of a small part in a TV drama that Carla was associate-producing. Despite the ten-year difference in their ages the two had become friends right away, and it was when Chrissie failed to get any other work after the series was over, and Carla decided to take a redundancy pay-off from the TV company, that they'd first come up with the idea of creating their own show.

The initial concept of *There and Beyond*, the travel programme with a difference, had been Carla's, but they'd worked equally hard on nurturing it, shaping it, producing and selling it. Though, as executive producer, Carla held the senior position, they were very much a fifty-fifty partnership, and Chrissie's past fame – and notoriety – as well as her courageous struggle to overcome her adversities had provided them with some useful publicity at the outset, which in its turn had opened more investors' doors than they had even dared hope for. In fact, at the beginning, it had seemed they couldn't go wrong. The money had poured in – and God knew they needed it, for the idea of putting a dramatized insert into each programme, illustrating the chosen country's history or culture, was outrageously expensive. But it was an idea that had captured the imagination of more than one broadcaster, and it hadn't been long before they'd wrapped up a deal with the BBC who, at the time, had promised an early evening transmission on Channel One. Boy, had the champagne flowed that day!

What Carla wanted to know now was, when was it going to flow again? They already had four dozen bottles of it, pyramid-stacked in the fridge, just waiting for that magic day when the programme finally hit the air. In fact, she was staring at it right now, as she took out a carton of milk to lighten her coffee.

'No, it's not bad news,' Chrissie beamed, as Carla came back into the office. 'BA have just come up with an offer of two free flights to Dar es Salaam provided we go next week. From there it's only a short hop over to Zanzibar.'

'Next week!' Carla cried. 'What's the rush? And how did you manage to talk them into that when we don't even know if we've got a second series yet?'

Chrissie shrugged. 'That's their offer. And think of the

location. Zanzibar! That wonderfully exotic mix of east and west cultures, all those harems, and the slave trade . . .'

'You don't have to sell it to me,' Carla laughed. 'I'm all for it. But unless you've got some way of knowing what the future holds . . .'

'I think we should research it anyway.' Chrissie was nothing if not decisive – she was also rash, and Carla had to admit that both characteristics had a good record of paying off.

'You go,' Carla said. 'Get a local tour guide to help you out. I'll man things here, and carry on trying to strongarm some kind of commitment out of the Beeb.'

'That's what I thought you'd say,' Chrissie grinned, 'so I've already reserved my seat. How's Richard, by the way?'

Before Carla could answer Chrissie was reaching for the phone. 'Oh, Jackie Sumner called,' she said, as she started to dial. 'She's got some kind of deal going with a costume place that might work for the next series. Apparently if we give them a credit, they'll hire out for free. I told her you'd get back to her. Hi, it's Chrissie Fields here,' she said into the receiver. 'Can I speak to Funny Sodd?'

Carla laughed.

'Who?' Chrissie said, giving Carla a wink. 'Sogg? Funny Sogg? Oh, Sunny Fogg. That'll be him.' She paused. 'Yes, and that'll be me.'

Carla sat down at her desk and started to unload her briefcase. A couple of minutes later the door opened and Davey, their silken-haired, smooth-tongued Australian assistant, who spent the best part of the day performing miracles of scheduling with his love life, dragged himself in.

'Coffee, drugs, anything will do,' he droned.

'Hi Davey,' Carla said cheerily. 'See you got yourself another early night last night.'

'You're not kidding,' he responded. 'Eight o'clock we went to bed . . .'

Carla smiled. 'Spare me the details. Did you pick up the post?'

He nodded and pulled a handful of letters and junk mail out of his backpack.

Carla looked quickly through. Damn! Nothing from the

Beeb. Well, it was certainly going to shake them up if she and Chrissie managed to get an offer from another broadcaster. Though the question they'd be faced with then was would the BBC sell?

They'd cross that bridge when they came to it.

'Davey, get on to George Biggins and ask him if he can make three more copies of programme five,' she said, turning on her computer. 'That's the one in Thailand. And ask him to do it at the same rate he did the last ones. Oh, and give Margie a call back about the advertising rates in Condé Nast. You'll find them in the usual file. I updated it yesterday.'

'I had another call from Simon Flowers about a launch party,' Chrissie said, hanging up the phone. 'He's still prepared to give us a fifty per cent discount, if we take care of the publicity. I explained that we're still waiting for a transmission date, but he's OK with that. He just wanted us to know that the offer stands.'

'Tell him I love him,' Carla responded, tapping in her password to go online. 'Does he know we've got over a hundred people on the guest list?'

'Yep. Dear God, Davey, what's happened to you? You look horrible.'

'I can't go on like this,' Davey groaned.

'What's her name?' Carla asked, without looking up.

'Sherry.' His handsome face was troubled, his wiry physique was sagging. 'I'm shagged out,' he confessed.

'Aptly put,' Chrissie commented. Then, 'Just out of interest, have you ever gone to bed with a girl without having sex?'

Davey was bemused. 'What?' he grunted. 'Isn't it the same thing, just a different way of saying it?'

Both Carla and Chrissie burst out laughing, which seemed to confuse poor Davey all the more.

Still chuckling, Carla began reading through her email and typing in quick responses. 'When did you say you're going to Zanzibar?' she asked Chrissie.

'Next Tuesday. How long's Richard in the country for this time?'

'Don't ask. At this rate I'll be moving into our new flat on my own.'

'I'd offer to help,' Davey assured her, 'but I'm taking Sherry

16

to Brighton that weekend. When is it, again?'

'You're outrageous,' Carla laughed, throwing a pen at him. 'Has my solicitor called, by the way?'

'Oh yes, she did. Last night, after you'd gone. Said you might be able to exchange a week earlier than scheduled. And the bank called to say that they need your signature on something, so can you go over there. They need Richard's too.'

Carla checked her watch. 'He's probably still asleep,' she said. 'I think it was a pretty rough trip this time.'

'Is he ever going to give it up?' Chrissie asked.

'What do you think? The man's addicted to danger.'

'And you're addicted to him.'

Carla didn't deny it. Of all people, Chrissie knew how close she and Richard were.

'So what are you planning to do while he's here?' Chrissie said.

'We'll probably go down to the country for a couple of days, see my mother and brother and his family. Spend some time just the two of us.'

Chrissie was only half listening, as she went on with her work.

'How's it going with Bob?' Carla asked. 'Any news?'

Chrissie shook her head. 'He's not going to call. He never does. It's always me who ends up calling him.'

'You don't have to,' Carla reminded her. 'In fact, he's such a pig I wish you wouldn't.'

'It's all right for you, not yet thirty with your whole life ahead of you,' Chrissie retorted. 'In my case, I'm going to be forty next month and there isn't exactly an abundance of available men out there, especially not ones as perfect as Richard.'

'There's always me,' Davey chimed in.

'Well, you can't seriously think the Bob thing's going anywhere,' Carla said bluntly, 'so I don't know why you're wasting your time. Damn it, you're a beautiful woman, Chrissie. Absolutely stunning, in fact, with more personality than anyone I know, so why can't you just call it a day with that slimeball and give someone else a chance?'

'Let's get off the subject,' Chrissie replied, a deep flush

17

spreading over the softness of her cheeks. 'I'm going over to the library to see what more I can dig up on Zanzibar.'

After she'd gone Carla regretted being so harsh, though she knew that it was the only way to get through to Chrissie – at least where men were concerned. It was astonishing really, that a woman like Chrissie, who had so much going for her in so many ways, had such disastrously poor taste in men. She just never seemed to get it right, and this Bob character, a photographer from her modelling days, who'd exhumed himself from her past a couple of years ago, was about as disastrous they came. He smoked pot all day, regularly forgot their dates, slept around all over the place, and behaved like he was the greatest gift to womankind, when what he was, in fact, was an abomination to mankind. Carla loathed him, mainly because she was afraid he might entice Chrissie back into the drug scene, for Chrissie's resolve wasn't always as tough as it appeared. With her concern about her age and becoming too old to have children, she was easy prey to any kind of temptation that might make the pain go away.

Around midday, after losing her temper with her contact at the BBC for his pathetic procrastination, Carla called Richard. She'd probably just blown every chance they'd ever had of getting the series transmitted now, but God damn the man, didn't he realize that people had invested good money – not to mention trust – in this series? And what the hell good was it to him, sitting around on a bloody shelf gathering dust? He was never going to make his money back that way. And the season for travel programmes was going to be over before much longer, so if they didn't get it on the air now they'd have to wait another year, by which time all the hotel rates, air fares, and God knew what else they'd quoted, were going to be out of date. And exactly where that left the prospect of a second series was anyone's guess.

Damn the man! Damn! Damn! Damn!

And damn Richard too, for not answering the phone – though it was hardly his fault that she'd just lost it with one of the most powerful men in British television. He was probably still asleep, and being as exhausted as he was might not relish her offloading on him so soon after extricating himself from one of the world's more serious problems. So she left a message for him to get himself over to the bank sometime today, and to let her know if he wanted to eat in or out this evening.

At one o'clock she went to meet a couple of friends for lunch at Mezza, leaving Chrissie a note to remind her that she was supposed to be there too. Several attempts to call Chrissie on her mobile had met with no response, mainly because, as Davey had pointed out, it was lying dead on her desk. Which was much the same state as Carla was going to be in, when Chrissie found out what Carla had just called their contact at the BBC.

'But he deserved it,' Carla explained to Jilly and Rosa over a much-needed glass of Pinot Grigio. 'He's been messing me about and putting me off for months now, and thanks to him it's looking very much as though we're going to miss the boat. Which means all the blood, sweat and tears of the past year and a half have been for nothing, and we can kiss goodbye to any future programmes and start looking for new jobs.'

Rosa Gingell, a thirty-something actress who looked like Ruby Wax on a bad day, made a suggestion. 'You should send Chrissie over there to speak to him personally. Men usually turn to jelly when faced with her. Men like that, anyway.'

'Already tried it,' Carla answered, looking across the crowded restaurant to see if there was any sign of Chrissie yet. 'It almost worked, he gave us a tentative date, then bottled out over the phone. I wonder where she is? Do you think we should go ahead and order? I'm starving.'

Jilly, another actress, who was almost famous for her appearance in a series of low-fat butter commercials, was starving too. 'I swear doing these diet ads is going to be the death of me,' she complained. 'I'm getting so I'm actually *afraid* to eat. Of course, if I was blessed with Chrissie's figure and didn't have to work at it, the way she never does, I could eat anything I wanted. But a girl's got to work, and God forbid I should be the other half of the commercial, the half with the cottage-cheese thighs.'

Rosa said, 'Where did you say Chrissie was? At the library?'

Carla nodded. 'She's off to Zanzibar next Tuesday,

researching for the new series. She claims that going through rehab taught her how to think positively, and all I can say is she must have been a star pupil, because she's determined to go, despite the fact we've got no idea if the programme'll ever get made.'

'I wonder sometimes if she doesn't try too hard,' Rosa commented.

Carla frowned. 'What do you mean?'

Rosa shrugged. 'Just that. She seems to overdo it a bit sometimes, and it ends up looking like a front, something that's not quite real.'

'Oh, I think it is,' Carla corrected. 'In fact, one of the most wonderful and amazing things about Chrissie is that despite how badly she's been treated by so many people in her life, she's just about the most genuine person I know, and she'd almost rather die than ever hurt anyone herself.' The last was a deliberate effort to stop Rosa's bitchiness going any further, but it obviously hadn't worked, for Rosa said, 'If you ask me, she's too generous and kind-hearted for her own good. And she still gets really bad depressions, doesn't she? I mean, now and again?'

'Occasionally,' Carla conceded. 'But she's got it under control.'

'That's good,' Jilly said, 'because I'd hate to think of her suffering again, the way she did before.' She paused, awkwardly, then went on, 'You know, I hate to say it, but whenever I've seen her lately she has seemed a bit low. Does she seem that way to you?'

'No,' Carla answered, feeling guilty that she might not have noticed.

'I've noticed it too,' Rosa chipped in. 'I was with her the night before last, at Susie and Patrick's. She definitely wasn't herself then. She hardly said a word all night.'

Carla was feeling worse than ever. 'She seems all right to me,' she said lamely. 'I mean, probably this transmission business is getting her down, but . . .'

Rosa continued, 'You know, I thought it must be Bob up to his old tricks, but I saw him a few days ago and he said he's been trying to get hold of her for weeks, but she's not returning his calls.'

Carla was confused. 'She's not? But I thought . . . We were just talking about him this morning, she made it sound as though . . .'

'If you ask me, it's the big four-oh,' Jilly said decisively. 'She's always been scared of getting old. And who can blame her? Can't say I'm looking forward to it myself, though I've still got a few years to go.'

'Yes, well, let's just hope that's all it is,' Rosa said, in such a dark tone that the others looked at her in surprise.

'What do you mean?' Carla demanded, trying not to be annoyed.

'Well, there's always a chance she might be, you know, *ill*.'

Carla's face paled. 'What on earth makes you say that?'

'Well, it happens, doesn't it? Women do get sick, especially at her age. I mean, you've only got to look at the breast-cancer rate.'

'Oh Rosa!' Jilly snapped. 'You're always so hung up on people getting ill. If there was anything seriously wrong with Chrissie, especially something like that, then you can rest assured Carla would know.'

'How? If she didn't tell her?'

'I just would,' Carla replied hotly. 'I see her every day, for God's sake. She wouldn't be able to hide something like that.'

'I'd say breast-cancer was pretty easy to hide,' Rosa retorted. 'I mean you can't exactly see it, can you?'

'Don't be obtuse,' Jilly chided. 'Carla's right, she would know if there was anything seriously wrong, even if Chrissie didn't tell her, because she'd be sure to notice when Chrissie's hair started dropping out, which it would if she had cancer and they gave her chemo. Or is it radiation that makes your hair fall out? Whichever, cancer's not something you can keep to yourself, and knowing Chrissie the way I do, well, I'm not saying she'd go round broadcasting it, but she'd definitely tell one of us. No, you mark my words, it's the big four-oh that's getting her down, and the fact that she so desperately wants to have kids.'

Eager to think it was nothing more than that, Carla solemnly picked up her glass, and silently berated Rosa for planting sinister suggestions. In fact, she should know better than to respond, for it was just like Rosa to create doubts and

21

problems where none existed, which was the reason Chrissie had always resisted casting her in *There and Beyond*.

'My God! What's wrong with you lot? Did somebody die?'

'Chrissie!' Carla cried, spilling her wine. 'Are you all right? I was starting to wonder if you'd been hit by a bus.'

'I got engrossed,' Chrissie answered, pulling up a chair. 'Honestly, Zanzibar is just perfect for us. It's *so* fascinating, you're going to love it. I brought a stack of books back with me, and left them on your desk. I'll have a glass of whatever they're drinking,' she said to the waitress.

Carla was looking at her closely, and was relieved to see that she seemed anything but ill.

Evidently Jilly was in agreement. 'You look fantastic,' she told her. 'Have you discovered some secret elixir?'

'She always looks fantastic,' Rosa warmly concurred.

Carla blinked. This was bizarre, considering the conversation they'd been having a minute ago. 'Are you going to eat?' she asked, passing Chrissie a menu.

'No, I grabbed a sandwich on the way back from the library and I'd already eaten it by the time I found your note reminding me about lunch. Incidentally, Richard called while I was in the office to say he can't make dinner tonight, he's got a meeting with someone at *The Times*.'

'Oh bloody hell,' Carla said crossly.

'Don't shoot the messenger,' Chrissie responded, holding up her hands. 'He said you can get him on his mobile if you need to speak to him. So, Rosa, what's new with *Emmerdale*, did you get the part?'

'Still haven't heard,' Rosa answered. 'My agent's away and his assistant's bloody useless.'

As they launched off into the usual round of actor talk Carla sat quietly listening, while still wondering if Rosa's ghastly suggestion that Chrissie was ill might actually be true. Certainly Chrissie didn't look it, but that wasn't necessarily anything to go by, and the fact that Chrissie seemed exactly the same to her as she always did could mean that Chrissie was trying harder with her to hide it. But no, it didn't make any sense. They'd never hidden anything from each other before, and as Chrissie had no close family to speak of, it was always Carla she turned to in times of crisis.

So, discarding the horrible idea of Chrissie's imminent demise, she rejoined the conversation, which had just returned to Chrissie's upcoming trip to Zanzibar.

'Are you going to be able to see this chap at Channel Four before you go?' Carla asked.

'What have you got going with Channel Four?' Rosa bristled, always on the lookout for a part.

'Nothing more than a prayer at the moment,' Chrissie answered. 'Though we do have some money in the kitty towards the next series, which means . . .'

'Enough for about half a programme,' Carla interrupted. 'No use to man nor beast.'

Chrissie's smile faded. 'Are you saying I shouldn't go to Zanzibar?'

'I'm saying that it could be a waste of money,' Carla responded.

'So what, we just give up?'

'No, of course not. We should just be concentrating our efforts on getting the first series on air. Then we can talk about Zanzibar.'

'They're giving me a free flight,' Chrissie reminded her sharply. 'And you said yourself, it'll make a fantastic programme, so let's at least get it researched.'

Carla shrugged. 'OK. If that's what you want.'

Chrissie's eyes were still harsh.

'Don't look at me like that,' Carla laughed. 'I said OK.'

Chrissie relaxed, as a more familiar light returned to her limpid blue eyes.

The subject changed again then, and Carla only fleetingly wondered what Chrissie might have done if she'd really put up a fight about her going to Zanzibar. It seemed Chrissie was pretty determined to go, even though she had to know it would make more sense to wait. However, they rarely fought over anything, and since it really was a great location, Carla had no intention of using her executive-producer's power of veto, if she even had such a thing.

Chapter 2

By the time Carla and Chrissie left the office that evening the rain was bouncing so high off the pavements they were obviously going to get drenched.

'God, will you just look at it,' Chrissie grumbled, putting up her umbrella and standing aside for a raincoated punter to squeeze past into the dance club.

They stood in the doorway, staring dismally out at the solid, honking mass of traffic and madly scurrying commuters. After a while Davey came down to join them and stood there too.

'So,' Carla said finally. 'Who's the lucky girl tonight, Davey?'

'It's Sherry again,' he answered, already sounding depleted. 'The girl's insatiable. Problem is, I'm just too damned good.'

Chrissie grinned. 'Do you ever think of saying no?' she suggested.

'Wouldn't be polite, would it?' he retorted, and, hunching his shoulders, he took off down the shiny wet street towards Shaftesbury Avenue.

Laughing, Chrissie said, 'Where are you going now?'

'Over to the new flat to measure up,' Carla answered. 'Want to come?'

Chrissie shook her head. 'Can't. I'm going out for dinner.' They stood a couple of moments longer, until Chrissie said, 'So, are we going to stand in this doorway all night?'

'Rosa saw Bob,' Carla suddenly blurted. 'He said you weren't returning his calls.'

'What?' Chrissie cried with a laugh. 'Well, that's rich,

coming from him. The bastard hasn't rung me in at least a month. When did he tell her that?'

'Last week, I think.'

'The man's got a short memory, is all I can say. Now, I'm about to brave this rain. Are you coming?'

'Just a minute,' Carla said, taking hold of her arm and stopping her. 'I want to ask you something.'

Chrissie looked startled, then, Carla thought, almost defensive. For some reason it made her nervous. 'If there was anything wrong,' she said softly, 'I mean, you know, if you ... Well, you're OK, are you?'

Chrissie's eyes showed her confusion. 'Of course I'm OK. Why do you think I wouldn't be?'

Carla shrugged. 'It was just that Jilly and Rosa thought you'd seemed a bit down lately, and well, maybe sometimes I get so preoccupied with Richard, you know, worrying about him and everything, that ... You'd tell me, wouldn't you, if there was anything wrong?'

'Of course,' Chrissie said, squeezing her hand. 'You're my closest friend. Who else would I turn to? But there's nothing wrong, I swear.' She smiled, reassuringly. 'Absolutely nothing.'

'So,' Carla said, when ten minutes later they descended into the Underground station, shaking out their umbrellas, while trying to dodge other people's, 'who are you having dinner with?'

'Oh! Uh, my cousin Elaine and her husband. I think we're going to the Ivy. Why don't you join us if Richard's going to be late?'

'No, he's hoping to be back by nine, and God knows I get to see little enough of him as it is. But give Elaine and Don my love.'

Carla would probably have forgotten about the conversation then had she not, to her astonishment, bumped into Elaine on the King's Road a couple of hours later. Carla had just finished measuring up at the new flat, and had popped into the Conran Market to get a few supplies before heading home. Elaine, it seemed, had been carrying out the very same errand.

'But aren't you having dinner with Chrissie?' Carla said,

looking at the delicious deli-prepared meals in Elaine's basket.

'No. What makes you say that?' Elaine replied, looking genuinely confused. Then, clapping a hand to her head, 'My God, don't tell me I arranged it and then forgot.'

'I think you must have,' Carla laughed, 'because she only told me a couple of hours ago that she was having dinner with you and Don tonight.'

Elaine was shaking her head. 'You know that's weird, because I haven't spoken to her in over a week. Maybe Don arranged it and forgot to tell me.'

'That'll probably be it,' Carla said, lifting an arm to wave down a passing taxi. 'Anyway, nice seeing you.'

Carla was almost home before she opened up her mobile phone, and without really knowing why, got a number for the Ivy and called it.

Yes, Chrissie Fields was there, they'd get her to come to the phone.

Carla rang off quickly. She didn't want Chrissie to know she was checking up on her, and why else would she be calling except to say she'd changed her mind and was coming over to join the party. But what party? Who was Chrissie there with, if not Elaine and Don? It was so bizarre to think that Chrissie might have lied, that Carla was already out of the cab and paying the fare before she noticed that the lights were on in the flat. Immediately her heart lightened, for obviously Richard had managed to get home earlier than he'd expected. She was being so keen to see him that the mystery slid effortlessly from her mind as she ran up the stairs to join him.

'What's all this?' she laughed, opening the door to find the table laid out with starched white linen, glinting silver cutlery and flickering candles. 'And what are you cooking? It smells heavenly.'

'The meeting got cancelled,' he told her, coming out of the kitchen to greet her, 'so I thought I'd give you a treat.'

Tall though she was, Carla always felt deliciously swamped by his superior height, and wonderfully feminine in the encompassing fold of his embrace. 'Mmmm,' she murmured after he'd kissed her lingeringly on the mouth, 'I've been thinking about that all day.'

It was all the encouragement he needed to kiss her again.

'You know I hate it so much when you go away,' she told him, feeling incredibly turned on, 'but I can't help wondering if that's what keeps it so good.'

His eyebrows arched. 'You think we couldn't keep it up all the time,' he teased.

'Actually, I think we could,' she replied, and moaned softly as he pressed his erection against her. Then, easing gently out of his arms, she went to take off her coat and change into something a little more appealing than the navy sweatshirt and jeans she'd been in all day.

'How's this?' she said, appearing at the kitchen door a little while later.

He glanced up from the stove, and the look that came into his eyes when he saw her almost melted her bones. 'Oh, Christ,' he murmured. And turning off the gas he came towards her, his eyes burning with desire as they swept over the beauty of her body whose only covering was the same shimmeringly transparent robe she'd worn last night. When he reached her he stood looking down at her, allowing his eyes to speak the words in his heart.

Then he drew her to him, pressing his mouth to hers and pushing his tongue deep inside. 'Can dinner wait?' she asked hoarsely.

'Oh yes,' he answered, and taking her hand he led her back into the bedroom, where she'd already laid out the special sheets they used for this particular kind of love.

After watching her robe slip to the floor, he undressed himself too, then lying her down on the bed he took a long, agonizingly sweet time to coat her entire body in one of the thick, perfumed oils he'd brought back from the East. His hands were hard, and soft, probing and demanding, and maddeningly elusive to the parts she most wanted him to touch. Her nipples throbbed and ached for his fingers; her legs longed to open so that he could fill her full of himself. But it was an almost unendurable time before he finally began the most intimate part of the massage. And when at last her legs were apart and he was rubbing her lovingly with oil, she

27

started to climax with such slow and sensuous contractions that they seemed to spread their pleasure to the very depths of her body and beyond.

Then he was lying beside her, holding her tightly in his arms. He was so hard that she knew if she touched him he would come. And he wasn't ready to yet. She wasn't ready for him to, either. And rolling him on to his back, she spread his arms first, then his legs and after tying his wrists and ankles to each of the bedposts, she began rubbing her body all over his, until he too was covered in the thick, musky oil. Then she knelt over him and gripped the head rail, as she rubbed the flavoured oil he'd massaged between her legs over his face. His tongue moved into her, sharply, commandingly, and she cried out for more – and more.

Then she moved off him, and went to sit between his legs, facing him. She began to caress and fondle herself, showing him all the ways she liked to be pleased. After a while she removed her fingers from herself, and ran them wetly over his penis, down between his legs, then deep into his anus. His eyes closed in unspeakable ecstasy.

Then she swung herself over him, sat astride him and began to ride him towards a climax that he had no way of stopping or controlling. She knew how desperately he wanted to touch her, and yet how powerfully it turned him on to know he couldn't. She rode him hard, knowing he was watching his cock plunging into her. He spoke in harsh, crude words that inflamed her further, then, as they both shuddered into the throes of a tremendous climax, he spoke the most beautiful, lyrical words of love that she had ever heard. And he continued to recite them, fluidly, passionately, then utterly soothingly, as, exhausted, she lay on his chest and closed her eyes.

She might have slept then, she wasn't sure, all she knew was the grumbling of his stomach finally reached her and made her laugh. She eased herself gently from him and stood looking down at him.

'Just think, I could keep you tied up here and never let you go,' she said.

'Do you hear me objecting?'

She smiled, then almost said, 'Do you suppose one day I

might regret not doing just that,' but stopped herself. She had to stop tormenting herself, and him, with so much fear and imagined disaster. If she didn't, then there was every chance that the power of her own thoughts was going to make it happen. He'd told her that. He'd warned her just how effective thought could be. And she knew it, which was why she had to stop doing it.

After they'd showered, they ate dinner and talked about the new flat, which was so ludicrously expensive she could hardly bring herself to think of the price, for despite her modest success she was really a very long way from being able to afford such an exclusive address. Unlike Richard, who'd inherited a large sum of money when his mother had died, and whose earnings were so far and away above Carla's that she doubted she'd ever match up.

'It's not a contest,' he told her, when she brought the subject up. 'It doesn't matter which of us is putting the most into the flat, we're both going to be owning one hundred per cent of it. Well, us and the bank.'

'I know you keep saying that,' she responded, pausing to take the sliver of duck he was offering her, 'but you do understand that if . . .'

'Carla,' he interrupted.

'No, listen. If we can't get it together with a new series . . .'

'I'll take over the repayments completely,' he said. 'Now, when are we going to see your family?'

'The day after tomorrow, I think. I'm trying to push my meeting with Sky on to next week, so we can have a long weekend together. Chrissie's flying to Zanzibar next Tuesday, so I'll have to be back in the office by then. Do you know Zanzibar, by the way? Can you give her any contacts?'

'Never been there,' he said. 'But I'll ask around. Someone's sure to come up with something. How is she, by the way?'

'OK. Well, actually, maybe not. I don't know, something's going on with her that she's not telling me about. At least I think there is.'

'What makes you say that?'

'A couple of things, actually. Rosa and Jilly were talking about her at lunch time, saying she hadn't been herself lately,

29

which I hadn't noticed . . . But then tonight, I think she lied to me about who she's having dinner with.'

'Why would she do that?'

'God knows. And, Rosa, in typical Rosa fashion, has put it into my head that she might be ill, though that hardly explains a secret dinner date. The other theory they came up with is that Chrissie's hitting some kind of mid-life crisis now she's about to turn forty, and I just couldn't bear the idea of her going back into one of her depressions.'

'Forty's not so tough,' he commented. 'Look at me, I'm handling it OK.'

'Only a man could give that response,' she admonished. 'For a woman who wants children and doesn't have a boyfriend, it's tough.'

'What about . . . What's-his-name?'

'Bob. I don't know what's happening there, but God forbid she should ever have children with him. Unless she wants to go it alone, of course, because with Bob Simcoe that's what it would mean.'

He nodded thoughtfully, then, dismissing the subject, he said, 'Did you give notice on this place yet?'

'Yep. The inventory's being done the week we move out. I've managed to get some props guys I know to do the move.'

'We can afford a removal company,' he reminded her.

'I know. But I like doing a deal. And these guys need the work. What are the chances of you being here for the move?'

He thought about it. 'I'd say pretty good. I'm going back in the middle of next week, so I should be out of there by the end of the month.'

Carla's fork was back on the plate, her heart was in free fall. 'Next week!' she cried. 'Oh Richard, I thought you were going to be here at least a fortnight. I mean, apart from everything else I need you here to help organize things, and to give me support with this transmission issue, and to be there when I'm choosing fabrics and furniture . . . All right, all right, don't look at me like that. This Kosovar family's need is greater than mine. I know that. And you owe them. I just wish . . . Well, I just wish I could be really bloody selfish for once and say *I matter too*.'

'You matter most of all,' he said, surprised. 'It's just that your needs are . . .'

'Less urgent, I know. Not even approaching desperate.'

He was smiling, and, resting his chin in his hand, he gazed into her eyes and said, 'I keep asking myself, how did I ever get so lucky? A woman who understands me, loves me and ties me up and fucks me.'

Picking up her wine she took a sip and said, 'Yeah, I'd call that lucky.'

'So when do I get to tie you up and fuck you?'

'Oh, I'd say, round about . . .' She looked at her watch, 'Now.'

Laughing, he brought her mouth to his and kissed her. Then, reaching out for her, he pulled her on to his lap and held her close as he carried on kissing her.

Later, after they'd made love again, they lay in each other's arms, talking for a long time about their future, their pasts, and the extraordinary feeling they both had that maybe they'd known each other before, in another life that had somehow bound them together for all eternity.

He was very good at making it all sound credible, and she was always fascinated by the way he could bring the metaphysical to bear over the mundane. After all, she didn't really love him more than any other woman had loved any other man, it just felt that way. And the feeling that they had arrived on this planet, at this point in time, just to be with each other, was a feeling that millions of other lovers had shared throughout history. She just wished that whenever she compared them to a truly great love story, which she actually believed they were, she didn't always manage to come up with one that had a tragic end.

'If you only see things in terms of this life,' he said, 'then there can never be anything but a tragic end, because we all die, and on the whole we think of death as tragedy.'

'What else is it, if you leave someone behind who loves you?' she asked.

'Maybe a blessing.'

She shook her head. 'Never that.'

He smiled, and, cupping her face in his hand, he said, 'Believe me, there are times, for some, when death is a blessing.'

'Don't,' she whispered, 'it makes me think of all the terrible things they could do to you, if they caught you, because then yes, death would be a blessing.'

Valerie Craig was an attractive woman in her mid-fifties, with dark, bobbed hair, lichen-green eyes and the same startlingly sultry mouth as her daughter's. Also like Carla, she was five foot eight, and in good shape, though was perhaps a little heavier around the hips, and smaller in the bust. By the time Valerie was twenty-five she'd given birth to all three of her children, Mark first, then Greg, then Carla. Her husband, their father, had vanished with his female boss when Carla was only two years old, so Valerie, with the help of her mother, had brought the children up alone. It had never been easy, mainly because money had always been tight, but they'd managed, and perhaps as a result of the hardship they'd always been an extremely close family. At least until Greg had married Eva, an embarrassing social climber from Essex, who deeply resented Greg's relationship with his mother. Over the past several years Eva, or Evil, as Mark and Carla preferred to call her, had managed to make life so unbearable whenever she and Greg came to visit, that it was a relief all round when he'd finally stopped bringing her.

Now Greg only ever came for a couple of hours at Christmas, when Valerie insisted they see each other alone in order to avoid the bitter scenes that invariably erupted whenever he, Carla and Mark were in the same room. Spineless was a word that got thrown around a lot during those visits, along with tart, jealousy, bitch, and a whole lot worse. Mark and Carla were extremely protective of their mother, couldn't bear to think of anything, or anyone hurting her, so it stood to reason that they'd attack Greg and his wife, when it couldn't do anything but hurt Valerie to be virtually estranged from her youngest son.

Five years ago, just after Mark and Sonya's second child was born, Valerie had given them her three-bedroomed house on the outskirts of Bath and moved into the tiny cottage she'd grown up in, where her mother, Beatrice, still lived. Granny was everyone's favourite, for Granny's love of mischief surpassed even that of her grandchildren and great-grandchildren, and it was hilarious watching her being scolded by Valerie, or stuffing herself in a cupboard to hide when Maudie Taylor, the nasty old lady with whiskers, came knocking. It had been a great blow to them all when Granny died, but most of all to Valerie, who still missed her sorely and spoke to her, in her mind, all the time. Now Valerie lived alone at the cottage, and for a long time no-one had understood why she stayed, when the village was in the middle of nowhere and Valerie's part-time work as a nurse in a children's hospital, and intense studies to become a child psychologist, meant she had to make an eighty-mile round trip into Bristol several times a week. Then one Sunday morning, not long ago, while Carla and Richard were on a romantic weekend break in the Cotswolds, they walked right into the reason why when they went down for breakfast and found Valerie and Graham Foster, the crime writer, on the next table, apparently enjoying a romantic interlude themselves.

Of course they'd all known for ages that Graham had a crush on Valerie, heaven knew she took enough teasing about it, but it had never occurred to Carla that her mother might actually be involved in an affair with a married man. *Quel horreur!* The woman who had vowed, repeatedly, that she would never do what had been done to her, was actually sleeping with another woman's husband. However, Graham had been extremely quick to inform Carla and Richard that his wife knew about the affair, and had given it her blessing, so there was no question of deceiving anyone, nor was there any discussion of divorce or marriage, mainly, Valerie insisted, because she'd been a single woman for a long time now, was too used to her independence to give it up, and too afraid that marriage might spoil what she and Graham had.

'And Betty? She really approves?' Carla said, stunned that any wife could.

'Believe it or not, yes,' Graham smiled, taking Valerie's hand in his, though he still appeared anxious about what Carla might be thinking.

'I've talked to Betty myself,' Valerie said, as Carla glanced at Richard to see how he was reacting. 'I don't want to go into the intimate details, but rest assured, we wouldn't be doing this if anyone was getting hurt.'

Looking at Graham's gentle, concerned eyes, Carla thought she could guess the truth, and her heart went out to him, for Betty was probably one of those women who didn't enjoy sex, and was only too happy for her husband to seek his pleasures elsewhere. Carla almost hugged him then, for knowing Graham and how honourable and kind he was, he'd probably never been unfaithful before, had no doubt suffered quietly and with his unfailing dignity for years on end, before Valerie had come into his life. And how happy and youthful they looked together now, the two of them. So happy, it almost brought a lump to Carla's throat.

After that, though Valerie and Graham didn't exactly flaunt their affair, they no longer tried so hard to hide it, and very soon it was as though Graham had become a member of the family, in much the same way as Richard had.

When Carla and Richard arrived at Valerie's late that Friday afternoon, Mark and Sonya's children were already there, and since it was an unusually sunny winter's day they were on the grass next door playing rounders. Valerie was playing with them, so was Eddie, the dog, and since Valerie had Eddie as a fielder she was winning. However, the moment the kids spotted Richard and Carla bats were hurled over shoulders and their two little bodies came haring across the green to be swept up, swung round and roundly embraced. Not to be outdone Eddie was jumping up and down, licking anything he could get his tongue on, then in a final spurt of glee he grabbed his own tail and ran round in circles.

'Where're Mark and Sonya?' Carla asked, finally getting to hug her mother.

Valerie nodded towards an upstairs window. 'Siesta,' she answered.

'Who's Esther?' the five-year-old Kitty wanted to know, much to everyone's amusement. Turning to Richard, Valerie wrapped her arms around him, saying, 'How are you, darling? Welcome home.'

'It's good to see you,' he said, hugging her. 'We've just called in to see my old grandpa, he said you'd been over.'

'Last week,' Valerie confirmed. 'He seems to be doing well.'

'So he should be, with all those women vying for his attention over there,' Richard laughed. Since his grandfather had gone into community housing about twenty miles from the village Valerie had become a more regular visitor than Richard, and in a lot of ways a more welcome one, considering the old boy's eye for the ladies.

'Could you bear to take a look at my thesis later?' Valerie said, as they strolled back towards the green. 'Your comments were really helpful last time.'

'I'd be happy to,' Richard answered, laughing as the children started dragging him off to join their team.

'You've got to play with us,' Courtenay, the seven-year-old, told him. 'And you've got to whack the ball so hard that even Eddie can't find it.'

'You can play on Nana and Eddie's team, Auntie Carla,' Kitty announced. 'It's our innings. Eddie, where d'you put the ball?'

The game went on until well after Mark and Sonya had finished 'seeing Esther', by which time a few more villagers had been roped in to play, then it was all down the pub for lemonade and crisps, and a thousand million pushes on the swings.

Choosing a table next to the roaring log fire, while Richard went to get the drinks, Valerie said, 'I've been thinking about what to get Chrissie for her birthday, and thought maybe we could treat her to a weekend at a health farm.'

'Great idea,' Carla agreed, holding her hands out to the fire. 'I take it you're intending for us to go with her.'

'Of course. How is she, by the way? Did you get to the bottom of that Ivy thing?'

Carla rolled her eyes. 'It turned out to be much what I expected. She was actually meeting Bob, but didn't want to tell me because she's ashamed of the way she lets him treat her. Needless to say he stood her up again.'

'She'd have had some explaining to do if you'd accepted her invitation and gone along,' Valerie remarked.

'With Richard around she knew she was pretty safe. She's off to Zanzibar on Tuesday,' she added, as Richard arrived with their drinks.

'Zanzibar!' Valerie exclaimed. 'How exotic. Now I'm going to embarrass myself by having to ask where it is, exactly?'

'East Africa. Off the coast of Tanzania. Did you get the photos Chrissie sent you, by the way?'

Valerie groaned and laughed. 'I certainly did. Has Richard seen them?'

'Seen what?' he asked, slipping an arm round Carla as he sat down next to her.

'The photos from the ski trip Mum, Chrissie and I went on in February,' Carla answered. 'No he hasn't seen them. They're hysterical.'

'Well, at least she'll go skiing with you,' Richard grumbled. 'I can't get her to come with me.'

'Because you're so brilliant,' she retorted. 'I never get to see you, whooshing your way down the black slopes, while I'm making a total idiot of myself on the end of some gorgeous instructor's training pole. But I'm getting better. Chrissie's terrible. Mum's pretty good, though. She managed to arrive at the bottom twice, still on her feet.'

'Do I stand a chance of getting us all to go together one of these days?' Richard wanted to know.

'I think you could,' Valerie responded.

'We could ask you-know-who if he wants to come too,' Carla suggested.

'What a great idea,' Richard agreed. 'If he skis as well as he writes, I could have some company.'

Valerie's eyes were dancing. 'Sssh,' she warned, glancing round the pub, 'someone might hear.'

'Everyone knows,' Carla reminded her. 'Is he coming in tonight?'

'He should be. If he can get away.'

'What's his wife like?' Richard asked. 'I've never met her.'

'Very unassuming, very shy,' Valerie answered. 'But she's a great support to him with his writing, so much so that I think he's rather come to depend on her now.'

'Are you sure she's not writing them for him?' Richard joked. 'That sort of thing's happened before, when someone's too shy to take the credit.'

Valerie's eyebrows rose. 'You've met him, and fenced your intellectual duels with him, so what do you think?'

36

'Point taken,' Richard conceded, picking up his drink.

'Now, what about you two?' Valerie said, giving a quick wave to a couple of neighbours who'd just come in. 'How's the new flat coming along? I was in London with you-know-who the other day, so we drove past to have a look. My goodness, it's impressive.'

'OK, Mum, we're off now,' Mark said, coming in from the garden where Sonya was attempting to prise her children off the swings. 'You coming over tomorrow?' he asked Richard and Carla.

'Around twelve?' Carla said. 'We'll take a boat trip down the river, shall we? And have lunch in the pub over at Bathampton, provided it's not too cold, or raining.'

'Great. Sonya's seeing to the kids, so I'll say goodnight for her,' and stooping to kiss his mother and Carla, he shook hands with Richard and left just as Richard's mobile phone started to ring.

'I thought you were going to turn it off for the weekend,' Carla grumbled.

'I thought it was off. I'll just take this one call, OK?'

Since the pub was starting to get noisy he took the phone outside, and by the time he came back Graham Foster had arrived, whose wry, wicked sense of humour and warmth of spirit often made Carla wonder what it would be like to have him as a father. It was how he behaved, sometimes stern, always affectionate and unfailingly indulgent. And as he and Richard, with their gigantic intellects, got along like a house on fire, their cosy family image couldn't have been more perfect.

'By the way, who was on the phone earlier?' Carla asked, as she snuggled down next to Richard in her mother's lumpy guest bed later.

'A guy from CNN. He's in Italy, just got out of Kosovo. He's going to meet me next Thursday and come in with me.'

Carla was silent.

He reached out for her hand, and for a while they lay quietly side by side staring out at the moon.

'I'm sorry,' she said finally, 'but I've got such a bad feeling about this.'

'I'll be back by the end of the month,' he whispered.

Again she was silent. The end of the month was less than two weeks away, but it provided no comfort, for her instincts were like those of an animal who might have no idea what the danger was, just that it was imminent and unavoidable. 'Is it out of the question for me to come with you?' she said finally.

'Completely,' he answered. 'You don't know the territory, or the MO. You'll just put us both in danger.'

Of course, she already knew that. The question had been pointless. Almost as pointless as asking him not to go. For a while she toyed with the idea of going to Zanzibar with Chrissie, anything to fill the time until he came back. But someone had to be in the office in case that idiot at the BBC managed to make a decision, and one of Chrissie's fortes was going in first to forge the great deals they would need later when the crew arrived. In the meantime she, Carla, could start roughing out a script. Why not? After all, if Chrissie could think positively about their future, why shouldn't she?

Which meant that she could believe Richard really would come back, and that he would make it by the end of the month. She turned to look at him in the moonlight. 'You know it's because I love you so much that I scare myself like this,' she said.

He smiled. '"Eternity was in our lips and eyes, Bliss in our brows bent,"' he quoted, and kissed her.

Oh God, Antony and Cleopatra – another great love story with a tragic end.

Chapter 3

Chrissie left the following Tuesday; on Thursday Carla drove Richard to the airport. She was in a good mood because one of the executives at Sky was interested in buying *There and Beyond*'s broadcasting rights from the BBC, and it was possible the BBC might agree to sell.

'It's going to be tight,' she told Richard, 'but there's a chance I can tie this up in time to get the series transmitted straight after Christmas. God, I hope so. I can't wait to tell Chrissie.'

'Have you heard from her yet?'

'No. I probably won't, unless there's an emergency, because it costs about ten US dollars a minute to call out from Zanzibar and her mobile's up the shoot. I can fax the local tour operator who's helping her though, if I need to get hold of her. Have you got your mobile? I'll be able to get in touch with you, won't I?'

'It's right here,' he answered, patting a breast pocket. 'It won't be turned on all the time though. But if more than a couple of days go by without us speaking, I'll manage to get hold of you somehow.'

Her heart twisted with unease, but not wanting to dwell on it, she said, 'Shame about Chrissie's phone. I'd like to speak to her, if only to put my mind at rest, because I've got a horrible feeling she's taken that damned Bob with her.'

'What makes you say that?'

'It's just a feeling. But if I'm right, and he's carrying drugs . . . Well, I suppose the best we can hope for is that he only gets himself arrested. Oh great, look at the traffic,' she declared, as they left the M4 and headed towards Terminal 3. 'With any luck you'll miss your flight.'

But of course he didn't, and even if he had, he'd only have taken the next one.

'I cleared out all my old files yesterday, so they're ready for packing,' he told her, as she walked with him towards the departure lounge. 'Be ruthless with the books, I've got far too many, I could do with shedding some.'

'We'll have the space in the new flat,' she reminded him.

He smiled. 'Of course.' Then taking her in his arms, he kissed her tenderly on the mouth.

'Call me when you get to Italy,' she said.

'Of course. I love you.'

He kissed her again, then she stood watching him walk in through the gate, showing his passport and ticket, then turning to wave before he merged in with the crowd.

With Sky's interest in airing *There and Beyond*, and the flat purchase starting to move forward, Carla was kept busy over the next week. Richard rang as regularly as he could, and Chrissie managed a quick shrieked call of congratulation when she received the fax telling her about Sky's fantastic offer that the BBC had now accepted. Carla's fear that Bob was in Zanzibar too was put to rest when she called his London number and he answered, though she started to worry again when she went to collect Chrissie from the airport, and discovered her looking worse than death. Not that she had any real experience of these things, but if she had to imagine the way someone on drugs looked, this would be it.

'I'm sorry,' Chrissie said, leaving Carla to wheel her luggage out to the car, 'it must have been something I ate. I had the most awful flight, I hardly dared leave the loo.'

Carla didn't feel now was the time to ask if she was suffering a relapse, she was too horrified by what it might mean, and thankful that Chrissie had made it through customs without being detected, presuming she was carrying, which please God she wasn't.

'So how was the trip?' Carla asked, when they were in Richard's BMW, heading back into London.

'Fantastic,' Chrissie answered, forcing a smile. 'It's going to be one of our best programmes yet.'

'I've been reading up about it,' Carla told her. 'I've had a few ideas for the dramatizations, but I want to hear yours first.'

Chrissie nodded, and yawned. 'I'll have to get some sleep,' she said. 'By the way, have Sky actually committed to a transmission date?'

'I'm speaking to them later. It's not finalized yet, but I've put Simon Flowers on standby for the launch party, and the publicists are reworking the guest list. Just make sure you get yourself better fast, because it could happen any time.'

Chrissie smiled weakly, and let her head loll back against the seat.

It was two days later that Carla's life fell apart, so completely, and so devastatingly, that nothing, not even her worst nightmares could have prepared her for what was about to happen.

The first blow came just after eight thirty in the morning as she was preparing to leave for work. The flat was a mess with packing boxes everywhere, and the remains of a rushed breakfast still on the kitchen table. She had a meeting with the lawyers at ten to finalize the transfer of broadcasting rights. After that, the six transmission dates through January and February should be set in stone. Chrissie was meeting her at the lawyers', so was a friendly journalist who was going to announce the new deal in that evening's *Standard*. She was so excited she'd hardly slept, and now she was in grave danger of being late if she didn't get out of the door in the next two minutes.

Gulping down the rest of her tea, she made a quick check in the mirror, brushed a couple of stray hairs off her black Hamnett trouser suit, mussed up her hair because it looked better that way, then grabbed her thick winter coat. She was already halfway out of the door when the telephone rang.

'Damn!' she muttered.

She waited, listening to the machine as Richard's voice announced their number and asked whoever it was to leave a message. The bleep sounded, then came the last person she expected to hear: her brother Greg. He never called, ever. She hadn't even realized he knew her number.

Reaching for the receiver she snatched it up, 'Greg. I'm here. What is it?'

'Carla, you'd better sit down,' he said gravely.

A gully of fear instantly opened up inside her. She stayed standing, even when his words reached her and the room started to spin. She tried to speak, but there was no air in her lungs. Her legs were like lead. Dimly she heard him telling her that he was on his way over, but the sound was distanced by the wall of horror that had suddenly risen up around her. At the end of the call she stayed where she was, holding the receiver, until it finally slipped from her fingers and fell to the floor. Then her legs buckled and she sank down onto the edge of a chair.

She was still there, eyes staring sightlessly ahead, heart thudding like a distant drum, when an eternity later there was a knock on the door.

She stood up and went to answer it.

'Can I come in?' Chrissie said.

Carla let go of the door and walked into the sitting room. Everything was wrong. It was as though time had slipped its rails, and the day, as it was only minutes ago, was now on a parallel journey with the one she had been thrown into. Chrissie shouldn't be here. They were supposed to be meeting at the lawyers'. She should be on the train, speeding through the dark, underground tunnels towards High Holborn, not trapped here in this alien other world floundering towards . . . 'Did Greg call you?' she said, her voice croaking. 'Is that why you're here?'

'Greg?' Chrissie repeated. 'Your brother Greg?'

Carla started to speak, but the words wouldn't come. Her hands were icy cold, her heart was like a scythe.

Chrissie watched her, apprehension darkening her eyes. Did Carla already know why she was here? Was that why she was looking so pale, and acting so strangely? But she couldn't know. It simply wasn't possible. 'I know we should be with the lawyers,' she said, 'but . . .' She broke off as Carla fixed her with wide, haunted eyes. Unable to bear it, Chrissie looked away. If she knew, why didn't she say so? 'There's something I have to tell you,' Chrissie said, still unable to look at her.

Carla sat down.

Chrissie sat on the edge of the sofa opposite. 'Oh God,' she suddenly blurted. 'I don't know . . . There's no easy way . . .' She looked at Carla, barely able to see her through the tears swimming in her eyes. She tried to smile, but her mouth shook, and she bit her lips. 'I . . . I'm going to have a baby,' she finally managed.

Carla looked at her. For some reason this didn't seem to be the fantastic news it should be, so she said nothing.

'It's Richard's,' Chrissie said.

Carla continued to stare. The words didn't make any sense. Chrissie hadn't just said that she was carrying Richard's child. Greg's call, and this strange state she was in, had affected her hearing.

'Oh God, I'm sorry,' Chrissie said, starting to cry. 'I wish to God . . . I tried to stop it, we both did . . . But now there's the baby and . . .' She pressed a hand to her mouth. 'Oh Carla, I'm sorry,' she sobbed, 'I'm so, so sorry, but I couldn't go on lying to you, and Richard . . . He feels so bad about hurting you . . . He couldn't bring himself to tell you . . .'

Carla's eyes were unblinking. Suddenly this new day was exploding into a terrifying nightmare beyond anything she could make herself believe. She was being sucked into a spiral of madness and couldn't move to stop it . . .

Chrissie was speaking again, saying something about Kosovo, that he wasn't there, had returned to London . . . 'Oh Carla, I know how much this must be hurting you,' she sobbed, 'but you're my best friend, I can't go on lying to you.'

Carla looked over at the door as someone knocked. Dully she got up to answer it. This time it was Greg.

'Carla? Oh God!' he cried, catching her as she staggered against him.

'It's OK. I'm OK,' she breathed. Her face was ashen, her limbs were shaking. 'I'm ready to go. I'll get my bag.'

She went into the bedroom, leaving her brother alone with Chrissie.

'Hello,' Chrissie said, using her fingers to wipe away the tears as she stood up.

Greg's face was pale, and his eyes were red. 'Hello,' he replied, awkwardly. Then almost as an afterthought, 'Thanks for being here.'

Chrissie was confused, but before she could speak Carla came out of the bedroom.

'OK,' she said to Greg.

'Where are you going?' Chrissie cried, belatedly realizing that something was very wrong with the way they were behaving.

Carla looked at Greg. 'You tell her,' she said brokenly. 'I'll wait in the car.'

As the door closed behind Carla, Chrissie turned in panic to Greg. 'What?' she cried. 'What's happened? Where are you taking her?'

'There's been an accident,' Greg answered. 'Our mother's dead.'

And now here she was, almost a year later, curled up on the sofa in her mother's house with Eddie, still not knowing how she had managed to survive that terrible time. It was probably only thanks to her brothers, and Sonya, that she had. Left to herself . . . Well, she had a pretty good idea what she'd have done, because the pain had been so bad, and her mind so unstable, that for months either Mark or Sonya had stayed with her at the house, afraid to leave her alone.

Tonight was the first time in a while that she had allowed herself to relive those final weeks of her relationship with Richard. In the early months she'd gone over it obsessively, searching for the signs she must have missed, the little nuances or hints that should have warned her what was coming, but she'd never found them, and nor could she now. Right up to the last she had believed utterly in his love, and a part of her, that poor, sad, deluded part that continued to long for him even now, still did. The last words he'd spoken to her, on the phone from Kosovo, were to tell her he'd be home in two days and that he couldn't wait to see her. But of course the call hadn't been from Kosovo, it had been from Zanzibar where he'd been with Chrissie. And he never did come back.

It had taken months to make herself believe that the lies and deception were real. Day after day she called him on the phone, begging him, often hysterically, to come back to her. In the end he refused to speak to her any more, so in a crazed

44

and desperate state she'd driven up to London and banged on their door, screaming and pleading with them to let her in. They must have called Greg, because her brother had come to get her, and take her back to the village.

She hadn't spoken to Richard since that terrible day, nor to Chrissie. The memory of it burned shamefully through her now, but there was no denying how desperately she longed to turn back the clock to a time when she still had her mother; when Chrissie was still her best friend, and Richard wasn't the stranger he was now. She still woke in the night, convinced it was all a dream, but it took only seconds for the terrible truth to engulf her, and then all the bitter, unanswered questions, and raw, battered emotions would trap her in wakefulness till dawn. She thought she'd known him so well, but the man she knew would never have behaved the way he had. The man she loved would never have told such lies about rescuing a family in Kosovo; lies made obscene by how smoothly and movingly they'd been told. And his pretence of loving her – for that was all it could have been, a pretence – was so convincing it had never even occurred to her to doubt it. Yet all the time he was making love to her best friend. For how long, she still didn't know, but it seemed that even as they were planning their future, he'd been planning another with Chrissie. How could he have done that? How could Chrissie? How had either of them faced her, or her family, knowing how treacherously they were betraying her? The pain, the grief, the loss, had all been so harsh they had practically driven her out of her mind, but in the end it was the betrayal that had almost destroyed her. The betrayal, and the dawning realization that the man she had loved so deeply, who she had truly believed was her soulmate, was nothing more than a coward and a liar, who had lacked even the courage to tell her himself that their relationship was over. At least Chrissie had been able to do that. But how she hated Chrissie now. How desperately she wanted to make her pay for getting herself pregnant by the man she knew Carla loved.

Hugging Eddie closer, Carla buried her face in his fur, and let the tears flow. Dear Eddie, he was always there with his comfort, never complaining, no matter how wet she made

45

him, or hard she squeezed. And her grip always got tighter when she thought of Chrissie. Apparently the shock of discovering that she'd told Carla about the baby just minutes after Carla had learned of her mother's death, had almost caused Chrissie to miscarry. Carla could only feel it a shame that she hadn't. She wished nothing good for Chrissie now, she wanted her to know only the pain and grief Carla had felt when she'd lost everything in the world that mattered.

Trying to choke back the tears, she pulled Eddie in closer. The grim comfort of churning up the hatred was only ever short-lived, and as Eddie licked her face she thought of her mother, and how much she had adored this daft, beloved creature. Oh God, she missed her mother. How desperately she had needed her back then to help get her past all that horrible pain – but how desperately she had needed Chrissie and Richard too, to help her over the grief of her mother's futile, senseless death. She'd been out walking Eddie, early in the morning, along a path they all knew well, and was only a few minutes from home. If it hadn't been raining she might only have twisted her ankle, but because the ground at the edge of the bank was wet, it had given way as she fell, so she'd lost her balance and crashed down into the stream where she'd hit her head on a boulder. The blow had killed her outright.

'Oh Mum,' she sobbed. 'Why, oh why, did it have to happen?'

She didn't remember much about the funeral now, probably because, as Sonya had told her later, she'd spent much of that time sedated. She didn't know until a long time after that Richard and Chrissie hadn't even sent their condolences. Under other circumstances they'd have been there, but as it stood they'd cut themselves out of her life completely. They were married now – Richard, who her mind and body still ached for, was married to her best friend. *Oh God, oh God, how could she bear it?* They lived in Chrissie's flat in St John's Wood. Chrissie had given birth to a baby girl earlier in the summer, but Carla didn't know her name, nor did she want to. If she had cable or satellite TV, she'd probably see Richard on the American news from time to time, but she couldn't afford either, and God knew it was bad enough watching any news and knowing he could be there, without the risk of actually seeing or hearing him. Mark and Greg had seen him though, on more than one occasion, for they'd taken charge of her affairs in a way that she had simply been incapable of at the time.

Greg had really come through back then. It was a shame it hadn't lasted and that he was now back under his dreadful wife's thumb so that they hardly ever saw him again. But at the time of their mother's death, when the three of them had needed to grieve together, he had been there. He'd also been the one to extricate Carla from the purchase of the flat in Chelsea, managing to get her entire deposit back, which he'd used to buy Chrissie out of the company. So now Carla owned *There and Beyond*, the first series of which had still to be transmitted, since no-one had completed the deal with Sky. But Greg and Mark had guessed that when the worst of it was over the programme could prove a lifeline for Carla, and in the event, they were probably right. At least it gave a focus to her days now, even though the very thought of returning to London filled her with such dread she never considered it for long.

As for the flat she had shared with Richard, Mark and Sonya had organized the removal of all her possessions, bringing her clothes down to Somerset and putting everything else in storage. Carla had no idea if she'd ever be able to look at any of it again, certainly she wasn't ready to yet. She'd thought she was, for days it had seemed as though she was getting close, but the email she'd received earlier had told her just how far that was from the truth.

It was still there, on the computer, though she had no intention of rereading it now. She didn't need to, she could remember what it said. If she'd looked a little more closely at the sender's address she'd have known right away that it was from Richard, for who else would use the screen name Micromegas, Voltaire's classic piece on the smallness of man in the cosmic scale? Had she realized in time that the message was from him would she have deleted it? She'd like to think so, but knew she wouldn't have. And now she had read it, it had opened up all the pain and hurt again, along with all the confusion and anger. But worse was finding out how deeply she still felt about a man who had deceived her so cruelly.

'Dear Carla,' he had written, 'I hope you are well and recovering from the terrible loss of your mother. I think about you all the time, and both Chrissie and I miss you terribly. It's because of that that we would like you to consider being godmother to our little baby girl, and that way come back into our lives. *Quoi que vous fassiez, écrasez l'infâme, et aimez qui vous aime*. Richard.'

Voltaire again. Whatever you do, stamp out abuses, and love those who love you.

Her heart caught on a fresh wave of pain. It was incredible, inconceivable that he could have written such a message. Stamp out the abuses! Be godmother to their daughter! That he could actually think she would do it was breathtaking in its delusion. He must have lost his mind – or he just didn't have any idea of the extent to which he had hurt her. But how could he not know? He'd seen her pain, he'd heard it, he'd even been afraid to confront it. So how in God's name did he have the audacity to contact her now, with insinuations that his treachery and her heartache were of no importance in the superior scheme of the universe? Stamp it all out and forget? Love those who loved her? Dear God in heaven, didn't he understand the kind of damage he had caused? Was there no awareness of the hatred his duplicity had spawned?

Yet even as the heat of all those bitter memories fermented and boiled in her veins, she was asking herself why they had felt it necessary to invite her back into their lives; what was missing for them that they thought they needed her now? And why had Richard found it necessary to convey his love?

'Oh God, no, no, no,' she cried, squeezing Eddie so tight that this time he squealed. 'How could I even consider believing it after everything I've been through? Why would I even want to?'

Forcing herself up, she went to lock the doors before going to bed. She was never afraid here, but the email had put her on edge and left her feeling, strangely, as though she wasn't alone in the house. She was overemotional, of course, but knowing it was no comfort.

As she went into the old-fashioned kitchen with its cracked-tile surfaces, big china sink and steamy niche windows, her heartbeat was cruel. Eddie was right behind her, seeming to sense he was needed, as she looked at the oak Welsh dresser where photographs of her mother, smiling and loving, looked back at her and brought tears to her eyes. Everything in her ached for her mother. The pain of her loss was so deep it hadn't even begun to heal. She wondered if it ever would.

She moved closer to the Aga for warmth and tried not to think of the fuel it needed – fuel she couldn't afford. Pride wouldn't allow her to admit how desperate she now was for money, not just for the programme she was trying so hard to resurrect, but to live. She'd been a long time without any kind of work that paid, and the small insurance policy that had matured on her mother's death, which had been split between her and her brothers, had been used up months ago. Now all she had was the slim possibility of a cheque from Channel 4, from which the most she could pay herself as a producer was a couple of hundred pounds, plus the small sums she earned as a script-reader for Jed Forsyth, the director who'd helped out her and Chrissie by directing three episodes of *Beyond*'s first series, for next to no money.

Meanwhile, her overdraft was well into five figures, the old Toyota she now drove needed a new gearbox, there was rain coming in through one of the kitchen windows, and if she didn't pay the electricity bill by next Wednesday they were threatening to cut her off.

Night after night she lay awake worrying. And that night proved no exception, for around one in the morning, after no more than two hours' sleep, she was staring despairingly into the darkness. The sound of rain on the roof reminded her of the leaking window. She should go and stuff towels in the cracks, but it was cold and she didn't want to get out of bed. She wanted to lie here and cry enough tears to bring her mother back. Her heart was full, and shuddering with its burden. Her nerves were tense and every sound was making her jump. Outside, at the end of the garden, she could hear the horse chestnuts creaking in a listless wind. An occasional spiky fruit plopped onto the roof of the shed. This was her home. Everything was the same as it always was, nothing had changed, except, since the message from Richard, everything was different, and for some reason she no longer felt safe. He and Chrissie were still out there somewhere, alive and in love, while she was here, hopelessly trapped in the pain of knowing how happy they were, and how afraid she was.

Chrissie stood a few feet from the bath, gazing at the water as it gushed from the tap and turned the fizzing ball of salts to foam. She really had no idea if she had the energy to get in, but she was going to try. For her own sake, as well as Richard's, because there was a chance the hot, scented water might soothe some of the tense exhaustion from her bones. She knew if she asked, Richard would come and bathe her, but would she be able to make love afterwards? Dimly she remembered that this was the point of her taking a bath, to wash away the smell of the baby, and to try to make herself attractive to her husband, whose patience surely had to be running out by now, though he was hiding it well.

The baby was asleep at last, though there was no knowing for how long, and right at that moment Chrissie wouldn't have minded it being for ever. Of course she didn't mean that, but maybe if someone offered her the chance to sleep for ever, she'd take it. Never in her life had she known such tiredness. It crept through her body like a drug, turning her limbs to lead and her brain to dough. Ryan Isabel Mere, who on occasions gurgled and laughed like any other baby, sucked her toes, waggled her fingers, and flirted with her daddy, was, for her mummy, a monster from hell.

That was how it felt when she refused to do anything but scream, morning, noon and night. *Waaah! Waaah! Waaah!* It seemed never to stop, and pushed Chrissie to the brink of madness. One day she was going to go over and it terrified her to think of what she might do. So far it was Ryan herself who kept pulling her back, by reminding her how cute and angelic and adorable she was when she finally settled against the breast and greedily sucked the milk she'd been refusing for hours. But what was going to happen if one day Ryan forgot to be adorable and just went on screaming? Chrissie supposed she just had to believe that the abrupt lapses into sweetness would keep on happening, even though she had no idea what suddenly changed inside Ryan, or what had caused all the screaming in the first place. She'd consulted untold doctors, health visitors, midwives, obstetricians, paediatricians and homeopaths, none of whom had considered there to be a problem, so all Chrissie could conclude was that somewhere, deep inside her baby's subconscious, Ryan hated her.

'Hey, what is it?' Richard said, coming into the bathroom and finding her crying. She tried quickly to pull herself together, but when he took her in his arms and began to rock her, there was nothing she could do to stop the tears. He was so kind and patient, but how fed up he must be by now of finding her in this state. He never said so, but he had to be. Anyone would. The baby's tantrums rarely seemed to bother him, but then he was away such a lot, and Ryan was never as bad with him.

'I'm sorry,' she sobbed. 'I suppose I'm just tired.' She lifted her head and gazed up into his gentle, worried eyes. 'I wanted us to . . . It's been so long.' Then she broke down again. 'I'm such a terrible wife, and a hopeless mother. I can't get any of it right, and I love you both so much . . .'

'Sssh,' he soothed, pressing his lips to her hair. 'We love you too. And there's nothing terrible or hopeless about you. You're doing a wonderful job, with both of us.'

She clung to him tighter and wondered how much longer she could go on like this. When his arms were around her, and he was being as tender and loving as he was now, she felt stronger, more secure, and almost brave enough to ask him the terrible question that burned her heart with its silence. Would he give it up? Stop travelling to distant and dangerous places, so that she didn't have to live half her life in terror of him never coming back? It was so awful, the waiting, the worrying, the constant dread of the phone ringing, then not ringing. And all the time Ryan screaming and crying in the background. How desperately she longed to ask, but what would she do if he said no?

'Come on,' he said, starting to untie her robe.

When she was naked she felt glad of the steam, hoping it would blur the sagging heaviness of her belly, and the silvery puckering around her waist and thighs that was never going to go away. She'd always had such a perfect body, now it was pale, worn out and flabby. Her hair, too, had lost its bounce,

51

and her once lovely shining blue eyes were bloodshot and shadowed almost beyond recognition. How could he desire her like this? What, in God's name, kept him coming back? It had to be Ryan, because no man in his right mind would want her in this state.

She was crying again, unable to stop.

Lifting her in his arms he carried her to the bath and laid her gently down in the water. 'It's OK,' he whispered, starting to sponge her. 'Everything's going to be OK.'

She closed her eyes and prayed for him to be right.

It wasn't until late the following morning that she finally woke up, in bed, with the curtains closed and only a hazy recollection of him lifting her from the bath, drying her, then carrying her to their bed and tucking her in. It wasn't the first time he'd done that, nor was it the first time he'd slept in another room so's not to disturb her.

Dismayed by how she'd let him down again, she pushed back the covers and swung her legs over the edge of the bed. The house was quiet, the only noise coming from the muted hum of the traffic as it roared up and down the distant main road. Going to the window she peered out at the rain-soaked gardens that formed the centre of their exclusive Knightsbridge square. The smart town houses were three-storey Regency dwellings, with a secluded mews at one end, and another garden square at the other. They'd been here for six months now, in this beautiful home, with its blue front door, black railings, white stucco front and large, high-ceilinged rooms.

Everyone had said she was crazy moving while she was suffering such a difficult pregnancy, but worse would have been continuing to live with the fear that Carla might turn up any minute and start threatening her again. God knew she understood Carla's pain, she didn't even blame her for wanting to kill her, but by the sixth month of her pregnancy Chrissie just hadn't been able to cope with it any more. Anyone who would listen knew how agonized she felt about falling in love with Richard, and how desperately she wished it hadn't happened, but it had, and in the end there just hadn't been a way to spare Carla all the pain she had gone through. Chrissie had tried a hundred times to tell her how sorry she was, how she'd never meant it to happen, but Carla had never been in a calm enough state to listen. And who could blame her for that, when she'd lost her mother the way she had, and when the terrible, terrible timing of Chrissie's visit that morning had sent Chrissie over the edge too?

Chrissie wasn't sure now whether it had been her or Richard's idea to move, but once the subject was raised it hadn't taken long to find this house, and as far as Chrissie knew Carla still didn't know where they were. It had been awful asking all their friends who might still be in touch with Carla not to reveal their new address, for it had felt like a whole new betrayal on top of the one they had already committed. Even worse was finding out that virtually no-one was in touch with Carla now, though not because they hadn't tried, but because Carla didn't want it. It made Chrissie's heart ache to think of her all alone in that cottage, cut off from the world she had known, estranged from the friends she had trusted, probably afraid now of trusting anyone ever again. The isolation was almost certainly a way of protecting herself from any more hurt, like hearing someone tell her how close Chrissie and Richard were, or how they'd been seeing each other for almost a year before Carla had been told. But no-one knew that, possibly not even Carla, because she'd never asked and Chrissie had seen no reason to tell her. And, as time went on, Carla would have been afraid of hearing about the birth of the baby, or how proud Chrissie and Richard were of their beautiful daughter. It would all be much too painful, and Chrissie knew that the day would never come when Carla would welcome any news of her and Richard.

Unless, of course, Richard himself delivered it. The very thought of him being in touch with Carla made Chrissie feel sick, for she could easily guess what he would say: that his marriage to Chrissie was a mess, and would never even have happened had she not forced him into it by getting pregnant. It wasn't true, she hadn't done it on purpose, at least not consciously, but looking back . . . Maybe she had always been this afraid of losing him. Maybe she really had believed that having his baby was the only way to sever the bond between him and Carla. God knew she hadn't wanted to hurt Carla, but how was she to avoid it when she loved Richard so much herself? Never in her entire life had she known a man who could make her feel so adored, and special, and necessary to his existence, as Richard could. For her there had been only pain and rejection and the most brutal betrayals. Twice she had tried to take her own life, terrified that the future might hold even worse than she'd already known. Not until she'd met Carla and they'd begun developing their programme had she dared to start believing that life might be worth living again. It was Carla who had turned everything around, who had shown her what a success they could make of their lives, and what triumph could be theirs if they dispensed with caution and believed in themselves and their dreams. Carla, with all her confidence and spirit, her energy and ambition, the laughter that was so infectious, and passion that was so inspiring. She was always exhilarating to be around, so demanding of herself and others, yet so generous too, with her affections, her praise and most of all with the way she drew those she cared for into her family and gave them a sense of belonging, the way she had with Chrissie.

And stealing Richard was the way Chrissie had repaid her.

Would the guilt ever go away? Would there ever come a day when Carla might forgive her? It was hard to imagine, almost as hard as conquering the fear that Richard regretted his decision and wished he was still with Carla. Intellectually she had been much more his equal, and spiritually Carla had always believed they were one. It was nothing short of hell for Chrissie to think of that, but even worse was that he'd never said he didn't love Carla any more, he'd only admit to loving Chrissie too. So was it any wonder she was in such a crucifying state of anguish, so terrified of losing him, not only to the dangers of his job, but to the much greater threat of his seemingly indestructible love for Carla?

By the time he came back with the baby Chrissie was dressed, made up and looking as attractive as she could manage considering the lankness of her hair, and the swollen bags around her eyes. But the unbroken sleep had helped, and the way her heart melted when she saw him with his tiny daughter, so entranced and enslaved by her, boosted her too, for surely not even Carla mattered more than Ryan.

'Sssh, she's sleeping,' he whispered, gingerly lifting the

pushchair up over the three front steps and into the house.

'I don't know how you do it,' Chrissie grumbled, though she was smiling, and pleased that he could.

After closing the door, and slipping off his Barbour, he turned his attention to Chrissie, allowing his eyes to fill with the love she prayed so desperately that he really felt. 'Is this for me?' he murmured.

She nodded, and hoped that the dress she had chosen, which was much too tight for her really, didn't make her look ridiculous rather than seductive.

'You look beautiful,' he told her.

She smiled. 'Beautiful enough to distract you from the computer for a while?' she teased.

His mouth came down on hers and as he pulled her hard against him, desire suddenly washed through her with an urgency she hadn't felt in months. Or maybe it was panic? But did it really matter, when he was responding with an equal passion?

Whisking her into the dining room where packing boxes were still stacked up around the walls, he pushed her down on the floor, shoved her dress to her waist and yanked down her panties. As he entered her his mouth was crushing hers, and as he rode her, he gazed into her eyes and told her over and over how much he loved her. And when he came, she came too, her arms and legs around him, and the belief in his love, for the moment, shadowing the doubt. But this one overzealous encounter on the dining-room floor wasn't enough, their needs had been neglected for too long, and Richard's exotic tastes had to be indulged.

Smiling shakily, she got to her feet, pulled down her dress so he wouldn't see her nude in the daylight, then, telling him not to move, she went to get the rope. When she returned he was still on the floor, his trousers open, a new erection already beginning. She knelt down beside him, and began telling him exactly what she was going to do to him when she had him at her mercy, but even before she'd finished looping the rope round one wrist Ryan started to scream.

'It's OK,' he said when she looked at him in panic.

But it wasn't, she knew in her heart that it wasn't. 'I'm sorry,' she mumbled.

He kissed her, then, leaving her kneeling on the floor, he went to pick up the baby. She knew she should go too, that Ryan would be hungry and her breasts were so full they hurt. Looking down at the front of her dress she saw the large, damp patches the milk was making. Milk she should give to her daughter, but there was too much resentment, hatred, confusion and despair racing around in her head to make it safe for her to move.

Richard came to stand in the doorway. Ryan was in his arms, whimpering. Wasn't he angry at having their love-making interrupted that way? Didn't it matter to him?

'Are you going to feed her?' he said softly.

Dumbly she nodded, and got to her feet. For once, as she took the baby, Ryan didn't cry, though the tears in Chrissie's eyes were blinding. She loved her daughter more than she'd ever loved anything or anyone in her life, but she was afraid of her too, and the conflict was tearing her apart.

'It shouldn't take long,' she said to Richard, starting up the stairs.

But by the time she came back more than three hours had gone by, and the door to his study was firmly shut. He hated being interrupted while he was working, so Chrissie wandered out to the laundry room, and hoped that the washing and ironing might take her mind off the jealousy she felt of all the hours he spent on the computer, because, God knew, there were times when that machine seemed to be turning into the biggest threat of all.

Chapter 4

The rain that had slammed down in torrents for the past week had finally stopped, leaving the morning basking in a crisp, shimmery sunlight, and the fields that sloped to the woods at the heart of the valley rolling in a white, gauzy mist. Behind Carla's cottage the birdbath her mother had installed was being put to vigorous use by a pair of jays, while Eddie watched from a window and tried to contain his excitement.

In the end Carla let him out and smiled as he bounded towards them, expecting to join in the fun. In an instant the birds had fled, and spotting a squirrel scurrying along an overhanging branch of the horse chestnut, he got himself into a frenzy trying to work out how to jump up there. As she watched him, Carla let her mind wander back over the chat she'd had with Graham at the pub last night, when, not for the first time, they'd discussed the email she still hadn't answered.

Graham's advice, on the whole, was to do nothing until she was ready, which made sense, of course, but this past day or so she'd started to feel annoyed with herself for her indecision. Still, at least she wasn't feeling quite so spooked any more, though certain questions Graham had asked her last night were coming back to her now and causing her insides to shudder in other ways.

'Do you honestly think Chrissie knows about that email?' he'd said gently.

Her heart had jumped, and her eyes showed her pain as she dealt with what that might mean.

'Of course, I'm only guessing,' he continued, 'but I think there's a good chance she doesn't, and that Richard has attempted this in the hope of jolting you into a response.'

It had been so hard, yet so wonderful to hear that. 'But why would he do that?' she said.

'I think you know,' he answered. Then he said, 'Would you take him back? If he wanted to come?'

Her heart turned over. How could she answer that when even she was appalled by how desperately she wanted it? So, forcing a smile, she'd said, 'Sonya thinks I should just ignore the email. Part of me thinks I should too.' Even as she'd said it her heart had folded in two, for though she knew Sonya was right, she simply couldn't bear the idea that he would never be in her life again. No matter what he had done, or that he was married to someone else now, after all these months of hoping and praying with such utter and painful desperation that he would get in touch, how could she just ignore him when it was as though God himself had relented?

Graham's face was creased with concern, and not for the first time Carla noticed that his beard had acquired more grey since her mother's death. 'I suppose it depends what you're thinking of saying if you do respond,' he eventually answered.

She shook her head. 'I'm not sure. I mean, I certainly don't want to be godmother, but I don't want him to think it's because I'm still angry, or hurt.'

'Then what do you want him to think?'

Carla's cheeks coloured as she looked away. The truth, the *real* truth, was that she wanted him to think he'd made a terrible mistake with Chrissie and that he should come back to her. 'If Chrissie doesn't know about that email . . .' she said. 'In fact she can't know. She'd never . . . I mean, put yourself in her shoes. You remember what it was like back then, the terrible things I said . . .'

His gentle eyes showed that he remembered too well, and Carla's cheeks flushed. As dear a friend as he was, and as forthright and honest as she was trying to be, she was still embarrassed by how she had behaved in her demented state, when she hadn't only threatened to kill Chrissie and Richard, but their baby too. 'I wouldn't do it,' she said softly.

'Of course not. I know that.'

Carla stared down at her drink. After a while she said,

'How does he know I'm not going to ring up Chrissie and tell her what she can do with her invitation?'

'He doesn't. But you know Richard, the man thrives on danger.'

Her heart was back in her throat. Yes, that was the Richard she knew. The one she missed and longed for, the one she could never stop thinking about, and would do almost anything to have in her life again . . .

The sound of voices coming from the next-door garden surprised her back to the present, and gave her a momentary jolt of unease. What was anyone doing next door? Unable to see over the dividing wall, which was no longer visible under its burden of ivy and brambles, she listened for a moment, but the voices stopped almost as soon as she heard them, and the sound of a door creaking closed returned the two gardens to their usual quiet. Carla walked a few steps down the path, ducked under the washing line, then looked up at Gilbert Marne's house. It was gloomy and neglected, with two broken windows and a small, jagged hole in the roof. There appeared to be a few more bricks missing from the chimney too, and the creepers were so dense now that she guessed the downstairs windows wouldn't be visible at all. If someone was there with a view to buying, they were certainly going to have their work cut out restoring the place to any kind of glory.

Going back inside she moved quickly along the hall to the front door, glad she hadn't taken in the paper yet this morning so she could use it as an excuse to see who was visiting next door. To her surprise, the only car outside the two cottages was her own. Then she jumped as a voice said, 'Good morning.'

'Oh, Reverend,' she gasped. 'I didn't see you there. How are you?'

'Jolly good,' he answered, moving his ample bulk right out of Gilbert's front door in order to make room for someone to follow.

'Oh, hello, Mrs Taylor,' Carla said, smiling past her dislike. 'Not thinking of buying, are you?'

Not as skilled as Carla at disguising her feelings, Maudie Taylor's pinched, whiskery face remained embedded in rancour as she said, 'I heard intruders in here last night. Did you hear anything? I told the Reverend, we don't want squatters moving into our village. Did you hear them?'

'I didn't hear a thing,' Carla answered, 'and I was awake for most of the night.'

'Well, I heard them.' Maudie turned to the Reverend. 'All that nonsense about ghosts,' she snarled. 'It was squatters, I'm telling you.'

'Well, there's certainly no-one here now,' the Reverend responded. 'No sign of anyone having been here either.'

'Are you saying I imagined it?' Maudie challenged, a nasty gleam in her eye.

'Not at all. Must have cleaned up after themselves. Some squatters are like that.'

Carla hid a smile as she waved to Beanie and Lloyd Lamar, Dumbbell's owners, who were driving past in their new Volvo Estate. Maudie glared at her, then stalked off down the path, leaving a quivering air of hostility in her wake.

The Reverend smiled benignly. 'Lovely morning,' he commented to Carla.

'Lovely,' she agreed.

He nodded, then after leaning over the wall to pat Eddie who'd come to investigate the voices, he set off after Maudie, who was now waiting outside her own garden gate.

Enjoying the unexpected warmth of the sun Carla remained where she was for a moment, gazing along the village, which rambled in an uneven sort of crescent around to the church, forming the kind of shape an American dentist would want to straighten into a perfect smile. Actually, calling it a village was overblowing its status, for it really only qualified as a hamlet, which, along with the four bustling villages that surrounded it at a distance, made up the parish of St Martin-in-the-Glades. However, despite its mere dozen cottages, and few facilities, like the church, the pub, Teddy Best's shop and an old-fashioned red telephone box, everyone always referred to it as the village of Cannock Martin. The few tourists who passed through generally only paused long enough to fatten up the ducks and admire the church, before pressing on to the quaint little tea shops and craft displays elsewhere in the parish. So, on the whole, theirs was a sleepy little outback unbothered by strangers, and few ever got to find out about the colourful troupe of Cannock's inhabitants.

Seeing Joe Locke, the pseudo-devil-worshipper, lugging out his dustbin reminded Carla that she had to put out hers, and by the time she was back with it Faith, the post lady, was standing at the gate growling at Eddie. It was a game Eddie loved, since it was the only time he was allowed to growl and bark at a human and get away with it.

'Hear the ghosts was howling again last night,' Faith remarked, her long, crinkled face with its random dabs of powder and cherry red lipstick appearing almost puppet-like in the sunlight.

'Shrieking,' Carla confirmed, dragging the dustbin into place. 'Didn't get a wink.'

'Oh, so that's the reason for the dressing gown at nine o'clock in the morning. Maudie just told me you had a fancy man here.'

Carla's eyes widened, partly with surprise, partly indignation. 'Did she really say that?'

'Not a one to gossip, me,' Faith told her, digging into her sack for Carla's mail.

'But.'

'But that's what she said.' She was all business now, as though the passing on of gossip was as serious a duty as the delivery of mail. 'Said she sees him coming out of here regular, like.' She winked in a conspiratorial fashion. 'So, come on then, who is he?'

Managing to swallow her annoyance, Carla said, 'Can't tell you, I'm afraid. He's a married man.'

Oh, Faith liked that – a lot. 'Really,' she said darkly. 'See what you mean. Got to keep it under wraps if he's married. Well, you don't need to worry about me, my lips is sealed. Won't tell a soul.' She glanced both ways over her shoulder, then leaning in closer said, 'No-one from round here, is it?'

Carla tapped the side of her nose, and turning back inside closed the door quietly behind her, knowing very well that the rumour of her married lover would be all over the village before the church clock could strike the half-hour. She wasn't sure now whether she was pleased she'd done it, or not, but it was hardly important, since the only man who was ever in and out of here was her brother, and well Maudie knew it. But it was all soon forgotten when she flicked through the mail to find an envelope bearing the Channel 4 logo. Her heart did several flips, as, in a state of mounting unease, she wrestled with the decision of whether to open it or not. She knew that it very probably contained a cheque, and a new broadcasting contract, since she'd done the deal a week ago – the day after she'd got the email from Richard – and had no reason to believe they had changed their minds. The trouble was, once she took their money, there'd be no going back. A return to London would be imminent, and the setting up of a new series would be obligatory. Which would be great if she was ready for it. Maybe she was, but her confidence was so low it was hard to believe that she still had what it took to produce. And what about the courage to go it alone? It was all so intimidating, but she had to admit it was exciting too, at least it was until she thought of how lonely she would be, back in the city, avoiding her old friends and too nervous to make new ones. However, the alternative, of just giving up, sending the cheque back and forgetting about her programme, simply wasn't an option, because she'd never forgive herself if she did that, and she knew it.

The cheque and contract were exactly as discussed, and the relief that flooded her heart was immeasurable.

'Thank you, God,' she whispered, the genuineness of her smile feeling strange on her face. 'Thank you, thank you.' Then she picked up the phone to call Sonya, who'd worked so hard to help her achieve this that the celebration had to be hers too.

After joining in with Sonya's shrieks of delight, as though Sonya were teaching her how to do it, she ran upstairs to shower and dress, then she was back on the phone again, speaking to Graham.

'Congratulations,' he said warmly when she told him. 'That's the best news you could have given me. So how long do we have to wait to see the first programme?'

'Three weeks!' she cried. 'Only three weeks. Can you believe it? They've put it straight into the schedules, just like they said they would. Oh please God everyone's going to like it, if they don't there won't be a second series and if there's no second series . . .'

'One step at a time,' he said, laughing. 'And everyone's going to love it. Now, can I buy you a drink this evening, to celebrate?'

'Of course. Oh God, I'm sorry, I've interrupted you working, haven't I? How thoughtless. I just got carried away . . . Oh, there goes my other line. I'll see you at the pub later.'

After taking a call from the garage quoting her an exorbitant price for a new gearbox, she quickly wrote out a cheque for the electricity – an expense she could justifiably put down to the company – then turned on her computer to search out the preparations she'd made in anticipation of this momentous event in her life. Of course, when she'd been drawing them up, she'd just been going through the motions, pretending to herself, and everyone else, that she really would make a comeback, while never actually believing she would. Yet somehow it seemed to be happening, and all those dreaded dark thoughts and memories of how it had been the first time around, when Chrissie had been there to share it, would just have to be overcome.

No doubt easier said than done, though nothing looked less surmountable right at that moment than the issue of promoting and marketing the series in three short weeks. Almost everything else she could handle herself, but such crucial matters simply had to be handled by experts, and there was no money to cover it. Of course, Channel 4 would do their bit, but Carla needed someone on her payroll to oversee the entire picture, the way the publicists had the first time around. Well, paying someone to do this wasn't an option, so it seemed she had no choice but to take it on herself. She still had the old publicists' files so maybe she'd better start researching the names of those she needed to speak to at all the relevant places. The list was endless, the incentives she could offer non-existent, and the task of making any of it work was so daunting that already it was dulling the shine on the thrill of actually getting this far. And what if no-one liked the programme? What if it turned out to be a dud? Then it would all have been for nothing, and she was going to have wasted a lot of important people's extremely valuable time.

But on she ploughed, making phone call after phone call, setting up meeting after meeting, as though going to London was something she did every day, and organizing the transfer and shipment of over a hundred cassettes as though they were coming free with cornflakes. Thank God the money was now available to cover that at least, or it would be as soon as she got round to depositing the cheque. Maybe she should leave that to Sonya, while she concentrated on re-editing the shows to reflect the current year's prices, information she had still to co-ordinate, and tried to come up with some extraordinary inducement for the men in suits to part with their money for a follow-up series.

By the end of the day her adrenalin finally started to wane, but she had every reason to feel proud of what she'd managed to accomplish. The email from Richard had only crossed her mind about three dozen times an hour, and each time it had spurred her on to even greater heights of determination and belief in herself. It was amazing just how much inner strength it gave her to know that she was on his mind, and that he wanted her back in his life. It was changing everything, for without that unexpected boost to her self-esteem she honestly didn't know if she'd have gone so far as actually closing the deal with Channel 4, and she certainly wouldn't be seriously contemplating a return to London.

At six thirty she poured herself a glass of wine, then returned to her computer, intending, with her newfound energy, to respond to Richard's email at last. However, it seemed taking that step forward was going to be even harder than she thought, for she still wasn't clear what she wanted to say. The last thing she needed was to find out that she was wrong about him again, and that all he was really after was her forgiveness so that he and Chrissie could wrap up their guilt and get on with their lives. It would be another rejection, and she just couldn't take it. Besides, while he was waiting, she was the one in control, and it had been the other way round for so long that she truly didn't want to give it up so soon.

Remembering that she had agreed to meet Graham at the pub later, she decided to go in search of her mother's unfinished thesis. It was something she'd resolved, a while ago, that she would give to Graham, since it was he who had talked her mother into furthering her studies, and who had helped her with much of the research. So too had Richard, which was one of the reasons she'd been unable to face looking at it before. She guessed it was probably in the spare bedroom, where Sonya had stored all the personal papers and photographs in the weeks after the funeral. It was a room Carla rarely went into, and whenever she did, to get towels or sheets from the airing cupboard, she left again quickly. The evidence of all her memories was shut up in this room, for Sonya had stored not only her mother's and grandmother's papers here but hers too. Three women, three different generations, and an emerging pattern Carla never liked to dwell on, for, after being deserted by the men they loved, both her mother and grandmother had come to live here, and both had died here alone.

As she pushed the door open, the landing light spilled across the patchwork bedspread and on to the red-carpeted floor. There was nothing to be nervous about, it was only the room she'd slept in a thousand times as a child when Granny was here, and as a grown woman when her mother was here, often with Richard. That thought alone was enough to stop her where she was, but pushing it aside, she reached down to ruffle Eddie's ears, then turned on the light. Everything was exactly as it should be: freshly made bed ready for when her niece and nephew came to stay, Granny's Edwardian-style dressing table, with a glass top and swing mirror; a few family photographs from years ago, toys that the kids kept there; the Hoover; a clothes horse; and the tall double-fronted wardrobe where the memory boxes were kept.

In typical Sonya fashion all three sets of papers were separately stored, so that Carla soon realized that everything in the first box she opened belonged to Granny. For a while she flicked curiously through the photos, smiling and remembering, until feeling herself sinking a little too far into the sadness of nostalgia, she put the photos back and set the box aside. Returning to the wardrobe she raised the lid of the second box. Recognizing the photo albums that were lying at the top as her own, she dropped the lid and lifted the box clear of the small wooden tea chest at the bottom. Inside the chest she found her mother's diaries and personal records, old letters, treasured drawings from her children in their early years, dozens and dozens of photo-wallets, old school reports, award certificates, medals, all kinds of memorabilia, and, in a large brown envelope, the first hundred and seventeen pages of the thesis she'd been working on during the year before her death.

Carla's breath was shallow, and the grief very close to the surface, as she opened the envelope and pulled the pages free. Beside her, Eddie whined, then laid his head in her lap and sighed. Seconds ticked by as she struggled with her emotions, seeing her mother's dark, shining eyes, and the smile that was so beloved. She had been so proud of this thesis, had been working so hard for the degree that would open all kinds of new doors. She'd got so far . . . Carla's eyes closed as she tried to squeeze back the pain. She swallowed hard. It was an awful, bewildering feeling, holding this unfinished work. It was like seeing the futility of life in material form, for what did any of it matter now that it had been so randomly and needlessly cancelled? The abruptness of her mother's death was as pointless as the incomplete paragraph on the final page, which in itself was as perfect a symbol as Jung could have given.

She flicked slowly through it, occasionally pausing to read the typewritten lines. She could see her mother, sitting night after night at her treasured Olivetti laying down the interpretation of her findings, the recommendations drawn from her conclusions, the challenges inspired by her learning. Carla's heart ached with a heaviness she could hardly bear. She recalled so vividly the eagerness in her mother's eyes whenever she'd discussed her thesis with Richard. His broadness of intellect was such that he could easily debate the issues her mother raised, and in ways that often stretched her mind around entirely unexpected areas of learning. It had created a bond between them, one that Carla had been so proud of, and could almost feel as she sat there now, remembering. A knot of emotion began tightening her throat as she thought of how much her mother would have missed him too, and how devastated she would have been by the unexpectedness and depth of his betrayal.

With a tremulous sigh, she let the pages fall closed. This document was such an intrinsic part of her mother, and so manifest in its power to evoke happier times, that she knew already she wouldn't be able to give it away, not even to Graham.

Opening the large brown envelope again, she was about to slide the thesis back inside when she noticed a small, handwritten page that had been squashed in the bottom. Pulling it free, she smoothed out the creases and held it up to the light. It appeared to be part of a letter, written in her mother's untidy, forward-sloping hand, but with no first page it was impossible to know who she'd been writing to. It was only as she read it that the steady beat of Carla's heart began decreasing to a slow, dull thud of horror.

'. . . and ever since she told me I've been agonizing with myself, day and night, over what to do. Of course, the truth will have to come out, there is no question of that, but I cannot feel happy with the responsibility she has left me with. That we have all been so taken in is what makes it so much more troubling, because lies and deceit on this level, and covered so well, are very unsettling indeed. But I don't want to get into the calling of names, or apportioning of blame, there will certainly be time enough for that later. How I go about dealing with it now is uppermost in my mind, but of course Carla must be told first, so I would ask you to be there with me when I break it to her. I know that like the rest of us, she has no idea . . .'

Carla's face was ashen when finally she looked up. There was no more, it was where the single page ended, but she didn't need any more to understand what it was about. Her mother had *known* about Richard and Chrissie. Chrissie had told her, then left her with the responsibility of breaking it to Carla, and this letter was to Richard, asking him to be there when she did. Or was it to Graham?

She stared blindly down at the page. It had to be to Richard. Her mother must have slipped the letter into the thesis when she'd asked him to look at it, and he, without realizing, had left this single sheet behind. So what had happened then, after he'd read it? Presumably he'd refused her mother's request, because Chrissie had broken it to Carla in the end, before knowing that Valerie was dead. But surely to God he wouldn't be so callous, or cowardly, as to turn her mother down, then hide behind Chrissie . . . No! Not even the fact that Chrissie had come to see her on that fateful morning, or that Richard had never spoken to her since, could make her believe that he'd refused her mother's request. So maybe he'd never seen the letter, though if he hadn't, she could only wonder where the rest of it was now.

Her heart was pounding as she loaded everything back into the wardrobe and left the room. A few minutes later she was at her computer, typing an email to Richard. It was brief, and straight to the point. 'Did my mother know about you and Chrissie? Did you get her letter asking you to be there when she told me?' After clicking on send, she sank back in her chair, and breathed deeply in an effort to calm her shaking nerves.

'I think I was probably in shock,' she told Graham later, after she'd recounted what had happened. 'Reading that letter was . . . Well, it was like it was happening all over again. I might have overreacted, I'm not sure, but if she did know about Richard and Chrissie . . .' She turned to look at him. 'Did she?' she asked, swallowing hard. 'She'd have told you if she'd known, wouldn't she?'

He shook his head helplessly. 'She never mentioned it,' he answered.

Carla's eyes went down. '. . . Carla must be told first,' her mother had written, so no, she probably wouldn't have told Graham.

They were sitting by the fire in the pub, the only ones in, apart from Teddy Best and Joe Locke who were playing cards over in the corner, under a darkly dramatic painting of a coach and four horses in full flight. 'So you think the letter *was* to Richard?' she said.

'It would certainly seem to be,' he responded.

After a while she laughed dryly. 'You know, I've had so many horrible thoughts going round in my head since I read it. So much hate and anger . . . It's like I'm right back at the beginning . . .' She took a breath and expelled it in another humourless laugh. 'What a day. There I was heading off down the road to a new future at the start of it, and now this jolt back to the past at the end of it.'

Reaching out for her hand he gave it a reassuring squeeze.

'The past often jams out a foot to trip you up,' he responded. 'I sometimes find it's a way of stopping you moving ahead too fast when there are still issues to be dealt with.'

Carla picked up her drink.

'Deal with them now,' he said, gently, 'that way you can leave him behind, and move on with the rest of your life.'

Carla's insides churned. She couldn't even think about those words, for there wasn't a bone in her body or a wish in her heart that wanted to move forward without Richard, and she couldn't imagine a day ever dawning when she would. Though precisely how they were going to fit into each other's lives now he was married she hadn't yet worked out. Maybe she'd have a clearer idea once she knew if he'd received her mother's letter, though now she was recovering from the shock of it, she had to ask herself what difference it would make if her mother *had* known about him and Chrissie? None. It had all still happened. Chrissie was now his wife, and they were the proud parents of a bouncing baby girl. Each of those facts twisted her heart with a seemingly unending pain, for how hard it was to think of their joy and togetherness this past year while she'd struggled alone in the depths of despair. Could she ever forgive that? Did she even want to? Would she hate him if she found out he had been afraid to face her, even with her mother? In truth, the answers changed with the irregular pattern of her moods, but one thing she did know was that she was still a long way from being ready to let go.

So all she said to Graham was, 'It certainly prompted me into answering the email, and not with anything like the response he might be expecting.'

Graham's eyes twinkled, which made her smile. 'What'll be interesting now,' he said, 'is to read his response. And by the way, please don't worry about the thesis. I understand perfectly.' Then his face suddenly brightened as the door opened and Perry and Fleur Linus, Cannock's new-age geriatric couple who had kitted out their old motor-home like a spaceship in the hope of contacting other planets, and whose approach to logic was like a search for the Holy Grail, came bundling in from the cold. 'Oh good, I'm just in the mood for a spot of alien folklore,' he declared, rubbing his hands. 'How about you?'

Chapter 5

Carla was hurrying down the stairs, trying not to fall over Eddie who was bounding along with her, seeming to think all this speed was a game, instead of a rush to open the door before whoever was knocking managed to break it down.

At last she fell against it, slid back the chain and dragged it open. 'What the . . . ?'

'Surprise!'

Carla blinked, blinked again, then her whole face lit up. 'Oh my God!' she gasped. 'Avril? Oh my God! Oh my God!' And throwing her arms round Sonya's cousin, who'd been her best friend all through sixth-form college and university, and was how Sonya had come to meet Mark, she began dancing up and down in pure joy. 'When did you get here?' she cried. 'Why didn't anyone tell me you were coming?'

Avril's pretty, suntanned face was beaming. 'Because it would have spoiled the surprise,' she laughed. 'How are you? You look fabulous.'

Carla grimaced. 'But look at you! When did you become a film star?'

'Oh, that was last week,' Avril airily responded.

'And where's Sonya? How did you get here?'

'She dropped me off on her way over to her mum's. She'll be back around lunch time. So, do I get to come in? Hey, Eddie!' she shrieked, spotting him lurking behind Carla's legs. 'Don't you remember me, you little squirt? How are you?' And swooping down on him from her great height of five feet five inches, she gathered him into a whole body hug. Not entirely sure what to make of this Eddie licked her face a couple of times, then looked to Carla for approval. Seeming to

70

get it, he swiftly motorized his tail and set about removing Avril's make-up with one of his more hearty welcomes.

'You look so sophisticated and gorgeous,' Carla told her, glancing back over her shoulder as Avril followed her along the hall to the kitchen. 'America obviously agrees with you.'

'America agrees with anyone if they've got money,' Avril responded. 'Oh God, I'd forgotten how much I love this cottage. It feels so much like home. And is that tea! A huge round fat teapot full of tea? Tell me it's Typhoo. And is that toasted Hovis I can smell?'

Carla was laughing. 'You haven't changed a bit,' she told her. 'Except for the clothes and suntan. And the hair. I love it all sculpted round your face like that.'

'Isn't it cool?' Avril agreed, patting it. 'Had it done by the same girl as does Sharon Stone. Do you think blonde suits me?'

'It should, it's your natural colour.'

'But I've been dark for the past few years. Well, you saw me at the . . . Anyway, we'll definitely have to get to work on you. When did you last visit a hairdresser, or manicurist, or colour specialist, or any kind of ist? Oh, let me take my coat off first,' she gabbled as Carla offered her a mug of steaming hot tea. 'Are you ready for this?' And unfastening the top button of her black velvet swing coat, she swept it from side to side like Salome's last veil, then cast it with a flourish on to the back of a chair.

'Oh my God, you look sensational,' Carla murmured. 'What a figure!' and she laughed as Avril, dressed in skintight black leggings, thigh-high boots and deeply plunging black top, waggle-danced round in a circle.

'How about it?' she demanded, smugly. 'Cost a fortune, but worth every penny, wouldn't you say?'

'You mean, you had it done surgically?'

'Where do you think I've been these past five years?' Avril demanded, gliding her hands over her voluptuous shape. 'You don't get anywhere in LA without gigantic tits and a tiny ass, and I sure as hell didn't uproot my lardy old British butt just to go over there and sit on it. So yeah, course I had surgery.'

Carla was still laughing. 'The look might have changed, but

71

you're the same wonderful Avril, and I can't tell you how fantastic it is to see you.'

'Yeah, I thought it might be,' Avril responded, going to stick a slice of bread in the toaster. 'Oh, Eddie, Eddie, Eddie, you want a piece too,' she crooned. And after adding another slice for him, she inhaled deeply and closed her eyes as she said, 'Oh, it's so good to be standing here in this kitchen with you, and knowing what I know.'

Carla was confused, though grinning. 'Which is?' she prompted.

Avril winked, and picked up her tea. Then in a genuinely sombre voice, she said, 'I'm really, really sorry about your mum. Sonya said you don't remember much about the funeral, which doesn't really surprise me, because you didn't even seem to know who I was when I got there. I wanted to stay longer, but I'd just got this new contract with one of the major studios for a new action-thriller that was worth megabucks, so I had to fly back. But I had to come. She was very special . . . I know I should have written, or called, but you know how it is, and Sonya's kept me up to speed with how you've been doing.' She suddenly grinned, showing her expensively straightened and capped teeth in an extremely infectious smile. 'So, don't you want to know how long I'll be staying?' she demanded.

Carla laughed and shrugged. 'Amongst other things,' she answered.

'So ask.'

'OK. How long are you staying?'

Avril's chin came up. 'For as long as you need me,' she declared.

Carla's brow wrinkled.

'I'm a PR expert, aren't I?' Avril boasted. 'And according to Sonya that's just what you need right now. So, give me the story.'

Carla blinked, not entirely sure she'd just heard right.

'The story,' Avril prompted. 'The scoop. What's the programme about?'

Carla was incredulous. 'But what about your office in LA?' she said. 'I mean, I can't possibly afford someone like you . . .'

'Yeah, yeah, let's make like that's all done with,' Avril cut

72

in. 'I'm a big shot West Coast hype-hustler whose good fortune and limitless talents don't mean a goddammed thing if I can't put them to use for a friend when she needs them. So, where do we start?'

'But what about your other commitments? Surely you can't just . . .'

'Carla, honey, with the money I've made I can do just about anything I like these days. And with the staff I've got, I can take off on a slow boat to ecstasy, or take Ecstasy on a slow boat, and believe you me, they can cope. So, I say we start by searching out the nearest health spa so's we can get you looking a bit more like your real gorgeous self. Oh, and would you believe, I just happen to have a couple of numbers right here,' she declared with mock surprise as she produced a leather-bound notepad from her Ferragamo handbag and used a fine silk ribbon to flip it open.

'I'm dreaming,' Carla mumbled. 'I've got to be dreaming.'

'Sure, the whole of life's a dream. Isn't that what Descartes reckoned? So what do we need here? Hair cut, restyled, highlighted. Face oxygenized, peeled, enzymed, exfoliated and rejuvenated. Body detoxed, mud-wrapped, massaged, steamed, pummelled and pampered. Nails trimmed, shaped, buffed and polished. Feet soaked, de-callused, salted, replenished and rubbed. Let me see, anything I've forgotten? Ah, the wardrobe. Well, we'll get on to that when we go up to London. Is that your car outside, by the way?'

Carla nodded.

'Can't be seen in that. Give it away. We'll rent something suitable for your new image as a stunningly successful independent producer who's sassy and connected enough to hire herself a gen-u-ine PR professional from the U-nited States.'

Carla was shaking her head and laughing in disbelief. 'Just when did you turn into my fairy godmother?' she wanted to know.

'I guess about the time you turned into Cinders. Which reminds me,' she went on, returning to her notepad: 'Prince Charming,' she wrote, 'must give him a call when I know what I'm calling him about.'

Carla's face was draining. 'You're not talking about . . .?'

'Richard? Good God no. We'll just move right on past him and start planning the stupendous launch party you're going to throw that'll get the whole town talking.'

This time Carla shook her head more vigorously. 'No party,' she said. 'I'm sorry, I don't want to appear negative, but apart from not having the budget, I should remind you that Chrissie's fronting the programme, so it's going to look very odd if we throw a party and don't invite her. And if we invite her, which I'm absolutely not prepared to do, we have to invite Richard, which there's just no way in the world I'll . . .'

'Got the message,' Avril chimed in. 'But don't worry, we'll work something out. Are you in touch with them at all? Does she know the programme's got a transmission date?'

'If she does it wasn't me who told her.'

Avril nodded. 'Do you want to use her in the publicity at all?'

'No.'

'OK. So what we need to do is find your front person for the next series and start promoting her – or him. Re-enter Prince Charming, who's sure to have some ideas. Ah, toast! Eddie, do you take butter or jam? I see, three dozen tail wags in less than three seconds, must mean both. And I do declare if Carla had a tail, then by the look of her she'd be wagging hers too. But before we get into circus acts, I reckon you, Carla, should get that pretty little butt of yours upstairs and dressed, while Eddie and I carry on fixing things here.'

In a something of a daze, and almost breathless with the speed at which Avril was managing to take over, Carla obediently trotted up the stairs, followed by the faithful Eddie who brought his toast with him, and slotted the shampoo spray on to the bath taps ready to take a shower. With it being too cold to remove her dressing gown until the hot water came through, she kept it huddled around her as she padded into the back bedroom to ferret out a clean towel. Noticing that the door of the wardrobe where the memory boxes were kept had fallen open, she pushed it closed, turned the key and emerged on to the landing in time to hear Avril gabbing away downstairs with Faith, the post lady.

'You might be getting mail for me,' she was saying, 'because I'm going to be moving in here for a while.'

'Oh, that's nice,' Faith remarked. 'She was getting a bit lonely here on her own. Until she got herself that new boyfriend, of course. Nice that. Shame he's married though, she deserves someone special if you ask me. Someone she can call her own.'

Carla didn't know whether to laugh or scream. The woman obviously had no shame, gossiping so outrageously right on her victim's doorstep.

'No! He's not married, is he?' Avril cried. 'I never knew that.'

'Told me so herself,' Faith assured her. 'Married he is.'

'Well I never. I knew he was on the run, and I keep telling her she shouldn't be harbouring criminals, she could get herself into trouble. But married!'

Carla had to stifle a laugh, as she had no problem at all imagining the three 'O's that had just formed on Faith's gullible face. 'On the run,' Faith echoed. 'What, from the police like?'

'Yeah, them too,' Avril confided. 'Anyway, better go before she hears what we're saying.'

'*You* are incorrigible,' Carla told her as she closed the door.

Avril laughed. 'Go get showered. I'll start ringing around to try and find us a decent rental car. Oh, before you disappear, what's the password to get into your email? I gave your address to my PA, so I'd better tune in for the latest crises.'

Carla froze. She hadn't checked the email herself yet this morning to see if Richard had replied to her message last night. It wasn't that she thought Avril would deliberately pry, or even that she felt the need to hide anything from Avril, it was simply that she wanted to read his answer first. However, it was going to look extremely odd if she were to refuse to give Avril a simple password in the light of everything Avril was about to give her. So, with a roll of her eyes, she confessed it was Eddie, and went off to take a shower.

By the time she came back downstairs Avril was at Sonya's desk heavily engrossed in striking a deal for some kind of Porsche that she wanted driven down from London, so that she could use it to 'drive *up* to London. *Moron*,' she added under her breath.

75

Seizing her chance Carla quickly typed in her password, waited through the squeal and crush of the Internet connection, and felt her insides flutter as the American-accented words, 'You've got mail,' issued from the speaker.

Her heart immediately tightened as she saw Richard's address, and dragging the mouse to the relevant line she clicked it open.

She was so convinced that it would contain an answer to last night's question that she had to read the short message three times before she could make it sink in. In the end she recognized it as another quote from Voltaire, this time, she thought, from the *Philosophical Dictionary*. 'The greatest geniuses can have false judgement about a principle they have accepted without examination,' the message said.

Was that an answer? If so, what exactly was he saying? Was it himself he was alluding to as the genius? And what principle was he referring to?

She felt a sudden flood of anger. To him this might be a game, to her it was anything but.

'Jerk!' Avril muttered as she put the phone down. Then with a happy smile, 'Cinderella's carriage will be here by one.'

Carla stared at her, then, remembering the Porsche, she started to laugh.

'So,' Avril said, screwing up her nose as she slipped on an extremely chic pair of Gucci sunglasses to shield her eyes from the dazzling glow of a Riviera sunset, 'is it Richard who's got the post lady all aflutter?'

Carla started, then, looking down at her drink, she said, 'No. The married man Faith's talking about is my brother, Mark, did she but know it. Or Graham, I suppose, as he pops in from time to time.'

'Graham? The writer? The one your mum was seeing?'

Carla nodded.

Avril sighed. 'Well, I'm glad it's not Richard,' she said.

Carla turned away and gazed out at the spectacular view. She hadn't quite got to grips with being here yet, since it had happened so fast that her head still felt as though it was back home in Somerset. First the Porsche had arrived, then Sonya,

76

then bags were thrown into boots, Eddie was whisked off by Sonya, and the next thing she knew she was zooming up the M4, being bundled through the airport, and was on a flight to Nice. From Nice they'd taken the helicopter hop over to the Principality, checked into the Hotel de Paris, and now here they were, sitting on the terrace of Monte Carlo's famously exclusive Thalassotherapie health spa, wearing sumptuous white terry robes after the two stupendously luxurious massages they'd just received, and sipping champagne cocktails as they watched rich men's yachts bobbing and gliding in and out of the harbour below. Part of her felt as though she might just as well die right now, since tomorrow couldn't possibly bring anything better, and even if it did she'd just feel overindulged. Another part felt disheartened by Avril's remark.

'Do you have any contact with him at all?' Avril asked.

Carla took a breath. 'Just a couple of emails.'

'Saying?'

Remembering the first one Carla's expression turned wry, as she said, 'He's asked me to be godmother to his daughter.'

Avril choked. '*What?*'

Carla smiled and picked up her drink.

Avril was still reeling. 'Is the man on drugs?' she demanded.

This time Carla laughed. Then she gave Graham's theory that the invitation was merely an attempt to establish contact.

Avril looked baffled. 'Bloody peculiar way of doing it,' she retorted. 'But then, I have to confess, Richard Mere was always a mystery to me, and from what I remember it sounds just like the perverse kind of thing he'd do. Anyway, go on. What else do these emails say?'

Carla told her first about the page she'd found in the thesis, then about the answer she'd received that morning.

By the time she'd finished Avril looked drunk. 'Do you want to run that last bit by me again?' she said.

As she quoted it again, Carla turned to gaze out to where the sun was disappearing in a fiery glow behind the dark pink crenellations of the Grimaldi Palace.

'How do you know it was Voltaire?' Avril asked. 'French classics wasn't your subject.'

Carla shrugged. 'He's used it before. I can't remember about what now, but he told me at the time where it was from.'

Avril seemed happier with that, then dismissed it with, 'But you still don't know if your mother knew about him and Chrissie?'

'No. But I don't suppose it's important now, is it?'

Avril's powers of analysis approached that from all angles before she said, 'No, I don't suppose it is. But I can see why it was a blow when you first read the letter. Must have brought it all back like it was yesterday.'

Carla looked at her and smiled, and right at that moment she couldn't imagine wanting to be with anyone else in the world.

Avril looked back, her small face made golden in the early evening light, her big eyes, thickly fringed with naturally curling lashes, only just visible through the dark lenses of her glasses. Though she'd hidden it well, she was still dealing with the shock of just how much devastation had been wrought on the vibrant Carla she used to know. Oh sure, Carla was making an effort to hide it, and were Avril anyone else she might be fooled, but she knew Carla too well. It wasn't only the gauntness of Carla's face and disturbing loss of weight that had changed her, a light somewhere inside her had gone out when that man had crushed her with his betrayal, and God help her, she seemed to think that these ludicrous emails were the way to getting it back. Avril could only be grateful that she was stepping in now, before any real harm was done, though not for a minute did she think talking Carla out of anything where Richard was concerned was going to be easy.

Still, now was definitely not the time to start trying, so in typical Avril fashion she said, 'Bastard. I hope his nuts drop off.'

Carla smiled, but didn't quite meet her eyes. 'So what about you?' she said. 'Are you seeing anyone?'

Avril's face broke into a grin. 'Honey, I'm so happy being single I need a therapist to help me deal with the guilt of it.'

At that Carla laughed, reminding Avril of how beautiful she actually was.

78

'I'm serious. Who needs all that shit?' Avril went on. 'My way I get to sleep at night. And do you see that guy over there, the Italian-looking one . . .'

Carla turned to the wall of windows that separated the indoor pool from the glossy white marble terrace they were sitting on. In their reflection she saw a good-looking man, probably in his forties, with greying black hair, powerful forearms, and a loose-fitting white shirt that enhanced the attractive darkness of his skin, sitting at a table two or three back from their own. 'I see him,' she said.

'I'm considering letting him screw my ass off tonight,' Avril confided.

Carla bubbled with laughter.

'What's so funny? I'm serious.'

'How do you know he's available?'

Avril rolled her eyes. 'Carla, didn't you learn yet that there's not a man on this planet who's not available if the offer's right? Look at Chrissie and Richard. No, OK, let's not look at them. Just take it from me, all you got to do is choose the man, then decide what kind of offer you want to make.'

Spotting the waiter hovering, Carla waved to him to bring more champagne. She was enjoying this. 'Go on,' she encouraged.

'I'm talking about sex, OK?' Avril warned. 'This is none of your *True Romance* stuff, cos frankly it's crap, and I just don't have time for it.'

'So how are you going to let that guy know you want to have sex with him?' Carla prompted.

Avril shrugged. 'I could go about it a lot of different ways,' she answered. 'Generally depends on how my schedule's looking. Tonight I guess you could say I've got time, and I kind of feel like dancing. Do you feel like dancing? We could go to Jimmy'z.'

'You're changing the subject.'

'Not really. I was going to invite him dancing. If you want to come too I'll ask him to line up a friend.'

Carla drew back. 'No, no, not for me,' she said.

'Oh come on, you've got to be dying for it by now.'

Carla shook her head, repelled by the very idea of anyone touching her but Richard.

'OK, no pressure. I'll just fix a time with Federico Fellini over there, then we'll go back to the hotel and have dinner. This may take a minute.'

Carla watched in growing amazement as Avril sat back in her chair, crossing her legs in a way to make certain her robe fell open to expose her thighs, and a glorious amount of cleavage. Then, after smiling at the man, she crooked a finger to beckon him over. Without hesitation he got to his feet, and as he came towards them Avril moistened her lips with her tongue in such an outrageous manner that Carla had to smother a laugh.

'Hi,' she said, as he arrived at their table. 'Do you speak English?'

'Leetle,' he answered, putting a quarter-inch distance between his thumb and forefinger.

'You know Jimmy'z?' Avril asked him.

'*Sì*. Jimmy'z.'

Avril sighed. 'Well, you know I want to go there, and my friend here, she doesn't want to go . . .' Removing her glasses she stared pointedly at the bulge in his jeans, then slowly raised her eyes to his face.

'I take you Jimmy'z?' he offered.

Avril smiled, then, after a shameless smirk at Carla, she set the time and place.

Jimmy'z was already swimming with beautiful people by the time Avril and her escort arrived – cool Swedish blondes too pert to be anything over twenty, luscious Italian babes complete with hairy armpits, sensuous *belles françaises* brazen with attitude, cute little American cupcakes, in fact every nationality, and every description of young, hot, female and available. All the takers had to be was male and rich, and they sure seemed to be out in abundance tonight. It was a bit like the twenty-first century's answer to slavery, Avril reflected, with the Principality's reputation capturing the girls, the harbours, nightclubs and casinos parading them, and the men of vast wealth coming in to buy.

As a space opened up at the bar, Avril pushed her way through and climbed up onto an empty stool. Her escort was right behind her, looking delectable in his tight black lycra shirt and Armani jeans. During the taxi ride from the hotel they'd stumbled through a few amusing attempts to communicate, but since she spoke no Italian and he virtually no English, they still didn't know much more about each other than the fact that they were going to be making the beast with two backs by the end of the evening. Actually, what else was there to know?

While her escort ordered a couple of kamikazes Avril watched the teeming mass of dancers and revellers with all their gorgeous suntanned flesh, and sleek healthy hair, and felt nothing short of thrilled that she wasn't those girls' ages any more. It was such a downer being young, insecure and poor, no matter how beautiful you were. Thirty, confident and rich was a much more satisfying place to be, so was away from home, since it offered her the freedom to explore and exploit her fantasies in a way she'd never risk back in LA, partly because of the fear of running into someone she knew, but mainly because of how many psychos there were out there.

Here was different, and her escort couldn't have been a more obvious gigolo if he'd had a price tag looped round his neck with condoms. She'd already slipped him a couple of thousand francs, to take care of the drinks – and at these prices he was going to need every centime – and later, depending on what she required of him, and how good his performance, she'd slip him anything between ten and twenty thousand more. Oh, life was so much simpler when you could pay. No messing about with all that commitment stuff, or waiting for calls that just weren't going to come, or humiliating yourself in ways that even Jerry Springer's guests hadn't thought of. No, no, no. Monogamy, devotion, heartache, just weren't her thing. She'd never been seriously involved with a man, and had no intention of starting now, especially not when she saw the kind of mess so many of her friends ended up in. Sure they got over it, eventually, but the pain, the misery, the utter devastation that tore them up like they were yesterday's trash, that just wasn't for Avril.

Shame Carla was buying into it, but then most did, though there weren't many whose mothers upped and died the very same day as the great love of their life and their best friend decided to go public with the coming of the stork. So it was no great surprise that Carla had been half-demented with grief; Avril wouldn't even have blamed her if she'd turned into a homicidal maniac. In fact, she'd probably have paid for her defence. However, mercifully, that hadn't been necessary, and it had to be said that Avril was a whole lot happier about helping to fund Carla's comeback than she'd have been throwing money at a murder rap. It was just this renewed contact with Richard that was bothering her. Not that she had anything against the man personally, until he'd taken the gold for asshole of the year of course, and now all this messing about with Carla's head via the email when he was in no position to offer her anything except a whole lot more grief . . . Well, Avril wasn't liking what he was doing one bit, because there was just no way Carla was over all the shock and pain of it yet, so this cryptic shit he was luring her in with was almost guaranteed to skew her judgement and could, ultimately, prove the death of her revival.

The question was, how to get Carla to jump on the man's face like it was going to trampoline her off to the stars? No doubt Avril would come up with an answer at some point, she usually did, but right now she was much more interested in downing a few more kamikazes, lapping up even more attention than her transparent black dress was already attracting, and spinning and rocking around the heaving dance floor, before going off to her own appointment with the stars.

By two in the morning she was breathless from dancing, several degrees right of tipsy and ready to leave. It was perfect timing for the fantasy she'd chosen to live out tonight, and though she wouldn't have minded swapping her Italian for the sombre, suited business guy who'd been eyeballing her almost since she'd arrived, she didn't much fancy the scene it might cause if she tried. So, after a seductive smile in the businessman's direction, she took her Italian's arm and left.

Her suite at the Hotel de Paris was a lavish enclave of Renaissance splendour, or was it *fin de siècle*? For all she knew it could be both, and more, with so much gilt and fancy wood-carving, thickly brocaded draperies, and imposing four-poster bed with enough swags and canopies and fringes to get lost in. She wasn't big on interior design, and antiques didn't do much for her either. All she was interested in was clean sheets, reliable plumbing, the technological where-withal to connect her to the outside world, and a spectacular view. In this suite she had it all.

After closing the doors that led into the suite's bedroom, she turned to the Italian who was oozing testosterone now that his real skill had been released from its zipper. Avril had taken it out herself, in the lift on the way up here, then she'd made him walk with her, arm in arm, along the corridor, like any married couple. They'd passed no-one, but at that time of night she hadn't really expected to, it just gave her a kick to think they might.

She smiled as a dozen tremors of lust eddied through her. She really got off on looking at a man with his cock out, waiting to be told what to do. And she'd made the right decision in leaving the businessman behind, because this guy's body was so hairy and hard that when added to his inability to speak English, she knew already she was going to be in for one hell of a session.

To her delight he proved an impressively fast learner, and in a matter of minutes she was naked and flat out on the massive leather-topped desk, while talking on the phone to her office, who were just getting ready to wrap it up for the day. As she spoke she watched him roll on a condom – trousers round his knees, shirt hanging open – then, grabbing her legs to pull her buttocks to the edge of the desk, he made ready to push his cock up inside her. Already it was blowing her mind, and to think it was only going to get better!

She didn't look at his face as he entered her, she just listened to her PA, and felt his hands massaging the huge, hard ampleness of her breasts. She was somewhere else, discon-nected from what was happening, yet getting so damned turned on by it she could hardly stand it. Then his fingers were squeezing her plum ripe nipples, pulling them and flicking them, as the motion of his hips began picking up speed.

'Just get on to Conrad and have him do it,' she told her PA, as Signore Italiano jerked her up and down the surface of the desk.

'He's out of the office through Friday,' her PA responded.

Avril arched her back, then almost gasped as the Italian shoved her knees up to her shoulders and began ramming violently.

'Get on to him at home,' Avril said, barely able to keep her voice steady. 'Tell him the commission's up five per cent, so it's worth getting out of bed for. *Oh shit!*' she suddenly cried, as the pasta man's thumb began delving around for the hot spot. 'I've got to go.'

'Hang on,' her PA said. 'I've got a message here from John Rossmore letting you know how to get hold of him.'

The Italian was banging her so hard now, she could barely speak. 'Put it on the email,' she gasped, then almost dropped the phone as he abruptly withdrew his cock, flipped her over, and getting onto his knees behind her drove into her again. Somehow she fumbled the phone back on the receiver, then grabbed on to the edges of the desk as he began galloping her towards the peak.

'Yes! Oh yes!' she cried, climbing fast now.

His hands alternately circled her waist and grabbed her breasts. Then the hair on his chest was scraping her back, and her legs were almost giving way beneath her. It was time to come, and knowing exactly what would do it, she turned her head so that she could see his face and managed to pant, 'By the way, what's your name?'

Chapter 6

'A crisis in India! What do you mean, *a crisis in India*? Just what the hell do you think's going on here?' Chrissie's eyes were glittering with fear as she glared across the kitchen at Richard. She'd been expecting this. For the past two days, since the riots had started, she'd been waiting for him to come and tell her he was going, and the entire time she'd been working herself up into a riotous state of her own over what she could do to stop him.

His handsome face was calm, his pale blue eyes showed how unsurprised he was by her outburst. 'Darling, it's what I do,' he said reasonably. 'Political uprisings, guerrilla . . .'

'Don't patronize me!' she spat. 'I know what you do, but how can you even think about going away now, when I need you here?'

He came further into the spacious, high-tech kitchen. The dull, drizzly weather outside was darkening the place, so he flicked a switch, flooding the white cabinets, black granite worktops and stainless steel sinks and cooker with too much light. This, and Ryan's room, were the only two in the house they had got round to renovating; the others, some with bare floorboards, others with half-painted walls and torn wallpaper, would remain works in progress until Chrissie made up her mind how she wanted them to look.

The heavy black travertine table was between them, bearing half a dozen baby bottles into which Chrissie had been expressing her milk. She was looking at him nervously, but defiantly, ready to defend her actions over the milk, and the assignment. But he was so good at arguing, and lately she'd been having trouble turning her thoughts into clear and coherent words.

As he walked round the table towards her, her eyes narrowed with caution, and when he raised a hand she cowered sharply away. 'No! Don't you dare hit me. Just don't . . .'

He stared at her in surprise. 'Chrissie! I've never hit you, so what are you talking about?' he demanded.

'But you want to hit me, don't you?' she cried. 'I know you do.'

'I don't want to do anything of the sort. Now please, for God's sake, try to pull yourself together.'

With a jerky movement she pushed back her hair. 'I *am* together. In fact, I'm very together, thank you very much.'

'Good. Then understand that I have to go. It's how I earn a living, and this house has taken up the best part of my inheritance.'

'I can earn a living too! So why don't you stay here and let *me* go out to work?'

'Doing what?'

Fury blazed in her eyes. 'I'm an actress, for God's sake! I can get work as an actress.'

His eyes went down, as he tried to work out the best response to that. But she hadn't finished.

'*And* I'm a director! I directed three episodes of *There and Beyond*, and if *you* hadn't sold *my* programme to *your* ex-girlfriend then I'd have something to work on now, wouldn't I?'

He took a breath. 'Darling, it was a decision we came to together, to sell the programme . . .'

'No! It was you! You decided, because you felt sorry for her and didn't want her to end up with nothing.'

'Nor did you. But Chrissie, it's all academic now, and it isn't getting us any closer to . . .'

'I can still act,' she cut in belligerently. 'I can ring up my old agent and tell him to get me some work.'

Richard's response was slow in coming. 'Do you think you can earn as much as I do?' he said in the end.

At that she snapped. 'Stop it!' she screamed. 'Stop making me feel inadequate and useless and ugly and . . .'

'You're none of those things,' he barked. 'I'm just trying to point out that the bills need to be paid, and my work as a foreign correspondent . . .'

'War! It's war you report, Richard, and I can't stand it! I don't want you to get killed. I want you here, where I can see you, and where Ryan can see you too. Do you want her to grow up without a father? Don't you care about her?'

Richard sighed, and pushed a hand through his hair.

She stood staring at him, sweat beading on her face, hysteria burning in her eyes. Somewhere, behind all this, she knew she was repulsing him, driving him away and making sure he'd never want her again, but there was nothing she could do about that. She was desperate for him not to go, not only because she didn't want him to get killed, but because she was terrified of what she'd do to the baby if he wasn't there to stop it. Even now, as they stood there confronting each other in the kitchen, Ryan was upstairs screeching, and Chrissie couldn't stand it any more.

'Then go!' The words erupted suddenly and bitterly from her mouth as her face twisted with anger. 'Go on! Go! We can manage without you. In fact don't bother coming back, because we can manage better without you.'

There was sadness and pain in his eyes as he looked at her, and a kind of helplessness in his tone as he said, 'Darling, you have to get help. I know it's not what you want to hear . . .' He broke off as she suddenly rushed towards him and began beating him with her fists.

'Stop treating me like I'm crazy!' she raged. 'It's you who makes me crazy. And her! That monster upstairs that never does anything but scream and shit and drive me up the wall every minute of the day and all you care about is a fucking crisis in *India*!'

Managing to grab her hands, he held them tightly against his chest and tried to force her to look at him.

But she wasn't seeing him. All she was seeing was the horror of her life billowing up around her in great big black waves, like the ones that had tried to drown her many years ago, when she'd been so afraid that all she'd wanted was to die. And like a horrible echo bouncing through distant, invisible caves, she could hear someone screaming, yelling abusive words and hissing like a snake, and though she knew it was her, it was as if it wasn't her, because there was nothing about it that she could control. All the venom and paranoia and fear and desperation was pouring out of her in a stream of manic frustration. On and on and on she screeched, more and more abuse and terror, until she was sobbing so hard that no more words would come and her legs were so weak she could no longer stand.

Pulling out a chair, Richard sat her on his lap and held her tight. 'Ssssh,' he soothed. 'Ssssh. I'm here. It's OK. Nothing's going to hurt you. There's nothing to be afraid of.'

Still she couldn't speak, as her whole body shook and shuddered in the aftermath of hysteria. Though she clung to him, and he held her too, she knew he wanted only to get away, to be as far from her and her unwashed clothes and dirty body as possible. There was no crisis in India. He'd made it up, so that he could get away from her and that screaming monster upstairs that she just wanted to pummel and punch and stifle and strangle.

'Oh God, Richard,' she sobbed. 'I don't know what's happening to me. I'm so afraid. I just . . . I just . . .' But there was no way she could make herself utter the words she was thinking, for no woman in her right mind would ever think such evil thoughts about her own child.

'Listen,' he said, tilting her chin up so he could look into her face. He smiled tenderly at the devastation her outburst had caused. 'If you really don't want me to go . . .'

'I don't,' she cried. 'Oh God, I really don't. I know it's selfish, and that you should go really, but I'm so afraid without you, and I know we need the money, but I was thinking, you said you were offered that advance to write a book? Well, couldn't you take that and then you could stay home and write it, and you wouldn't have to go to India and . . .'

He put a finger over her lips. 'I'm hearing you,' he said softly.

She gazed at him with wide, apprehensive eyes.

'Is that what you want?' he said.

She nodded.

'OK. Then that's what I'll do.'

For a moment she wasn't sure she'd heard right, then she could barely catch her breath on the sudden rush of relief. 'Oh God, Richard,' she gasped, throwing her arms round his neck. 'I love you so much. And I swear I'll get some help. I'll go to see a doctor, and we can get someone in to help with the baby. And I won't interrupt while you're working. I'll find some decorators, and I'll call my agent so that I can help out. Oh darling, I love you so much.'

Smiling, he smoothed her hair and said, 'I love you too.'

'Are you sure you don't mind about India?'

'I mind much more about you. And if me not going to India will make you feel better, then I'm not going to India. But I do want a promise from you that you will see a doctor, and that you will start looking for a nanny.'

'I promise. I swear. Cross my heart. Oh Richard!' Her breath ran out again, then her hands were flying about her face as she gasped, 'Oh God, I look so awful, how could you want to stay with me? But I'll lose weight, I swear and I'll join a gym, and I'll . . .'

'Enough,' he laughed, squeezing her. 'Now, I think one of us should go and see what's bothering our daughter, don't you?'

The light dimmed in her eyes.

'I'll go,' he said, picking up one of the bottles. 'You can stay here and make us a cup of tea.'

'Shall I get the rope?' she giggled as he reached the door.

There was a moment's pause before he turned back and said, 'No. Not right now.'

Her bottom lip came out, but he left, and then she was once again overcome by a huge onslaught of relief, and amazement, that she'd actually found the courage to ask him to stay. And he had agreed! In the end it had been so easy. And not even Carla had managed to get this far, so maybe he did love her more than Carla.

It was only a matter of seconds before the horrible fear that he might end up resenting her began blazing a trail through her triumph – and with such certainty that it left no doubt in its wake. In fact it had probably already started, because he had just turned down sex. Richard *never* turned down sex. He *loved* sex, so the only reason he'd passed up the chance was because he was really pissed off about having to stay, and so angry with her for making him that it had killed all the desire he had for her and left him despising her.

But for the baby's sake she had to keep him here. So what was she to do? Maybe a glass of wine would help. But no, he didn't like her to drink, and she'd already had two glasses today. Had he smelt it on her? Was that why he was insisting she see a doctor? He thought she was a drunk. But two glasses wasn't much, and in her heart she knew that what he was really worried about was how hard she was finding it to cope with Ryan. So she'd do what he said and get a nanny. The thought of someone else in the house made her instantly nervous, but if she got an older woman, someone he'd never look at twice in that way, it should be all right. And if she prepared a special dinner for him tonight, and cleaned herself up a bit, he might discover that he did still find her attractive after all.

She became so engrossed in her cookbooks and painstaking efforts to adhere to a complicated recipe for stroganoff that it was a long time before she realized it had turned completely dark outside, and that the house had been silent for some time. She glanced at the clock. Two hours must have gone by since Richard went upstairs, and it was ages since she'd last heard Ryan scream. Maybe she should go and check on them. It was safe to go near the baby when he was there. Nothing bad would happen then.

The kitchen was in the basement, so she had three flights of stairs to climb to get to the cosy little pink and white bedroom that belonged to Ryan. But she had only got as far as the ground floor when she looked up to see Richard coming down the stairs.

'Are you OK?' she said. 'I was just coming to look for you.'

'She's asleep,' he answered, 'and I have to confess I dropped off with her. So what have you got cooking? Smells good.'

Her eyes were playful. 'It's a surprise,' she told him.

He glanced at his watch. 'How long have I got before we eat?'

'Um, about half an hour. I thought I'd take a shower now, and . . .'

'OK. I'll just make a couple of calls and check on my email, then I'll open one of the bottles of Puligny that we had at the wedding.'

Though he was offering to open one of the special bottles of wine, which possibly meant that he considered this evening to be worthy of marking, what with all the new decisions and promises and plans they had talked about, her answering smile was still shaky, for she guessed that one of the calls he'd be making would be to cancel his trip to India. She wished she knew the right words to say, but none seemed appropriate, so she tried to look contrite and agreeable and full of understanding and appreciation as he left her at the foot of the stairs and walked into his study. He closed the door quietly behind him, and, not wanting to overhear the excuse he gave the NBC editor who'd called him with the assignment, she took herself off to shower alone. And maybe, since she wasn't screaming for once, she'd take a peek at the baby too.

Carla was in her old stone kitchen, with Eddie at her feet, and a fabulous new look gazing back at her from the mirror. She loved what the French stylist had done to her hair, cutting it and reshaping it into a scrunchy sort of bob, and the creams and lotions Avril had insisted on lavishing upon her had definitely perked up her skin, which had undeniably lost lustre this past year. Now it was glowing, and as she watched her lightly frosted lips curve with pleasure, she remembered how uplifting it was to look this good. In fact the world was starting to feel like a conquerable place, and her wonderfully slimmed-down thighs in their new Versace jeans, that Avril had bought in one of the staggeringly expensive boutiques of Monte Carlo, were just such a treat to behold that she couldn't stop admiring them.

Naturally she had every intention of paying Avril back, which Avril was making a pretence of believing, but for the moment Carla had to swallow her pride and accept that her friend was right, looking the part was often *the most important* part of creating the right impression. And impressions were everything when it came to persuading someone that the right place for their money was in your pocket.

During the two days in Monaco, and all the way back on the plane, they'd discussed little else besides the programme and its goals. Avril's energy was boundless, and her talent for inspiring was second to none. She'd now roared off back to London in the Porsche to start hitting on all her contacts for the favours she needed, leaving Carla's head spinning with ideas, and her hopes brimming over with the belief that the programme really was going to work.

Turning away from the mirror, she went to put on the kettle, possibilities for all kinds of new programmes tripping over themselves in her head. Though she was longing to get to work on them, she had to accept that for the time being at least they'd have to stay where they were, since nothing about the second series had been firmed up yet, nor would it be until she had funding. *Oh please God, please, please, please, let it happen.*

When the tea was made she found a few more tasks to do in the kitchen, then she remembered there were things she needed to sort out upstairs, after which she called Sonya to thank her again for looking after Eddie, then she toyed with the idea of ringing Graham to let him know she was back and available for a drink tonight. But that had to wait, because when she and Avril had driven past his house on their way into the village she'd noticed Detective Inspector Fellowes's white Toyota parked on the gravel outside. The detective was a regular visitor to the rectory, assisting Graham with his research and providing vital inspiration for stories. No doubt the two were deeply ensconced in the mapping out of some dastardly plot, so the last thing Graham would welcome was a 'guess where I've been?' call from her. She'd leave it until after six, and try him then.

In the meantime she'd run short of excuses to keep her out of the office. Ridiculous really, that she'd got herself into such a state of nerves about playing back whatever messages there might be on her machine. But while they remained there, and she remained here, she could continue clinging to the hope that one of them might be from Richard. Actually, she didn't really expect any of them to be, but that wasn't going to prevent the crushing disappointment when she found out that none were. Of course there would still be the email, so all

92

hope needn't be lost, it was just that she would so dearly, dearly love to hear his voice.

There was nothing on either the answerphone or the email.

For one horrible moment she thought she was going to cry, until she reminded herself that, really, it was her turn to contact him, since she hadn't yet replied to that bizarre quote from the *Philosophical Dictionary*. And actually, she did have some idea of what it might be about, though wasn't sure she had the courage to admit it, just in case she was wrong. But if she was right then it could only mean that his feelings for her hadn't changed, and he'd made a terrible mistake in going off with Chrissie.

Oh God, what were they going to do?

But the only real question right now was what was *she* going to do?

Send an email, of course.

Saying?

'I'd like a straight answer to my question, did my mother know about you and Chrissie?'

Or: 'Are you completely insane? Why the hell do you think I'd want to be godmother to any child of yours and Chrissie's?' Oh God, the awful feelings that stirred up inside her whenever she thought of him holding and loving a baby that wasn't hers . . .

But what if he was suffering as much as she was? What if he was trying to find his way back? It was going to be so hard, and maybe he needed her to give him the answers. Or at least to let him know that she wanted it too. But she couldn't risk it. Not yet. She had to be sure that she was reading this correctly, before she even thought about exposing herself that way.

So in the end she typed a message saying only, 'Richard, tell me what you really want,' and clicked on the send box.

As she sat back her heart was beating fast, as though she had performed some amazing physical task, rather than the more minimal feat of pressing a button. Then the phone suddenly rang and she almost leapt out of her skin. Was it possible for an email to get there that fast? She felt suddenly strange and disoriented. She hadn't spoken to him in over a year . . . Was she going to have to speak to him now, with no time to think?

Gingerly she lifted the receiver and put it to her ear. 'Hello?'

'Ah, good, you're back,' Graham's voice said. 'I saw a light on down there and hoped it wasn't anything sinister.'

A vying mix of disappointment and relief rushed through her. 'No, just me,' she responded, rallying swiftly. 'How are you?'

'Fine. How was Monte Carlo?'

'You know!' she cried. 'Who told you?'

He was laughing. 'You should know by now that you can't keep anything a secret in this village. So did you have a good time with your friend Avril?'

Carla had to laugh, for obviously Faith had been delivering more than the mail again. 'We had a wonderful time,' she said. 'It was just what I needed to boost up my energy before all the hard work begins. Are you free for a drink this evening?'

'Absolutely.' Then his tone seemed to sober a little as he said, 'I've some news for you that you might find, well, interesting.'

Carla's heart jolted. Was it something to do with Richard? Why did everything have to be to do with Richard? 'I want to give Eddie a bit of a run,' she said, 'then I need to shower after the journey back. So I'll meet you at seven?'

'Sounds good,' he replied, and rang off.

It was almost dark by the time Carla finally got out of the door with Eddie, having been caught up on the phone with Avril for ages, then with all the calls that had resulted from that one. There was no doubt Avril was a powerhouse when it came to getting things moving – she'd even written the spiel Carla should deliver when she spoke to all the contacts she was giving her, like TV reviewers, travel-magazine chiefs, newspaper columnists, chat-show researchers, and a whole host of others who were in a position to promote her programme. Avril already had a meeting lined up the next day over at Channel 4 to get the low-down on what kind of promotion they were planning, and though she didn't need Carla to be there, she did need her to fax over whatever material she had on each individual show.

94

'Everyone's asking about Chrissie,' she warned. 'She's the celeb, she's the show's front person, so she's the one they want to talk to.'

Carla's voice was stony. 'Out of the question.'

'We're way too late for the glossies,' Avril continued, 'but I think I can get some ad space in some of the weeklies, probably feature space too. But again, Chrissie's going to be the one they want.'

'How do we get round it?' Carla demanded.

'With difficulty, but I'm working on it. I'm also looking into renting an apartment so's we've both got somewhere to stay in London when we need it. I've told the agent to find one with a garden so Eddie's got some space too.'

Carla smiled. 'Thanks,' she said. 'He'll like that.'

'Any emails?'

It was a moment before Carla realized she was meaning for her. 'Yes,' she answered. 'Do you want me to read them out?'

'OK. My laptop should've turned up by now. I told them to FedEx it. Is it there?'

'I haven't seen it. Or, wait a minute, there's a card here telling us to call so they can redeliver. I'll do that tomorrow.'

After she read out the half-dozen or so messages that had come through for Avril, she made the calls that Avril had insisted couldn't wait, then went quickly back online just to see if there was any response yet from Richard. There wasn't, so she rooted out Eddie's lead from his overnight bag to take him out before it got dark.

She'd more or less failed in the last, as the sun had already gone down and only the final milky glow of daylight was lingering over the fields as she and Eddie headed off down the lane that led into the woods. She wouldn't go far, it was too spooky in the dark, and besides, after two days in the warmth of Monte Carlo, she was feeling the cold. One of the alternative shorter routes was along by the stream where her mother had died, but Eddie always got so distressed when they went that way, and she had to confess she didn't like it much either.

In the end, she turned them back onto the path that made a loose, rambling circle around the outskirts of the village. This wasn't a walk she took often, probably because of how close the path sometimes veered towards the backs of the cottages. She'd never stopped to wonder why that should be a problem, though tonight for some reason she did, and to her surprise she realized that it was because she'd wanted to keep a distance, both mentally and physically, from her neighbours. Of course she knew them all, and was never less than friendly when she saw them, but apart from Graham, she had avoided anything more than the most perfunctory contact ever since her mother had died.

Strange, but it was as if the past couple of days away were now serving to show her what a recluse she had become, not only from London and her old friends and old life, but from those she lived with now. Even the efforts to resurrect her programme had largely been made in the privacy of her home. She'd never discussed anything with anyone, except her family or Graham, nor had she allowed any but them to pass her front door. In fact, all this time she'd been keeping her neighbours at a stiff arm's length, treating them almost with suspicion, when they'd never done anything but be good and loyal friends to her, her mother and her grandmother. Indeed in their own way they were like family too, but she'd been so fearful of anyone ever mentioning Chrissie or Richard that she hadn't only cut herself off from those she knew to be in touch with them, she'd done the same with those who weren't.

Eddie suddenly started straining at the lead, and as Dumbbell, his girlfriend, abruptly popped from the bushes like a cork, a twig full of catkins snagged in her coat, Carla released him to go and play. Glancing over the hedge Carla saw Dumbbell's owners, Beanie and Lloyd Lamar, through the uncurtained windows of their cottage, Lloyd downstairs, watching the evening news, Beanie upstairs apparently piling fresh laundry into a cupboard.

She walked on, away from the village now, towards the old wooden footbridge that crossed the stream – the same stream that flowed and bubbled its way down to the spot where her mother had died. It was rare she could look at that stream and not imagine it running with her mother's blood, and tonight was no different. It was horrible. So painful and frightening to think of how something as simple as a fall had had such a disastrous result. She knew that the police had dealt very sensitively with the investigation that had necessarily followed, though Sonya had handled it all, so quite how large a role Detective Inspector Fellowes had played personally, Carla didn't know. She imagined he'd been a rock for Graham, which Carla was thankful for, because even now she could see the sadness in Graham's eyes, and almost feel his loneliness. She'd even wondered, once or twice, if he was ill, for there were times when he looked so tired and drawn that she was sure it was caused by more than the mere overwork he claimed.

Not even wanting to think about how awful it would be were she to lose him too, she crossed the bridge quickly, calling out to Eddie to smother the sound of the rushing water. Both dogs came scooting up behind her, growling and rolling in the grass, then bounding on along the path to where it ran between the back of Graham's house and the enormous apple orchard that belonged to a nearby farm. Large though it was, the old rectory looked so cosy and welcoming in the misty dusk, with lights burning in the downstairs windows and smoke curling from one of the tall redbrick chimneys. She'd only ever been inside once, when Betty was away on one of her regular hikes across the Pennines, or maybe it was the Pyrenees. Betty did a lot of walking, usually with her sister who lived somewhere up north. The house inside was exactly as Carla had expected: the sitting room dominated by a big old fireplace with an antiquated mirror above, rows and rows of bookshelves stuffed with classics, first editions, every conceivable type of encyclopaedia, and a wealth of other books, some of which had subjects Carla had never even heard of. The leather sofa and chairs were rubbed raw in places, the once expensive, but now threadbare rugs lay unevenly over the polished floorboards, and a lovely shiny brass fender embraced the hearth. The kitchen was in the classic old farmhouse style, with a long wooden table in the middle, the original range, lots of copper pots, all kinds of dried herbs and chipped wooden cabinets. It seemed such a shame that Betty was so shy, for the house cried out for people, and the one occasion Carla had visited, with her mother and Richard, they'd had a most entertaining evening feasting on the banquet Graham himself had proudly prepared, while cooking up all sorts of outrageous plots for his future books.

Looking over at the house now, she could see Betty and Inspector Fellowes in the kitchen, chatting and . . . Carla frowned in surprise, for Betty had just turned round and it looked as though she was crying. Inspector Fellowes, with his big, awkward hands and large physique was attempting to comfort her, then Graham appeared, and seemed to try to take over, but Betty pushed him away and Graham looked helplessly at the inspector.

Though intrigued to know what was happening, Carla pressed on, rounding the back of the church and grittily ignoring the cemetery. It was none of her business and she didn't want any of them to look out and spot her, as though she were prying. So she gazed out at the patchwork countryside to where the bushes were turning into large grey clumps in the darkness and the trees were stretching bare arms up to the moon. She inhaled deeply, loving the woodsmoke scent of autumn, and the wonderfully safe feeling she got from being in a place that she knew so well. What a godsend this village and its people had been this past year, but even so, she hadn't treated them properly. She had, now she really thought about it, probably shown little grace in refusing their invites, and even smaller consideration in backing away from their kindness and concern. Her heart began to sink with dismay as it all started coming back to her: the way she'd consistently refused the special bottles of wine Teddy Best brought her from France, to help cheer her up; her spurning of Beanie's offer of a free membership to the gym she owned over at Frome, to get her out a bit more. Even Perry and Fleur had stopped asking her to their UFO vigils, an honour, according to Graham, that was bestowed on very few. Just how much generosity had she thrown back in everyone's faces? Certainly more than she wanted to think about, and much more than anyone deserved. But her life was turning around now, and the very least she could do to make up for all the offence she must have caused was to invite everyone to a party at the pub for the first night of transmission. Who cared that she didn't have any money,

98

she'd find a way of paying; in fact, what was there to stop her taking it out of the budget she already had? After all, in its way it would be a launch party, and as such would be utterly qualifiable for a tax deduction.

Half an hour later, more resolved than ever to throw this party, she was standing at the bar, informing Jack and Sylvia of her plans. Their response couldn't have been more heartening, for Sylvia literally threw out her arms in joy, and Jack, in his more muted way, said, 'Just give me date, time and numbers, and the place'll be yours.'

'Damn right it will,' Sylvia confirmed, taking a tall glass from the shelf behind her. 'We'll have to talk about catering,' she said decisively, an impressive collection of gold bracelets clattering up and down her fleshy brown arms as she served Carla's drink. 'There's lots of stuff we can offer. Canapés and nuts and the like. Or we can do hot food, you know, chilli, or roast chicken, or toad-in-the-hole. Oh, it's a great idea. And doesn't her hair look lovely, Jack? Haven't seen you looking so good in ages. Where d'you get that done, then?'

'Monte Carlo,' Carla responded with a grin.

'What!' Sylvia cried. 'You mean *the* Monte Carlo! How posh. D'you hear that Jack, she's been to Monte Carlo. Never takes me anywhere like that,' she added to Carla. 'All I get is bloody Butlins or Benidorm, and these days it's hard to tell the difference.'

Carla laughed. Obviously Faith had managed to miss the pub when delivering Saturday's round-up of the gossip.

'Anyway, let's get back to this party,' Sylvia said, her hazel eyes sparkling with glee. 'We haven't had a good do here for ages, so we're going to make this one a bit special, aren't we Jack? And to think your programme's going to be on at last. We'll make sure our telly's working properly and we'll put it up in a place where everyone can see it. Oi, Teddy,' she called out, as the bell over the door jangled and Teddy Best came stomping in from the cold, 'did you hear that? Our Carla's going to have a party to celebrate her programme, and weem all invited. That includes you, you old skinflint, so you can give us a good price on some of that grub you got over there in that shop of yourn.'

Teddy's florid face was beaming. 'A party!' he echoed.

'Reckon I d'like the sound of that. And don't you be calling me no skinflint, Sylvia Clifford, cos I always gives you a good deal on everything, and well you know it. Give us a pint, Jack. And what's our Carla having?'

'I've already got one thanks, Teddy,' she answered, twisting round on the bar stool as he came towards her. 'Let me get yours.'

'All right, pint it is then. So what's this party all about? Changed your hair, I see. Very nice. Got a birthday coming up, have you?'

'I just told you, her programme's going out,' Sylvia said, rolling her eyes.

'That right? Well, that's some good news, innit? Your programme, eh?' And winking at Sylvia he added, 'What do you make of that then, us lot going to a showbiz bash? Reckon I'll have to get out me best togs for this one.'

'And those bracers you've got that light up,' Sylvia reminded him. 'But you'll have to remember to keep quiet while the programme's on so we can all watch it. Oh, here come Fleur and Perry. Hey, you two! Want to come to a party?'

Fleur's vague blue eyes blinked, as though she hadn't entirely grasped where she'd just landed. Beside her Perry was quietly wrestling with a dry umbrella. 'Party?' Fleur said. 'Oh yes, we love parties. And yes, we love Eddie too,' she added, as he trotted over to greet her.

Angie, the young solicitor who lived next to the pond, told Fleur about Carla's invitation while Perry ordered their drinks, and offered to provide some moody lighting for the special night. His kindly old face was glowing with the delight of being able to contribute, and Fleur's generally abstract manner seemed to be anchoring itself on all the ideas of what she might do.

Then as everyone else started arriving and were informed of the plan, they got into a kind of competition about what they could bring, or arrange, or stage, or generally add to the occasion, which Carla insisted had to include Maudie Taylor, even if she didn't end up coming.

'Oh, I think she will,' Graham predicted, having turned up in the midst of it all. 'She might not be the life and soul, but I can't see her missing such a great opportunity for a moan. And she likes a spot of the old rum, does Maudie. Remember last Christmas?'

Everyone, except Carla, laughed, for everyone but Carla had been there.

'Started making eyes at the Reverend, she did,' Sylvia explained. 'Christmas Eve it was. Never thought the old bag had it in her. But she's a bit fond of our Reverend, is Maudie.'

''Bout the only one she is fond of,' her husband grunted. 'She was in here giving me grief about serving kids under eighteen yesterday,' he went on. 'Course I never did, but try telling her that.'

'Try telling her to mind her own business, is what you want to do,' Joe Locke recommended.

'Listen to you,' his wife Gayle chided, 'you upped and ran away when she came over to have a go at you about the bonfire smoke the other day.'

'Did not!' he protested. 'I just went to get me amulets and elixirs.'

'What's that?' Jack wanted to know.

'For my devil worship,' Joe explained. 'She thought that was what the bonfire was about, and I wasn't about to disappoint her, was I?'

'You're terrible,' Angie laughed. 'She really believes you're into all that stuff, you know.'

'He's so bloomin' knowledgeable about it all, I reckon he might be,' Sylvia commented.

Gayle laughed fondly as they went on teasing him, until finally she told them, 'He's got this book in the shop, *The Satanic Bible*, and he sits there reading it all day for the sole purpose of tormenting Maudie Taylor.'

'She was up at the church nagging on about them squatters again yesterday,' Teddy told them, showing Jack his empty glass as a signal for another. 'Ask me, it's just an excuse to go and talk to the Reverend. Poor bloke. Don't know how he stands it. Going to have one on me now, Carla?' he offered.

'Why not?' she cried.

It was a good while after Joe Locke had put a third gin and tonic in her hand that she remembered Graham had something to tell her, so, insisting everyone excuse them, she dragged him over to their usual table and plonked herself down.

'So, come on then, what is it?' she teased.

He looked anxiously into her eyes, perhaps regretting mentioning there was anything at all. Then, seeming to realize he was alarming her, he said, 'I know it's none of my business, but has Richard asked you to meet him?'

Her smile instantly drained, as her heart gave a violent kick against her ribs. 'No,' she answered. 'Why do you ask? And by the way, it is your business.'

The momentary softening of his expression relayed his appreciation, then he was troubled again, as he said, 'Do you know if he's still driving a BMW?'

Carla's skin was prickling. 'No. Why?'

'Well, there was a silver BMW outside your place on Sunday, and Betty says the man who got into it looked just like Richard.'

Carla almost reeled at the way her insides responded, and for the moment all she could do was feebly echo, 'Betty?'

'She was outside clipping the hedge when she saw him,' Graham answered. 'She thought he could have been there for a while before she noticed him, because she wasn't looking that way. Then, when she spotted him, she came in to tell me. The car was already driving away by the time I got there, so I didn't see him myself, but she's pretty certain it was him. Has anyone else mentioned it? I wondered if anyone else saw him?'

'No-one's said anything,' she responded, looking over, but hardly seeing her neighbours all grouped at the bar.

'He didn't leave a note?'

She shook her head.

'Does he have keys to the house?'

Carla looked surprised.

'Betty wasn't sure,' he explained, 'but she thought she saw him closing the front door.'

Now Carla was more alarmed than curious.

'She could have got that wrong,' Graham said, in a hasty attempt to reassure her. 'It's hard to tell from our place, with us being at a bit of an angle. Maudie Taylor didn't say anything? She usually doesn't miss a trick.'

'I haven't seen her since I've been back, but we both know if she'd seen him she'd have been over to tell me by now.'

Graham puffed out his cheeks and contemplated his drink. Obviously he too was baffled. 'No more emails?' he said.

Carla shook her head. Then, remembering that she'd just sent one herself, she told him what it had said.

His eyebrows rose as he nodded approval. 'Sounds like a good move to me,' he said. 'Find out what he's really up to.' Then after a pause, 'Did you ever work out what that quotation from the *Philosophical Dictionary* might mean?'

Now that there was a chance Richard had been to see her, Carla didn't feel quite so embarrassed about confessing that she thought he was trying to tell her he'd made a mistake in marrying Chrissie. So she explained how she'd come to the conclusion, watching Graham closely as he listened, occasionally nodding, but saying nothing until she'd finished.

'Mmm,' he grunted when she did.

'In other words,' she said, putting it more succinctly, 'anyone, no matter how clever or principled, can find that they've made a mistake, even in doing what they thought to be the right thing.'

'Oh, indeed they can,' he confirmed with a smile. 'And what about any other possible meanings?'

She shook her head. 'I haven't been able to come up with any others,' she admitted. 'Why? Do you think it means something else?' She desperately hoped he didn't, because her explanation was the only one she really wanted.

'You know the man far better than I do,' he answered. 'But going with what I do know, I think there's a good chance you're reading it correctly.'

Carla's face softened with relief, and again she was smiling. 'So what should I do?' she asked.

He took some time to think about that, before finally saying, 'I don't think there's any more you can do until he responds to your last email, do you? It's a direct question, so let's hope you get a direct answer.'

'Do you think I should ask him if he was here at the weekend?'

Again Graham mulled the question over. 'You could,' was

his response. 'But why not wait to see if he tells you himself, when he sends his next message?'

Carla nodded, as all the possible reasons for why he might have come began playing through her mind.

'You still don't know his telephone number to call him?' Graham asked.

Embarrassed, she shook her head. 'He could always call me,' she said.

'And he hasn't?'

Again she shook her head. Of course, he could, for there was nothing to stop him, but in truth she wasn't sure she was ready to deal with that yet, so maybe she should just feel thankful he hadn't.

Downing the rest of his drink, Graham said, ' I'd better be getting home. Poor Betty was a bit upset with me earlier because I asked her to put off one of her walking trips until after Christmas. Selfish really, but I seem to work better when she's around.'

'So is she going?' Carla asked, standing up too.

His eyes were merry as he said, 'There's no stopping you women once you've made up your minds. And she enjoys spending time with her sister. So yes, she's going. Probably at the weekend.'

'So how's it going with Inspector Fellowes?' Carla asked, after they'd said goodnight to everyone and stepped out into the bitter night air.

His answering look was almost comically dubious. 'He's a good man. Even more of a stickler for detail than I am, but we're making progress. A couple more months and I might have a first draft you can look at, if you like.'

Carla was surprised, and highly flattered. 'I'd love to,' she told him.

His eyes shone with pleasure. 'OK, time to go,' he said. 'And don't worry about Richard having keys to the place, because I'm quite convinced Betty got that bit wrong.'

It was a reminder Carla could well have done without, as she and Eddie hurried back to the cottage, eager to get out of the cold, for even if her mysterious visitor had been Richard – and the silver BMW made it very likely, as it was the make of car he always drove – she was still extremely uneasy about the idea of anyone else having keys to her house. Except Betty probably had got it wrong, because certainly nothing was missing, or disturbed, and . . .

She stopped suddenly. Her heart was filling her throat and a horrible heat prickled over her skin. Sensing something was wrong Eddie looked around and growled, having no way of knowing that Carla's alarm was being caused by the FedEx delivery card she'd read out to Avril earlier. It had been on her desk, along with the rest of her mail, and she had absolutely no recollection of picking it up from the mat and putting it there herself. And as far as she knew, Sonya hadn't come to the house at all over the weekend.

Chapter 7

Avril's voice shrieked excitedly down the phone. 'Are you sitting down for this?' she demanded. *'Are you sitting down?'*

Carla winked at Sonya who was at her own desk, watching Carla on the phone. 'Yes, I'm sitting down,' Carla replied.

'OK, get ready, because this is like the biggest deal since Disney signed Mickey that we've got here. Guess who's agreed to direct the next series?'

Carla blinked in confusion. This wasn't something they'd properly discussed, and now Avril was telling her she actually had someone lined up to do it. 'Who?' she said warily.

Avril gave a little crow of delight before making the triumphant declaration, 'John Rossmore! OK, OK, I know what you're going to say . . .'

'He's an actor!'

'I knew you were going to say that. But he's big time!' Avril reminded her. 'And he wants to get into directing.'

'On *There and Beyond*?' Carla cried with an incredulous laugh.

'I'm serious,' Avril assured her. 'He looked at a couple of tapes from the first series last night, and he really wants to do it.'

Carla was staring at Sonya.

'What's happening?' Sonya whispered.

'But how do we know he can direct?' Carla demanded.

'Of course he can direct. He's done enough TV, for God's sake.'

'As an actor,' Carla reminded her coolly.

'They're making the changeover all the time in Hollywood.'

106

'This isn't Hollywood.'

'No it's Hicksville. Now come on, get a grip. This is an amazing piece of news that's going to make headlines in all the papers, which is something you could do with right now.'

'Aren't you forgetting one important point?' Carla said. 'There's no way in the world I can raise enough money to cover the kind of fee John Rossmore would want.'

Sonya choked on her coffee. 'John Rossmore?' she gasped.

'Wrong!' Avril declared. 'I've already talked it over with him, and he'll do it for whatever you can pay him. Come on, Carla. You've got a great product. Why else do you think someone like Jed Forsyth did it for a couple of biscuits and a pat on the head? You've got action, romance, period, location, thriller, comedy, and an absolute sweetheart of an executive producer . . .'

'But he's not a director,' Carla pointed out obstinately.

'So what? Neither was Chrissie, and you let her direct.'

'Yes, but she was also a partner in the company and she didn't come with his reputation. Everyone knows what a nightmare John Rossmore is to work with.'

'Listen, if he can get us the kind of publicity I *know* he can, think how much easier it's going to be raising finance for the next series.'

'And just what kind of publicity is he planning to do for the first series, considering he had absolutely nothing to do with it?'

Avril was clicking her tongue. 'Boy, you really have some to learn about how publicity works,' she said. 'John Rossmore is one of the very few actors in this country who appeals to men and women alike. Agreed? For the past three, or is it four years, since he made it big in whatever that bloody series was called, no matter what he does now people tune in, and if, for example, he happens to do a chat show and burbles on about this great new "travel show with a difference" that he's about to start shooting, the first series of which just happens to be going out that night, or whenever, and is so brilliant that everyone has to watch . . . Guess what, at least half of them will.'

Carla's enthusiasm still wasn't stirring. 'I'm sorry,' she said. 'I understand everything you're saying, but this is my programme, Avril, and I want it to stay that way. With someone as well known as John Rossmore involved . . . Well, the whole thing will end up turning into his . . .'

'Hey, listen to that ego!' Avril cried. 'But it's OK, I take your point. He's definitely a big fish, and you've worked too hard to get where you are to let him run off with all the glory. I just think you should at least talk to him, then see if you're still of the same mind. If you are, we can forget it and move on. But I'm warning you, if we don't take him, someone's going to root out Chrissie and she'll . . .'

'OK, I'll talk to him,' Carla cut in. Then added, 'Under no circumstances whatsoever do I want Chrissie involved in any of the publicity. Is that clear?'

'I hear you. Now, I've set up a meet for you and John tomorrow at three thirty. I won't be there, because I think it's better for you guys to get to know each other with no-one else around.'

'Where?'

'The Radisson Edwardian Hotel, at Heathrow. He's meeting you halfway.'

Carla looked at the receiver. 'Heathrow is *not* halfway,' she declared.

'It is if you're in Somerset and he's in Paris. Actually, it's closer to you, but he can only fly in for a couple of hours, because he's got some other commitment in Rheims the next day.'

Carla took a breath, then realized she wasn't sure what she wanted to say. In the end she came up with, 'How did you manage to get him?'

'I've known his sister for years,' Avril answered airily. 'She's out in Hollywood. An actress, but not doing quite as well as her brother. Now, changing the subject for a moment, any more emails from you know who?'

Carla's chest tightened. 'No,' she answered.

'So no response yet to the request for a straight answer?'

'No. But Graham told me last night that his wife thought she saw Richard here at the weekend.' As she spoke she was looking at Sonya, whose eyes immediately bulged with interest.

'No kidding,' Avril breathed. 'So what did he want? Any idea?'

'None. But there's a possibility he has keys to the place.'

Sonya's eyes almost popped as Avril shouted, 'What!'

Carla explained what Betty thought she might have seen. Then she added the mail's mysterious journey to her desk. 'Of course, it could have been me who picked it up,' she said. 'I was so spaced out when you dropped me off that I might have done it without realizing. It's just that I was pretty sure I didn't come into the study at all until quite a while after I was back. Still, no harm done. Everything's here, and well, I suppose I should think about changing the locks just in case.'

Sonya was nodding vigorously, then almost leapt out of her skin as someone knocked loudly on the front door.

While she went to answer Carla filled Avril in on her decision to throw a party at the pub.

Avril was thrilled. 'Do you want me to get some press in?' she offered. 'It'll probably only be local . . .'

'No, let's just make it a private thing,' Carla responded. 'Reporters and photographers will only turn it into a circus.'

'OK. Your call. Now you will be there to meet John tomorrow, won't you?'

'I will.'

'And leave your prejudice at home. Not all actors are egomaniacs, despite what you might read about them in the press.'

Carla turned round as Sonya came back in the door and held up a parcel from FedEx. 'Your computer's just arrived,' she told Avril. 'I'll bring it with me tomorrow, on the presumption that you'll be waiting somewhere in the wings while John Rossmore and I talk.'

Avril chuckled. 'You know me well,' she responded. 'Now, put me onto that cousin of mine, because there're a few things I need to discuss with her before I go. Oh, and by the way, the estate agent's taking me to see a flat in Chelsea Park Gardens later. Will Chelsea do for Eddie?'

Carla laughed. 'He'll work on it,' she answered, and passed the phone to Sonya.

Guessing Avril was about to school Sonya in ways to break down Carla's resistance to John Rossmore, Carla left them to it and went to check on Eddie out in the garden.

As she brushed him down and fussed him, she was mulling

over all the jitteriness and anxiety that had managed to slosh itself up on the shores of her newborn zeal. It was annoying, but true, that in total contrast to last night, she was now feeling almost reluctant to take any more steps forward. It all seemed to be going so fast, and she was afraid it might run her into a position she couldn't find a way out of. Like this situation with John Rossmore. She needed some time to think about that, but Avril wasn't allowing it, and apart from feeling railroaded, she was also angry that she hadn't put up a better fight. Then there was the apartment in London, which she'd known was coming, but she'd been tucked away here for so long, with no risk of running into Chrissie or Richard . . .

'Hey! Eddie!' She laughed as he started licking her face. Then, hugging him, she said, 'OK, it's the fact that there's no email from him this morning that's having this negative effect on me. So what do I do to get past it?'

Eddie immediately pounced on his ball and offered it as a solution.

'Oh, no!' she told him. 'I'm not throwing that so's you can go and get muddy again. So come on, in with you, we've got plenty to do and sitting here feeling sorry for me isn't going to get us very far.'

Returning to the office to find Sonya ready to take up arms on behalf of John Rossmore, Carla quickly grabbed the phone as it rang.

'Carla! Teddy Best. Thought I'd give you a call because I've just decided to go over to France this weekend and I wondered about some champagne for your party. I can get it a lot cheaper over there, if you want some.'

'That's a great idea, Teddy!' she cried. 'How much is it?'

His voice rang with pleasure as he said, 'Well, if you want some decent stuff I'd say about fifteen quid a bottle.'

'Perfect. Get two cases. Do you think that'll be enough?'

'Oh yeah. More than enough.'

Carla was about to ring off when she remembered he might be able to help in another way. 'Teddy, you don't happen to know any good locksmiths, do you?'

'Not offhand, but I'll make some enquiries and ring you back.'

Sonya was now on the other line talking to Sylvia about the

catering. Then Fleur popped over to have the proof for her personally designed flyer inspected, and while she was there Gayle Locke rang to ask if anyone had thought about music.

Realizing that this bash was going to start taking over, Carla made an instant decision to delegate all responsibility to Sonya, and was about to go off to Bristol for the first of the three sessions she had booked to re-edit the programme, when Graham called.

'The grapevine tells me that you're looking for a locksmith,' he said.

Carla was momentarily taken aback, until she looked out of the window and saw Faith across the road chatting to Maudie Taylor. Obviously Teddy had told her, and now she was informing the rest of the village that Carla needed new locks for her doors. And what could be the reason behind that? Faith would demand of all concerned. Carla could almost hear the tone of intrigue, bordering on scandal, that Faith was famous for, and was even mildly interested to know what answers she was coming up with. 'That woman!' she laughed. 'She was obviously a town crier in a previous life.'

Graham chuckled too. 'So, would you like me to talk to Barry?' he offered. 'He's sure to know a good one.'

'Inspector Fellowes? Of course, why didn't I think of that?'

'I'll get on to it and call you back,' he said.

As Carla rang off she was aware that her strongest motive for changing the locks was to punish Richard for not replying to her email yet. Which was so utterly absurd that she was surprised she could even admit it to herself. And just as bad was the conflicting reluctance to lock him out, when she didn't even know if it had been him in the first place. In fact, as far as she knew he'd never had any keys anyway.

'OK?' Sonya asked, looking up from the accounts she was working on.

'Mmm,' Carla responded. Then, suddenly galvanized, 'Couldn't be better! Now I'd better go or I'll be late.'

It was after seven by the time she returned that evening to find a lengthy note from Sonya informing her that Inspector Fellowes was sending someone over in the morning to sort out the new locks; that Avril had had a productive meeting with Channel 4 and was dying to tell her about it; that she had to call back everyone listed below, which included the *Radio Times*, Great Western Radio, the marketing manager of British Airways and a couple of provincial newspapers. There was also a party update that went on for a page and a half, and at the very bottom was a great big love-heart pierced through by an arrow bearing John Rossmore's name.

Laughing, Carla shrugged off her coat, and after giving Eddie a couple of biscuits, and making herself some tea, she went to turn on the computer. It was too late now to return any of the calls except Avril's, and before she did that she was going to check the email.

There were eight messages waiting to be opened, but none were from Micromegas.

Angry and upset, she slammed a hand on the desk and cried, 'Why did you ever have to come back into my life just to mess me around like this?'

As her words fell into the silence she turned back to the screen, knowing that the anger was about to desert her and leave her feeling only miserable and alone. It was all very well to be experiencing an upswing in luck regarding her professional life, but these new and confusing events in her personal life were definitely taking the edge off it all.

Then quite suddenly her heartbeat began picking up speed.

'Oh God, don't do this to me,' she murmured, sitting forward.

She'd been so intent on searching out Micromegas that she hadn't noticed a message from someone calling themselves *Bel Ami* – which didn't only mean beautiful friend, but was the title of one of Maupassant's classics.

Quickly she reached for the mouse and clicked the message open.

She read fast, too fast, so that she had to slow herself down and start again.

'You ask what I really want and I feel that to paraphrase Maupassant's Georges Duroy would express my thoughts better than I could do alone. "What was she going to do now? Whom would she marry? Had she any plans or projects, any settled ideas? How he would have liked to know! But why this concern as to what she would be doing? He asked himself the question, and realized that it sprang from one of those confused and secret motives that you hide from yourself and only discover when you start searching deep down inside yourself."

'In my search I have at last confronted my need to reconnect with the strongest part of myself. So I want to know about you; what you're thinking, what you're doing, what you wear, how you feel. Tell me everything, but spare me the pain of knowing that you love someone else now.'

Carla's heart was drowning in the words. 'Oh God, Richard, my love,' she groaned in despair. 'What have you done? What have you done?'

'Made a complete balls-up of everything, that's what he's done,' Avril responded when Carla repeated the question later, after reading her the email. 'And what a bloody cheek, asking you to spare him the pain of telling him you love someone else! Pity he didn't think about that before he went off screwing your best friend.'

'We've all made mistakes, Avril . . .'

'You call that a mistake! After all you've been through and you're calling it a mistake. That's like saying "I had a little smash" when you drove over a cliff and your car blew up. Email him back and plunge in the dagger by telling him you never knew what love was until you met . . .'

'Georges Duroy,' Carla supplied when Avril struggled for a name.

'No! Definitely not him. And though my recollection of that book might be dim, I'm sure I'm right in thinking that Duroy was a shallow bastard who couldn't keep his hands off anything in skirts. So I'm not as impressed with his choice here as you seem to be.'

Carla couldn't help laughing. 'What about him wanting to reconnect with the strongest part of himself?' she said.

'I can only think that Chrissie's cut off his dick,' Avril responded.

Again Carla laughed, but only because she knew exactly what he'd meant and was, in truth, so thrilled by this email that all the feelings she'd been struggling to suppress since he'd gone were now flooding freely back into her heart where they belonged. But she wouldn't discuss that with Avril, because by Avril's own admission she had no romance in her soul, and to be in touch with what was happening here a spirit of romance was vital. And even then it would be wrong of her to expect anyone else to understand the depth of her feelings for Richard, or his for her, when even they struggled to define it with words. The unusual power of their connection meant that though in a physical sense they could live without each other, as the past year had proved, he was obviously finding, just as she was, that it was only half an existence.

So the question now was, should she do as he asked and give him the succour of knowledge about her life? It would almost certainly mean continuing with the emails for a while, because she of all people knew how impossible it would be for them to stay apart once they had seen each other again, and he had other commitments now. Yet he had risked it on Sunday. She was puzzled by that, but not for long, as she realized that it must have been her lack of response to his email that had driven him to come and see her. Which only went to show how deeply he must be suffering. Her heart simultaneously sang and ached to know that he still cared so much. But while he was embroiled in a tangle of entirely different emotions that probably didn't as much concern Chrissie as his daughter, Carla was willing to accept that she had to be patient. In truth she didn't mind that so much, for her life was going to be so hectic and erratic in the next few weeks that right now probably wasn't a good time to be trying to sort things out with Richard. It was enough to have this contact with him that created no physical demands, yet enabled them to give each other the love and support they both craved.

It wasn't until she was getting into bed that she realized, with interest, that he appeared to have taken her forgiveness for granted. She cocked an eyebrow at that, but though on one level it might irk her, on another she was too happy to care that much. Besides, his betrayal with Chrissie wasn't only his fault, it was Chrissie's too, and as Avril had so eloquently pointed out when they were in Monaco, there wasn't a man on this planet who wasn't available if the offer was right. And Richard was no exception, as Chrissie had proved.

But thinking along those lines made her restless and

irritable, and prey to such a monstrous jealousy that it was already swallowing her up inside. She tried hard to avoid it, but it just wasn't possible when her mind was conjuring so many memories of their lovemaking, and her body, neglected for so long, was now desperate for the release. The mere thought of making love with another man was anathema, which was why the fact that he and Chrissie probably still shared the same bed, and could, for all she knew, be making love right at this moment, was almost impossible to bear. Pressing her hands to her head as though to shut out the images, she turned her face into the pillow to stifle her resentment of Chrissie, because Chrissie of all people had always known how much she and Richard meant to each other, that their relationship ran far deeper than most. Maybe it had been too much for Chrissie to bear, seeing Carla loved in a way she never had been, possibly even feared she never would be. So she had tried to take Richard for herself. Indeed she might well have thought she'd succeeded for a while, but there didn't seem much doubt now that she was about to learn the hard way that though you could seduce a man's flesh, you couldn't seduce his soul.

By the time Carla arrived at the Radisson Edwardian Hotel the following afternoon she was in the very worst of tempers. Not only had her poor excuse for a car whined and spluttered the whole way there, but the passenger window had jammed open an inch making the motorway noise intolerable, as well as turning the vehicle into a mobile fridge, and then the wipers had packed up during a brief but heavy storm, outside Reading, so that the only way to carry on living was to pull over to the side of the road and wait for God to get it over with. So now not only was she unprepared for this meeting, she was also late.

Late she could more or less forgive herself for, after all she had no control over the weather. But to be unprepared was inexcusable, particularly when she knew already that if she wanted to keep Avril on her side she'd have to hire John Rossmore, and if she was going to hire him she should at least be ready to wow him with some plans for the next series. Actually, the very idea of having to impress John Rossmore was really stoking up her resentment, because she just hated being put in a position where she had no say on her own damned project. But it didn't stop there, because there was also the fact that everyone was rooting for him, including her neighbours, since Faith had managed to get wind of his possible involvement and had delightedly spread it around. There wasn't much doubt that Sonya was the source of that little leak, having very probably been unplugged by Avril. So now here she was, about to meet a man whom she absolutely did not want on the team, but because of pressure from other sources, as well as her own professional pride, was having to put on a show for anyway. And what had she done to achieve that? Well, what she *should* have done, like any good producer, was spend the entire morning assembling a coherent and cohesive set of outlines for the next series to present for discussion. And certainly that was what she'd intended to do, but with the way her mind kept wandering to Richard, and how she was going to answer his email, all she'd actually managed was three fairly competent outlines which she'd boosted with several other ideas that she'd grabbed from the filing cabinet just before leaving.

It was no way to be meeting a new director, particularly when she needed to make it clear from the start that she was the boss. It would also be an advantage to appear in some way conversant with her own ideas, but since she'd had no opportunity to try them out on anyone before coming, she would just have to wing it and hope he didn't notice if she occasionally lost the plot. What was she talking about? The man was an actor, of course he wouldn't notice, all that was going to concern him was what *he* had to say.

Locking the car, and threatening to abandon it for ever in a ditch if it didn't get her home, she began battling her way across the car park, through sweeping gusts of wind that were gaily whipping up dust, diesel fumes, assorted rubbish and her skirt. What an utterly absurd choice of outfit to wear when she knew the airport was under constant attack from the elements, but hell, why wear a perfectly smart trouser suit, or long, heavy overcoat, when there was such fun to be had trying to hang on to her paperwork and hair while a voluminous grey voile skirt wrapped itself round her face?

116

Bracing herself against the thunderous roar of a jet taking off, and the pounding pace of passing traffic, she literally lurched round the side of the hotel, skimmed clownishly along the front of it, then finally flung herself in through the revolving doors. The sudden warmth and tranquillity almost dizzied her, as she stood there looking like she'd just dropped in from the local madhouse, while everyone else moved quietly and immaculately about their business. Not until later did any of this form itself into an amusing anecdote for Richard, because for the moment she was just too damned angry with herself, the weather and John Rossmore, to raise even a glimmer of humour.

After a quick trip to the ladies where she straightened up the short, double-breasted jacket of her suit, and tossed her hair into a more stylish form of dishevelment, she returned to the grand, thickly carpeted lobby with all its love seats, dark wood panelling and liveried porters, to seek out directions to the tea lounge. Discovering that it was at the top of the five or six steps over to the right, she walked briskly through the milling groups of tourists and businessmen, mounted the steps and found herself in an extremely pleasing baroque-style drawing room. The deep sofas and thickly cushioned chairs that formed each of the cosy niches were upholstered in tasteful fabrics; the lamps were elegant sculptures of bronze and marble, with white hessian shades and exquisite finials; and the small towers of petits fours and scones that were being served to the few guests were all presented on beautifully shining silver platters and crisp white linen.

Finding herself hungry and ready to be more amenable to Mr Rossmore just for choosing this place, she glanced around again to see if she could spot him. Considering his fame, and how comparatively small the lounge was, it shouldn't be difficult, but he was nowhere in evidence, and she was just *going to flip her lid completely* if it turned out that his plane was late and she was forced to sit here for three hours waiting, when she had not the slightest desire to meet him anyway, and when for two pins she'd . . .

'Hello. Carla Craig?'

She swung round to find him standing so close that she

117

might have bumped her nose had he not taken a swift step back. 'Uh, yes, yes,' she stammered.

'Hi, nice to meet you.' He held out a hand to shake. 'John Rossmore.'

'Of course,' she mumbled, taking his hand. Oh God, she hated men who looked like that, all glossy black hair, sculpted cheekbones and deeply intense brown eyes. He didn't even have the decency to look diminished by reality the way most screen actors did, because he had to be at least six feet tall, and was obviously in the great shape that every woman's fantasy should be in. 'Hello, how are you?' she asked tepidly.

'Fine.' He smiled, and she could tell instantly how used he was to winning people over with such a dazzling transformation to an already unspeakably handsome face. 'I was at the concierge's desk arranging a car back to the airport,' he explained.

She nodded, mutely.

Apparently unfazed by her hostility, he put a hand under her arm, saying, 'Come on, I've got us a good spot over by the window.'

Though she was aware of people staring as she allowed herself to be steered across the room to one of the more secluded niches, she was much more concerned with regaining the high ground, since he'd so neatly managed to wrest it for himself, and she still wasn't entirely sure how.

'Would you like tea, or something stronger?' he offered, waving her to a sofa.

'I'm driving,' she answered shortly.

'OK, tea it is,' he declared to the waiter who'd followed them. 'I'll take Indian and my guest will take . . .?' He looked at Carla.

'Jasmine,' she answered.

'Anything to eat, sir?' the waiter offered.

'Oh, I think so,' he replied, looking to Carla for confirmation. Receiving none, as she was busy opening up her briefcase, he said, 'Bring us the works.'

As the waiter went off, Carla clicked closed her briefcase and waited as one of the nation's heart-throbs shrugged off his much-worn Versace leather jacket, which he slung over one of the chairs, before sitting down on the sofa that was at right angles to hers. He was wearing jeans, and a bottle green collarless shirt with a white T-shirt underneath. Unremarkable on anyone else, yet contriving to look something else entirely on him.

He smiled at her again, forcing her to smile weakly back as she thought how he was neither quite as tall as Richard, nor as broad, though she'd concede that he was probably better looking, if you went for those kind of looks, which she certainly didn't. He veered too much towards masculine beauty for her taste, whereas Richard was much more rugged. However, he did exude a certain charisma, she'd give him that, and he was clearly making an attempt to be friendly, so maybe she should too.

Deciding to begin with some small talk, she said, 'What are you doing in Paris?'

He was about to answer when a phone started to ring in his jacket pocket.

'Oh hell,' he grumbled, reaching for it.

Well, there went any attempt on her part to be friendly, because the hell was she going to sit here snatching a few seconds of Mr Rossmore's precious time in between all his vitally important telephone calls.

'There, that should do it,' he said, switching the phone off and stuffing it back in the pocket.

Carla blinked.

'What were we saying? Ah yes, Paris. Actually, I've been there visiting an old friend, but the reason for flying back tonight is because I have to be in Rheims – how do you pronounce that blasted name? – in the morning. Would you believe there's an induction ceremony for the new chevaliers of champagne tomorrow evening, in the caves beneath Moët and Chandon, and . . . Well, I'm one of the inductees.'

Just like an actor, always talking about himself, she was thinking. 'How fascinating,' she said, grudgingly meaning it.

'Yes, it is,' he confirmed. 'Bit ritualistic, with all the cloaks and incense and swords, not to mention the kind of chants they go in for, but it's quite an event.'

Carla was wondering if he was about to pitch it as a programme idea, and knew she wouldn't be entirely averse if

119

he was. 'What exactly does a chevalier of champagne do?' she asked.

He grimaced. 'In my case, drink the stuff,' he answered. 'But I do have an interest in the different cuvées, and I've got quite a long association with a couple of the houses around Epernay. I do promotions for them and get involved in product placement on movies and TV series, that kind of thing, so I guess this is my reward.'

'So you actually get knighted?' she said. 'Like with a sword-tap on each shoulder, in front of some kind of altar or something?'

'Yes, that's how it happens. In front of an altar, in an underground cave that's entirely lit by candles.'

'Please don't tell me you have to prostrate yourself naked, or drink goat's blood, or something other-worldly like that.'

Laughing, he said, 'No, the clothes stay on and all that's imbibed is champagne, plus an extremely regal banquet that follows the ceremony. I could arrange for you to go some time, if you're interested.'

Startled, she nodded, then lifted a file from the small stack she'd put on the table. 'Yes, I think I would be,' she confessed. 'Would they be amenable to having cameras around?'

His head went dubiously to one side. 'That, I doubt,' he responded. 'But we could always ask.'

His use of 'we' immediately irked her, for it showed that he obviously considered himself to be already hired. She wondered if anyone ever said no to this man, and struggled with a sudden urge to become one of the first. Avril! She must remember Avril, and how none of this would be happening without her.

'I guess now's a good time to tell you what a great programme you have on your hands,' he said, managing to catch her off-guard again. 'It's innovative, imaginative, terrific entertainment and a genuinely quality product.'

What else could she say but, 'Thank you.' Then she added a little swipe with, 'I had an extremely good director for three of the episodes.'

'Jed Forsyth, I know. He speaks very highly of you too. And the other three were directed by Chrissie Fields, is that right? Or does she go under her married name now?'

Carla instantly stiffened. 'No, she still uses Fields,' she told him, without having the faintest idea if it was true.

'Her episodes are pretty remarkable too,' he said. 'And she does a great job of presenting. Will you be using her for the next series?'

'No,' Carla answered shortly. 'She's no longer a part of the company.'

Obviously realizing he'd stumbled onto thin ice, he rescued himself with, 'So who have you got in mind to replace her?'

'It's still up for discussion,' she answered. 'Avril's had a few ideas, but I haven't arranged any auditions yet. So now,' she continued, attempting to appropriate the interviewer's chair, 'what, if anything, would you change about the programme, were you in a position to?' Subtle, she thought, but a timely reminder that his own role was not yet confirmed, nor was it above hers, which was how he was managing to make it sound.

He was about to answer when the tea arrived, and several minutes passed as it was set out and poured, while a tower of exquisite delicacies was put in front of her and her mouth began watering so vigorously that she was afraid she might actually start frothing. When was the last time she'd eaten? she wondered. Last night? No, it must have been . . . Good God, it was breakfast yesterday morning. No wonder she was so famished. In fact, if the waiter didn't hurry up and push off, she might be tempted to shove him out of the way so that she could grab a couple of those dainty crab sandwiches before they got spirited away by someone else.

'At this stage,' John said, returning to a question she'd almost forgotten in her eagerness to get to the food, 'I don't think I'd change anything.'

Oh, sycophant, she was thinking, as the waiter finally dissolved leaving a clear path between her and the scones.

'That's not to say it's perfect,' he added.

She looked at him sharply, reminding him he was in no position to criticize, yet. Then she went on dolloping jam and cream on the side of her plate.

'I just think,' he went on, apparently not in receipt of her mentally transmitted warning, 'that we should wait for the first series to go out, or at least the first couple of episodes, see what the reviews are like, and the audience reaction. After all, it's pretty high-concept stuff, so we're going to have to see how it spins with the general public. If it goes over their heads, then obviously changes will have to be made to simplify it, make it more accessible.'

It was a moment before she could answer, since she'd been relying on the actor's love of his own voice to carry her through the particularly large bite she'd just taken out of a scone. 'And how do you suggest we do that?' she finally enquired, managing to block any escaping crumbs with a napkin.

He picked up his tea, and sitting back with it, lifted one ankle to rest on the other knee. As he began outlining the several ideas he'd had, she listened attentively and continued to eat. Then, noticing he wasn't joining her, she indicated the three tiers of food.

Shaking his head, but gesturing for her to continue, he carried on talking, and quite soon they were into a lively debate on the various shapes the programme could take. There was no doubt he'd really thought about this, and, on the whole, she wasn't as averse to his suggestions as she'd like to have been.

'OK,' she said, eventually, while getting ready to wolf down a thumb-sized eclair, 'let's move on to programme content for the second series.' Nodding towards the file she'd made up for him, she continued, 'That's for you. It contains ten or eleven outlines that I've drawn up, some obvious con-tenders for programmes, others less so, but our experience last time was that sometimes the less obvious turn out to be the most interesting.'

He was flicking through the pages, reading swiftly to see which locations she had in mind. 'Do you script the dramas yourself,' he asked, 'or do you get someone in?'

'I do it,' she answered, daring him to comment negatively now he knew that.

However, worse than negative comment was the slow, pensive nod he gave, and the failure even to raise an eyebrow. Such flaming arrogance! What did he know about scriptwriting anyway, when all he had to do was learn the damned lines? Already she was imagining the choice words she would use when relating this scene to Richard, hopefully in a way that would make him laugh and wish that he was with her in person to share the joke.

'Mmm, Argentina's an interesting choice,' he said. 'And Timbuktu. Incidentally, do you have any idea of dates yet?'

Busy with another scone she said, 'If we can get the money in place then I'm hoping we'll be in a position to start shooting at the beginning of January. Are you sure you don't want any of this? It's delicious.'

'No, really. But you carry on. And your schedule runs through to when?' he asked.

'Probably June. But obviously the pre-production is already under way. And the post-production will run on until sometime in September or October. Possibly even as late as November. Which means that you're looking at a whole year out of your normal schedule, which is probably much too long for someone in your position.' Why had she never thought of this before? It was perfect, because there surely wasn't an actor alive who would view such a long spell out of the limelight as anything but death to his destiny.

However, it seemed she was looking at such a person. 'I'd kind of figured it would be about that long,' he said, closing the file and looking at her.

What was going on here? He was seriously going to take a year out for a programme like *There and Beyond*? Deciding to dispense with all the interview pretence for a moment, she said, 'If you don't mind me asking, why on earth do you want to do this? I mean, being who you are, you surely can't be short of projects to direct. In fact, I'd've thought you'd be much more interested in taking on a feature film, or at the very least some kind of BBC drama, than this kind of series.'

'You're right,' he said, sitting forward to refill both their cups. 'I'm constantly inundated with scripts, but frankly I've not come across anything yet that I'd want to go out and raise money for, never mind put my name to. And if I'm going to get into directing I want it to be on something that's worthwhile and, well, quality – which I consider *There and Beyond* to be. Also, I'm keen to get out of acting, which I only got into by mistake, and don't particularly enjoy. However, it's earned me a pile of money, which I'm not complaining about, and it's given me a lot of advantages and privileges I probably wouldn't otherwise have had. But it's definitely time now to move on, and when Avril called me about your project, though I can't say I was particularly interested at the time, after I spoke to Jed Forsyth, then saw the first couple of episodes, I had a very different attitude.'

Unable to feel anything but pleased by such a generous compliment, Carla inclined her head gracefully, and accepted a third cup of tea.

'Of course, you might be averse to having someone like me on board,' he went on, 'which I wouldn't blame you for, because fame, as I'm sure you know, isn't always a blessing. But it does have its upside, which is why Avril contacted me. And as well as all the publicity I can bring to the table, you'd also be getting one hundred per cent commitment and co-operation, and a pretty good stock of actors who, to be blunt, would be more likely to stump up the goods for me than they would for you.'

'I'm not a director,' she responded tersely. 'So I wouldn't be asking them.'

'I'm sorry, I didn't put that very well. What I meant was they'd be more likely to do it for less than their usual rate if I ask them, than if anyone else were to.'

Mmm, well, that was definitely a bonus she hadn't considered, and certainly not one to be sniffed at. 'And if the twenty-million-dollar Hollywood offer comes along?' she challenged.

Apparently finding that amusing, he said, 'I'm flattered that you think I could command such a sum, but believe me, I can't.'

'But if it did?'

'Then I have to confess, twenty million would be hard to turn down.'

Not exactly the answer she was looking for, but she had to admire his honesty. 'Do you want that sandwich?' she offered, pointing to the last one left on the tray.

'No, really.'

She picked up the sandwich, and for a moment their eyes met, but not wanting him to think he could dazzle her the way he no doubt dazzled every other woman he came across, she looked quickly away.

'Going back to programme content,' he said, tapping the file he'd put on the seat next to him. 'I'd like to take a couple of days to look this over, then get back to you. Is that OK?'

Her head came up. No, it was not. At least not when he was making it sound as though he was the one mulling over a decision. As far as she was aware, she was interviewing him. OK, with a foregone conclusion, but he could at least pretend he was waiting for her decision, rather than the other way round.

He was still speaking. 'I was thinking it might help you to make your mind up about me if I could contribute something intelligent to the upcoming series. But I'm afraid I can't do that until I really know what you have in mind.'

Smooth, she was thinking. Very smooth indeed. And acceptable. 'Sounds like a good idea,' she responded. 'When are you back from France?'

'At the weekend. If you'll give me your number I'll call you on Saturday.'

'Would madam care for any more?'

She looked up at the waiter, then down at the empty tiers of the cakestand. She'd managed to scoff the lot. Embarrassed, she glanced at John Rossmore, who, with typical actor self-interest, didn't seem to have noticed. In fact, he was looking at his watch, obviously eager to get away now he'd gone through the motions of paying homage to her executive-producer status.

'Could you bring us the bill please?' he said to the waiter.

With practised ease the waiter cleared the table and narrowly avoided colliding with a bellhop who'd come to inform Mr Rossmore that the car was here to take him back to the terminal.

'I'm sorry this has been a bit rushed,' John said, turning back to Carla, 'but I was keen to meet you as soon as I could, and try to persuade you that I'm the right man for the job. I know there must be a hundred more questions you want to ask me, like what makes me think I can direct when I've never directed anything before . . .'

'Perhaps you can give me an answer to that before you go,' she cut in.

'Actually, I trained as a director,' he told her. Then without a trace of smugness he added, 'At USC in Los Angeles. I was there for a year in my early twenties. That might be more impressive were I not now in my late thirties, I know, but it's a great university and when you combine the skills I learned there with all the experience I've had of being around cameras and directors in both film and television since, well, hopefully some of that makes the grade as a qualification to direct *There and Beyond*.'

Pretty speech, she was thinking. And yes, USC certainly was impressive. So when, I wonder, do we get the truth about the violent temper and unbridled ego? Not to mention the womanizing, binge-drinking, obsessive gambling and alleged cocaine habit? All she said was, 'Good answer.'

After going through the formality of exchanging numbers and saying goodbye, she tried to insist on paying the bill which hadn't yet arrived. However, he wouldn't hear of it, and left her no choice when he dropped a fifty-pound note on the table and went off to get his flight.

'So?' Avril demanded, bounding in only seconds after he'd gone. 'How did it go?'

Carla was nodding slowly. 'OK,' she said. 'He gave a stunning performance of a meek, mild-tempered, eager-to-please new director, and almost had me convinced.'

Avril was grinning. 'You're a hard woman,' she told her. 'But don't you think he's gorgeous?'

Carla's eyebrows arched. 'No. But you obviously do.'

'How can anyone not? And he's such a charmer, don't you think? And those hands. Did you notice his hands?'

'No, I can't say I did.'

Avril gave a shiver of ecstasy. 'How can you not have noticed those hands? They're so long and slender and dark and masculine. I mean, everything about that man is just to die for. Anyway, how did you leave it?'

'He's reading the outlines I gave him and we'll speak on Saturday.'

'But do you think you can work with him?'

Carla rolled her eyes. 'Avril, don't tell me that between you, you and his agent haven't already got his contract drawn up because I won't believe you. And if you've already written the press release I'd like to see it first. It's all about favours,

126

isn't it? You do him one, he does you one. You're doing me one, so I do you one. And on it goes.'

'It's how it works,' Avril confirmed. 'But I swear I wouldn't be pushing this if I thought he was going to give you any trouble.'

'I'll remind you of that when he fires all the actors and goes on a bender in the middle of Baghdad during Ramadan.'

'You've got Baghdad on the agenda for the next series?' Avril said in amazement.

'No, but don't rule it out. In fact, never rule anywhere out, especially not now I'm in touch with Richard again, because he's got contacts all over the world, remember?'

Avril refrained from commenting on that by signalling to the waiter. She still didn't like this contact with Richard, because something wasn't right about it, apart from the obvious, but as yet she hadn't managed to figure out what. Until she did, she guessed she'd just have to keep quiet, for criticizing was only going to make Carla clam up, which wouldn't be a good thing at all. So, after ordering two glasses of champagne, she announced cheerily, 'We've got something else to celebrate. The *Observer* Colour Supplement want to do a three-page spread on the series, which should run to coincide with the third or fourth episode. A great midway boost.'

Carla was thrilled. 'You're a magician,' she told her. 'Just how do you do it?'

'Favours,' Avril reminded her. 'And now for the bad news, I'm afraid. I've had a call from someone on the *Daily Mail*'s Femail page saying they want to do a big feature on Chrissie, you know, everything from the bad first marriage, to the drugs, the attempted suicides, the . . .'

'I thought I'd made myself clear on that,' Carla said tightly. 'I don't want Chrissie involved in the publicity. End of story.'

'You don't have to see her,' Avril pointed out.

'That's not the point. The point is that this programme is mine now. It's all she left me with, though it cost me every penny I had to get it. It's thanks to her that I now drive a car that's not even safe to be on the road; that I live in a house that leaks and I can't afford to repair it; that I've spent the past year hating going to the supermarket because I can't afford

127

the kind of food I used to buy; I never go out, except to the pub, where half the time I avoid people because I can't buy them a drink; the only new clothes I've had in a year were the ones you bought me in Monaco, which was the only holiday I've had, which you paid for too. And those are just the practical things. What she took from me emotionally . . .'

'It's OK, I get the drift,' Avril assured her.

But Carla hadn't finished. 'She's put me in a place where near-poverty and pain are just the beginning,' she said, her voice shaking with feeling, 'because she didn't only rob me of the man I loved, she robbed me of my self-respect, my hope, my dreams, my trust, even my bloody sanity for a while. And now all I have is this programme, which I paid for with every last penny she could wring out of me. So *no*! The hell is she going to get any free publicity, public admiration, money, or whatever else she's seeking out of *my* programme. It's enough that she's going to be on the screen for six weeks, looking gorgeous, being professional and generally assumed Miss Perfect by a world that has no idea. OK, I know that someone might find their own way to her without going through you, but I want you, Avril, to do everything in that remarkable power of yours to stop them, because I've got no intention of sharing any more of my life with Chrissie Fields than I already have.'

Avril was soberly nodding her acceptance, and only stopped when the champagne arrived. Then, raising her glass to propose a toast, she said, 'To anyone else I'd say, power to you, or take it all the way. To you, Carla Craig, I say take it there, and beyond.'

Carla smiled and raised her glass too.

Avril drank first, lowering her eyes so she no longer had to meet Carla's. But it was OK, she didn't have to tell Carla she'd already accepted the Femail offer, she'd just get on the phone first thing in the morning and kill it all stone dead.

Chapter 8

'. . . so now Richard's taken a sabbatical to write a book about all the wars and troubles he's covered,' Chrissie was saying, 'and we've got ourselves a nanny – only a temporary one for the moment, because we're still interviewing – and boy have I got my work cut out, getting that house into shape. Can you believe we're still in packing cases? But Richard's so good about everything, and it all feels so much . . . Well, so much easier now, which is how come I managed to get away for lunch today. Oh, I'm so glad I came. I've really needed to get out, and I've missed you two so much.'

As she talked Chrissie was clutching her wine glass and turning her smiles on and off like a Belisha beacon, while Jilly and Rosa, as stunned by her appearance as by her performance, made slightly ludicrous attempts to smile back. They were at Joe's Café, the chic Draycott Avenue eatery whose spartan decor and unusual menu had kept it right up there on the list of places to be seen at. Indeed there were a few recognizable faces around today, but Chrissie hadn't noticed, for she was far too intent on telling Jilly and Rosa all about what had been happening since she'd last seen them.

'So how's the baby?' Jilly asked, flicking a handful of long crinkly blonde hair over one shoulder as she dug her fork into a cushion of grated carrot.

Chrissie gulped her wine, then smiled ecstatically. 'Oh, she's great. Lovely. Richard absolutely dotes on her, and she's so mad about him I hardly get a look-in.' She laughed, then laughed again. 'Really, you should see them together. It's so adorable. He's a different man since she came along. So gentle and kind and attentive. Not that he wasn't all those things before, but, I have to be honest, it hasn't been easy for me since Ryan was born. I had a really difficult labour – well, you know that, because you came to the hospital, but I haven't really felt up to seeing anyone since, and Richard's been so wonderful and supportive. Actually, it's why he's taken the sabbatical, he just knew that I didn't want him to go away again, so he said he'd give it up for a while. And it's such a relief, I can't tell you. It scares me to death every time he goes away. I mean, I just don't know what I'd do if anything happened and he didn't come back. Well, that's not going to happen now, at least not for a while. But anyway, listen to me going on about myself all the time. What about you? What have you been up to? I haven't heard any gossip in so long I'm just dying to catch up.'

Rosa's wide green eyes slid briefly to Jilly's, then back again. Not for a minute was she fooled by the happy wife and mother act, and she didn't imagine Jilly was either, but what else could they do but go along with it when Chrissie was obviously right on the edge, and God forbid either of them should push her over. 'Well, where would you like us to begin?' she offered. 'We've already covered work . . .'

'Oh yes, work,' Chrissie cried, sighing dramatically. 'What I wouldn't give to go back. We used to have such fun.' Her eyes defocused into the memory for a moment, then seeming to think she'd said something wrong she hastily continued with, 'But only when the baby's a bit older. I wouldn't dream of going back now. Though I do miss seeing everyone and when Richard's shut up in his study for hours on end I hardly ever have anyone to talk to.' She giggled. 'That's probably why I can't shut up now. I'm sorry. Go on, you were going to tell me about work. How's work?'

Rosa glanced at Jilly again, then without a single mention of already having had this conversation, she said, 'Well, in my case, as usual, there's nothing to tell. Zippo auditions, zero calls from agent. I'm thinking of changing, but I don't know who else would take me on when I haven't done anything for over five years.'

'What about men?' Chrissie said eagerly. 'Have you met anyone?'

'Hah! Be serious. You don't meet anyone at my age unless

they're already married, carrying more baggage than a jumbo jet, or gay.' Then with a spiteful little smile she added, 'Shame there aren't any more Richards around, I suppose, seeing he's so perfect.'

Jilly glanced at her sharply, then, as though to soften the edge, she smiled at Chrissie, and said, 'Aren't you going to eat anything? Those fishcakes are really good.'

'Oh, yes! Yes! I guess I'm just so excited about being here that I've forgotten to be hungry.' She scooped up a large forkful of fishcake and put it in her mouth. 'Mmm. Delicious. Now what about you, Jilly? Any new men in your life?'

Jilly rolled her eyes. 'Would you believe Steve and I are back together?' she said. 'Seems we can't live without each other. Trouble is, we can't live with each other either, so we'll see how long it lasts this time.'

'I think you two are made for each other,' Chrissie declared, taking another mouthful of food.

'Speaking of which,' Rosa said silkily, 'do you ever hear from Carla now?'

For a moment Chrissie's eyes widened like a child's as she watched Jilly glance fiercely in Rosa's direction again. But Jilly didn't say anything, so Chrissie quickly smiled, and, reaching for her wine again, said, 'No. Richard thought it was better not to have any more contact, after she, you know, threatened me.'

Jilly and Rosa nodded gravely, then, feeling it wise to change the subject, Jilly said, 'Did you bring any photos of the baby? I'd love to see her. She must be at least four months by now.'

Chrissie nodded. 'Yes, she is. Well, five actually. But I'm afraid I forgot the pictures. Richard put them out to remind me, but when I checked in the taxi on the way over, I'd forgotten to put them in my bag. I know, you'll have to come and visit. We haven't done much more to the house since you last saw it, but I'm getting to work on that in the next couple of weeks. In fact, if you know of any good interior designers . . . Oh no!' she gasped, as a waitress tried to take her glass. 'I haven't finished.' Then, noticing Jilly's and Rosa's astonished faces, she quickly let the glass go and said, 'I'm sorry. Please take it.'

An awkward silence followed, until reaching under the table for her bag Chrissie said, 'I'll just pop to the loo. If they take orders for coffee I'll have an espresso.'

Jilly and Rosa watched her weave a path through the tables, then drop down to the lower level, where she disappeared through a door next to the bar.

'My God,' Rosa murmured. 'What a state.'

Jilly's eyes were full of concern. 'Isn't she?' she agreed. 'I had no idea. Did you?'

'How would I? I've hardly spoken to her since the baby.'

'No wonder Richard's given up reporting for a while,' Jilly commented. 'Poor thing's in a really bad way. Do you think she's on anything?'

'What, you mean medication? She could be. Let's just hope it's legal.'

'Oh come on, she wouldn't go back to all that.'

Rosa shrugged. 'Some do. Anyway, she obviously didn't want to talk about Carla.'

Jilly's eyes widened. 'Are you surprised?' she said. 'And I don't understand you trying to bring the subject up when anyone can see how uptight she is.' She paused, then added. 'She looks absolutely dreadful, doesn't she? She must have put on at least a stone and a half. I've never seen her that size before.'

'Yet she hardly ate a thing,' Rosa pointed out.

'Could be nerves, if this is the first time she's been out for months.'

Rosa finished off her Perrier. 'Do you think anyone's told her about the programme going out?'

'Wouldn't she have mentioned it if they had?'

Rosa shrugged. 'I'm surprised no-one from the press has been in touch with her, you know, for interviews and the like. Mind you, looking the way she does she'd be doing herself a favour if she turned them all down.'

'Imagine what that would be like for Carla,' Jilly said, 'having Chrissie promote the programme after everything that's happened.'

'Oh, she'd survive,' Rosa sneered.

Jilly didn't respond to that, for she knew that Rosa's antipathy towards Carla lay in the fact that Carla had blocked her casting for any of the *Beyond* series. 'You know what, I think we should tell Chrissie about the programme,' she said. 'If she already knows, no harm done, if she doesn't, well, she has a right to know, don't you think?'

'Absolutely,' Rosa agreed. 'And imagine how she'd feel if she found out through a promo, or a reporter, or something? I mean, she's going to look pretty stupid if someone calls her up and she doesn't have the first idea what they're talking about.'

'Tell me,' Jilly said, going for a new angle on the subject, 'what do you think her relationship with Richard's really like?'

Rosa laughed and rolled her eyes. 'What's anyone's relationship with anyone really like?' she responded. 'But considering the mess she's in I wouldn't say it was great, would you?'

Jilly shook her head, then, after a moment's further reflection, she said, 'I wonder who started their relationship, her or him?'

Rosa shrugged. 'Does it matter now?'

'It might. I don't know. It could be why she's in such a bad way, because she can't forgive herself for taking him away from Carla. The trouble is she seems to genuinely love him. There again, so did Carla.'

'Well, we know which one of them he chose,' Rosa responded.

'Mmm.' Jilly mulled that over for a while, then said, 'You know, I always thought Carla and Richard had something really special, didn't you? I have to confess I even felt jealous of it sometimes, it seemed so, well, exclusive and . . . I don't know, deep, I guess.'

Rosa's expression was both sour and glum. 'I know what you mean,' she said, lamenting her own lack of success in the worlds of exclusive and deep. 'But then why did he go off with Chrissie?'

'Because she was pregnant? Maybe he loves them both.'

They sat with that for a moment, then Jilly added, 'You know what I think, I think Chrissie's afraid to trust him. After all, she, more than anyone, knows what he did to Carla, and if he's done it once, what's to say he won't do it again?'

133

'And leave her with the baby?'

Jilly shrugged. 'He could try to take Ryan with him.'

'My God, that would destroy her,' Rosa claimed. 'Except she doesn't seem particularly interested in the child, which is really weird when you consider how desperately she always wanted one.'

Downstairs in the ladies room Chrissie was locked inside a cubicle with a bundle of soft white toilet roll pressed to her face as she tried to stifle her sobs. She shouldn't have come here. She shouldn't have allowed Richard to talk her into it. But she'd felt so much better earlier. So strong and happy and excited about seeing the girls. She'd even managed to give Ryan a hug, but she'd put her down again quickly because she didn't like the way Ryan looked at her. Ryan thought she was a stranger, it was why she always screamed when Chrissie touched her. Babies didn't like strangers.

And Chrissie didn't like being away from Richard.

She should go home. She was afraid to be here any longer, but then the thought of going home scared her too, because he would be shut up in his study again, with the door closed keeping her out. When he went to the library, or to see old colleagues, he always locked the study door then too, so she couldn't go in. Why did he do that? What was he hiding? And what was he bringing home in those big brown parcels all the time? He said it was books, but she never saw them. It could be anything.

Everything was scaring her. She hated being so afraid, and wanted to stop, but she didn't know how to. There was a man who'd been watching her, and he terrified her too. She'd seen him twice now, once outside the house looking up at the windows, then again when she was flagging down a taxi to come here. Of course, he could be someone who lived on their square. But even that rational excuse didn't stop her fear.

'Oh God, please help me,' she choked. 'Please give me the strength to go back out there.'

At the table Jilly was checking her watch. 'She's been gone ages,' she said. 'Do you think I should go and see if she's all right?'

'One of us should. I'll order another round of coffee, hers has gone cold. Oh, hang on, here she is.'

134

'Hi, I'm sorry I was so long,' Chrissie said, all smiles as she bustled back into her chair. 'It's just that sometimes I get a bit, you know.'

From the look on Jilly's and Rosa's faces it was clear that they didn't know, nor could they find the right response to the swollen devastation of Chrissie's once lovely blue eyes and soft creamy cheeks.

'Are you OK?' Jilly finally managed.

'Oh yes, I'm fine,' Chrissie answered brightly, as though no such thing as a blotch had ever touched her face, and not a particle of mascara had even thought about smudging. 'Now where were we? I know we were talking about your West End run. I want to hear all about it. Which play was it? Who was in it with you? Who got off with whom?'

After an anxious glance at Rosa, Jilly, not sure what else to do, began telling her what she wanted to know. After a while Rosa chimed in too, then, like a train slowly gathering speed, the story started to become more animated and exaggerated, and then Chrissie was laughing, and seeming to enjoy it so much that they really got into their stride, and before long they were happily speeding her away from whatever had caused her to cry so hard, and taking her to a place where they could all forget for a while that she might just be on the brink of a breakdown, until Rosa suddenly said, 'Did you know that *There and Beyond* is being transmitted in a couple of weeks?'

Chrissie's face turned white, making it plain that she didn't.

Jilly kicked Rosa under the table, but Rosa didn't see how they could stop now, so she said, 'We guessed you might not have heard, so we thought that maybe it might be better hearing it from someone . . . Well, someone like us.'

Chrissie's eyes were darting about their still pink sockets as her head moved oddly from side to side. Then suddenly she said, 'Do you think Carla might want me to do some interviews? I haven't been in front of a camera for so long . . . But I could do it. If she wanted me to. I wonder who's in charge of publicity?'

'I heard she's got some hot shot publicity woman from LA helping her out,' Rosa said.

'Avril Hayden,' Jilly confirmed. 'You remember Avril, she and Carla went to university together.'

'Yes, of course I remember Avril,' Chrissie said, looking edgier and paler than ever. 'Maybe I should try to get in touch with her.'

Jilly nodded, uncertainly. 'Anyway,' she said, moving on, 'the really big news on the grapevine is that John Rossmore's supposed to be directing the next series.'

Chrissie looked stunned, then pinched with jealousy.

'But it's only a rumour,' Jilly hastily assured her. 'My agent mentioned it, but you know my agent, she gets everything wrong. And John Rossmore's an actor, not a director, so she's definitely wrong about this.'

'I really loved directing those programmes,' Chrissie declared. Then with an unconvincing show of nonchalance, she went on, 'Still, that's all in the past. I've got a baby now, and a wonderful husband, and such a hectic life that I'm wondering if I'll really have time to do any publicity. I'll just wait to see if anyone gets in touch with me, I think. Yes, that's what I'll do.' She looked at Rosa and Jilly, then, lowering her eyes to where her hands were tugging at a napkin, she said quietly, 'Yes, that's what I'll do.'

Rosa glanced at Jilly, then back at Chrissie as Chrissie picked up her bag and took five twenty-pound notes out of her purse and put them on the table.

'This is Richard's treat,' she said. 'He insisted.'

Jilly looked at the money. 'Please tell him thank you,' she said.

'Absolutely,' Rosa added.

'I will. It's been a lovely lunch. We must do it again soon. I'll give you a call, OK?'

After kissing them both she got her coat from the cloakroom, then went outside into the bustle of South Kensington to hail a cab.

It didn't take long to get home, and she'd barely closed the front door when Richard came out of his study to ask if she'd had a good time.

'It was OK,' she answered, taking off her coat. 'The girls were on form, and I kept my promise, I didn't have more than two glasses of wine.'

He smiled and kissed her.

'Did you know *There and Beyond*'s about to be transmitted?' she asked, looking up into his face.

He nodded, and searched her eyes with his own, before saying, 'There's a message for you to call Avril Hayden. She's doing the publicity. Elinor took it while I was out,' he added, referring to their temporary nanny.

'Where did you go?'

'Along to Harrods to sort out your birthday present,' he answered, squeezing her.

She turned away and started towards the kitchen. 'Where's the message? I should call Avril back. She might want me to do something.'

When he didn't answer she turned to look at him. 'What's wrong?' she said.

Letting out the breath he was holding he said, 'Nothing. Nothing at all. The message is on the board.'

Refusing to feel guilty about not going to see the baby who had a nanny now, she walked on into the kitchen to use the phone, and taking the number from the blackboard, she dialled it, then turned to gaze blindly out of the window, where their small patio garden was dying.

'Hi, Avril Hayden,' Avril's voice came down the line.

'Avril. It's Chrissie,' she said softly. Then, clearing her throat. 'Chrissie Fields.'

'Oh. Chrissie, yes,' Avril said. 'How are you?'

'OK. How are you?'

'Good. Thank you.'

'I got your message to call.'

'Yes,' Avril responded. 'Did you know that the programme's being . . .'

'Yes, I know,' Chrissie said.

'Right. Well, there's a chance that a couple of reporters, or feature writers or . . .'

'I'll be happy to do it,' Chrissie told her.

Avril was silent.

Chrissie's heart started pounding.

Avril said, 'The thing is, Chrissie, Carla, well, she went through a pretty rough time after everything that happened, and I think, perhaps . . .'

'It's OK. I understand,' Chrissie said sharply. 'You don't want me to do it.'

There was a long pause. Both knew the other was still there, but neither knew what to say. In the end it was Chrissie who spoke.

'I suppose this is better than killing me, which was what she threatened to do.'

Avril said nothing.

Chrissie put down the phone.

Several seconds ticked by, then, sensing Richard was in the doorway, she turned to look at him.

'Come here,' he said, holding out his arms.

When she didn't move he went to her, and held her tightly. 'It's all right,' he whispered, as she started to shake. 'You don't need them. We'll work things out for us, and you'll never need them again.'

Carla's laughter rang out as Avril did an hilarious imitation of Danny Williams, an *Express* reporter whom they both knew well, and, in equal measure, adored and detested.

'"So Avril,"' Avril was saying in a broad Welsh accent, while squinting one eye as though to keep a monocle in place, '"it's like this: we'll give you a full page for your story, if you promise me your next exclusive from Hollywood, with tits. Is that a great deal, or is that a great deal?" So I say, "Danny, make it a double page and I'll throw my tits in for free." And he says, "I heard you had falsies, but I didn't know they were detachable."'

'The man's priceless,' Carla laughed. 'So what did we end up with? Single or double?'

'Double, so's he can find out if they do come off. Now, that's not all,' Avril continued, going back to her reams of scribbled notes. 'Ah yes, are the master tapes in London yet? Channel Four needs them to put some promos together.'

'Sonya got Securicor to take them yesterday.'

'Great, so you're already onto that. Let me see . . .' She flicked through the pages, quickly reeling off everything Carla needed to know, and finishing with: 'I'm waiting to hear back from British Airways about buying the entire series to show on their in-flight video systems.'

Carla's mouth dropped open. 'You're kidding,' she murmured.

'Do I look like I'm kidding? We should hear in a few days. I know that's not really my territory, sales, but it kind of happened as a byproduct of something else, and who's going to say no?'

Carla laughed, and stuck her arms in the air for a luxurious stretch. They were in the cosy little sitting room at the back of the cottage, where a fire was shifting sluggishly in the hearth, and shadows from the rain-spattered windows speckled the gold and cream striped wallpaper above the dado rail. On the deep two-seater sofa, next to Carla, were printouts of the rough-draft scripts she'd been working on these past few days; covering the shaggy rug between her and the fireguard were examples of some of the magazines and newspapers Avril had been talking about, a slumbering Eddie, and a tray of cold coffee. Avril herself was slouched in the big comfy chair that everyone loved to sit in, her slim legs hooked over one arm, a clipboard resting on her knees.

'Now, on to the more personal stuff,' Avril said. 'I've spoken to most of the TV and radio shows that could feature you, and they're . . .'

'*Me?*'

Avril looked up. 'Of course you. If Chrissie's not going to be doing the interviews someone has to, and by my reckoning that leaves you. Which means you should prepare yourself to be asked about Chrissie, and whether or not she's going to be involved in the next series, what she's doing now, etc, etc. God knows what they'll ask, I just want you to be ready when they start getting to the down-and-dirty.'

Carla's expression showed how little she was liking this.

'Of course,' Avril said, looking down at the page in front of her, 'you can avoid it all by handing everything over to John Rossmore and letting him deal with it. We'll have no problem getting him airtime, obviously, and we can always fill him in on what does or doesn't need to be said regarding Chrissie. He's a professional at this, and you, little honey-pie, turned green the minute I mentioned it.'

The narrow escape was too recent for Carla's laughter to be anything but weak. Then, realizing she'd just been backed into a corner again, she fixed Avril with warning eyes, and said, 'He's on the team, OK? So don't keep doing this to me. I just have to tell him the good news, which I will when he calls.'

Avril's whoop of triumph startled Eddie out of his siesta and even made Carla jump. 'I knew you'd go for it,' she cried. 'I just knew it. So now I can get back to his publicity agent and start putting in motion everything we've been cooking up.'

'I'd like to talk to him first,' Carla said.

'Sure. When's that going to be?'

'Probably sometime today, if he keeps to his word and rings.'

'He will. Now, you're having dinner with us all tonight, aren't you? Sonya's booked a restaurant in Bath some-where . . .'

'I can't make it,' Carla interrupted.

Avril stopped in confusion. 'Why not?' she demanded.

Feeling a sudden tension in the back of her neck Carla glanced up at the bracket clock on the mantle, which had belonged to Granny, and was about as good at keeping time as she was at lying. So maybe she should just tell Avril the truth and be done with it. Actually, if she thought it would make sense to Avril she'd much rather do that, but it wouldn't, and the last thing she wanted was for them to end up rowing.

'I thought it was agreed, we're all going for dinner tonight,' Avril said, prompting her to speak. 'Mark and Sonya have got a babysitter. It's part of the reason I drove down here.'

'I know,' Carla responded. 'And I did intend to come, but with the way everything's going ahead so quickly . . .'

'What's that got to do with dinner this evening?' Avril demanded.

'I want to work on the scripts.'

Avril set aside her clipboard and swung her feet to the floor. 'OK, so now we've had the bullshit excuse, how about we go for the real one?'

'Let's just leave it, OK?'

'No. There're no prizes for guessing it's got something to do with Richard, so why not just come right out and tell me?'

'Because I'd rather not.'

'Are you seeing him? Is that why you can't come?'

140

'No.'

'So? What?'

'I don't want to discuss it.'

'Well, I'm sorry about that, because I do. I'm over here working my butt off to help you, and if this thing with Richard's going to start getting in the way . . .'

'We're talking about a family dinner,' Carla snapped. 'That's got nothing to do with what we're trying to achieve for the programme.'

Avril's eyes were harsh, but Carla could see the concern too, so in the end, knowing the tension was only going to get worse if she didn't come clean, she said, 'OK, this evening Richard and I are both going to read the same book between eight and ten. It's a way of being together, in our minds, knowing what the other is doing, and that we're thinking of each other.'

Avril continued to stare at her.

'It's the truth,' Carla assured her.

'Oh, I'm not doubting that,' Avril retorted. 'In fact it's so damned plausible where you and Richard are concerned it must be the rest of us who are wacko.'

Carla sighed. 'Please, don't let's argue over this,' she said.

'I don't intend to. I'm not even going to try to talk you out of it, because I can see that your mind's made up. But please don't think I'm going to lie to Sonya and Mark.'

Carla didn't bother to protest, for it was so damned difficult to make anyone understand the way she felt, or why she needed to do this, that there was no point trying. Maybe, once it was all sorted out, and she and Richard had found a way to be together again, it would be easier to make the others accept the strangeness now. But until then there was no reason to explain, or even share, the depth of their affinity with anyone but each other.

It was much later, after Avril had gone to meet Mark and Sonya, and Carla was thinking about taking Eddie out for some air, that John Rossmore called.

'Hi, is this a good time?' he asked.

'As good as any,' she answered, taking the phone back to the sofa and grimacing apologetically at Eddie who already had his lead in his mouth.

141

'I've been looking through the outlines,' he said, dispensing with preamble, 'and I've earmarked four that I'd like to get together and discuss.'

'Do you want to tell me which four?' she asked, curling her feet under her as she sat down, and allowing Eddie to join her.

'Argentina, Mali, India and Zanzibar.'

Carla froze. 'Zanzibar?' she echoed. Dear God, she must have scooped up the file with all the others when she'd rushed out of the house the other day. What an idiot! That wasn't supposed to have been there at all.

'To be frank,' he said, 'it's the one that's got me going the most, and probably strikes Mali off the list since they're both in Africa. I've always been intrigued by Zanzibar, the old trade routes, the slavery, spice plantations, sultans, piracy – for one small island it's got a heck of a history, fantastic cocktail of cultures, and your story notes about the black woman and the slaver have really grabbed me.'

All Carla could think about was the fact that she had no desire whatsoever to visit the place that had played host to Richard and Chrissie's betrayal. It would be like getting into their bed after they'd made love. Oh God, no! It was unthinkable. But how on earth was she going to tell John Rossmore that? Obviously she couldn't, which meant she'd have to come up with some other excuse.

'None of it's really been thought through yet,' she said feebly.

He laughed. 'You do yourself a disservice,' he responded. 'Your notes are almost as good as a script, and whoever went there – I guess it must have been Chrissie judging by the faxes between the two of you – she did a great job, because the details I've got here show that this programme's virtually ready for lift-off.'

Carla's hand was gripping the phone tightly as she steeled herself to tell him, without explanation, that it wasn't going to happen. But though she opened her mouth the words wouldn't come, because she knew already that his amazement would eventually lead him to talk to Avril, who would know immediately why she was refusing to go, and the last thing she wanted was to start a new series with John

Rossmore thinking she was an overemotional woman whose professionalism took second place to affairs of the heart. In fact she didn't want John Rossmore knowing anything about her personal life at all . . .

'You're not saying anything,' he told her. 'Have I overstepped the mark? I guess I should have asked you first if you're willing to take me on?'

'I think that's a charade we can end right now,' she retorted. 'Of course I'm willing to take you on, and I'm delighted that you find the Zanzibar story so compelling. However . . .'

'I was thinking you might like to choose the cinematographer,' he said, 'since I'm the novice here, and it could be more comfortable for you if you have someone you know on visuals.'

My God he was smooth, she was thinking, for he'd just outmanoeuvred her brilliantly by suggesting something that she was going to insist on. But how could she now, when it would appear so ungracious in the face of such humility? 'Cinematographer is a bit of a grand title for our little sketches,' she responded. 'Lighting cameraman or DP will suffice. And I'm sure you've got a lot more contacts in that field than I have, so please, feel free to make your own choice.'

There was a smile in his voice as he said, 'It's OK, I know I'm not going to win them all as easily as that.'

'I only put up an argument when I feel there's one worth making,' she replied.

'And then you win?'

'Usually.'

Laughing again, he said, 'Look, you might want to hit me for this, but why don't you try relaxing and accept that I'm on your side, and that it's going be my reputation out there too, once we get going. Speaking of which, I'm going to need some information and coaching from you and Avril before I start getting into interviews. Shall we set a date? We could also drop the flag on this Zanzibar project while we're at it, and talk about casting.'

Carla's heart thudded with a moment of panic. Committing to that now was going to put backing out later in the category of fat chance, and she was still hoping that after some time to think she might come up with a reasonable excuse to ditch it. But once again, what could she do but agree, when his enthusiasm was obviously genuine, and when she couldn't help but be flattered that he was so inspired by her ideas? 'Do you have any thoughts on that?' she heard herself asking.

'Several, actually. But I'd really rather do all this in person, and as we're obviously going to have to meet in the next day or so, it can probably wait. In fact, what are you doing this evening? Can you get up to London? Where are you?'

'Somerset. And I'm not free this evening.'

'OK. Then tomorrow. I could drive down there if it's a problem for you to come here. Where's Avril?'

'Here. So perhaps it would be a good idea for you to bring your publicity person here too.'

'Great. And don't worry about providing lunch for us all, if there's a pub nearby it'll be my treat.'

'Well, I suppose that's settled then,' Carla said tartly.

'Sounds that way,' he responded. And after jotting down her address and directions he said, 'See you around noon,' and rang off.

Sylvia was ringing the bell for last orders as Graham carried two gin and tonics from the bar to his and Carla's usual table. Several other villagers were in tonight, busily discussing the party as though Carla weren't even involved, while on the TV a spiky-haired comedian in tartan tights and lurex shirt struggled to make himself noticed.

'So,' Graham said, rubbing his hands together in a businesslike fashion as he settled down in front of the fire. 'Who do I get to hear about first, the famous film star, or the sharing of spiritual connections with Jean-Jacques Rousseau?'

Carla smiled wryly, and casting her mind back over the past two hours, she could almost recapture the utter calm she had felt channelling all her thoughts and feelings in the same direction as Richard's. For a while it had been as though he was breathing with her, thinking with her, joining her inside herself in a way that was maybe even more intimate than sex. How could she ever expect anyone to understand that, other than someone like Graham, who, as far as the human heart

144

was concerned, believed anything was possible, and virtually nothing was simple.

'The Rousseau experience was . . . surreal, and intense, and . . .' She shook her head in bewilderment. 'Just the physical act of holding the book, and knowing that somewhere out there he's doing the same, made me want to hold the book tighter, as though in some way he might feel it.' She didn't add that she'd taken off her sweater and bra and pressed the pages to her skin, just like he'd told her to, for that kind of detail was only for Richard. She'd already sent the email describing the thrill of the paper's coolness on her nipples, and the ache that had cried out inside her for him to be there, removing the rest of her clothes and filling her so full of himself.

'Reading the words,' she continued, 'absorbing them at the same time as him, is so soothing, as though we're linking psychically through a man whose philosophy is still alive, even though he's dead. It's all very esoteric and existential, I suppose, and hard to put into words, but now it's over I feel restless, unsatisfied, and almost desperate for more.' She sighed deeply and picked up her drink.

'Did he tell you whether or not it was him Betty saw last Sunday?' Graham asked.

'No, he didn't. Nor did I ask. But I will, and getting the locks changed was a bit of an overreaction on my part.'

'Well, it's done now. And I don't suppose you really want him going in and out when you're not there. Presuming it was him.'

Actually, she wanted nothing more than for him to come to her at the dead of night, slip into bed beside her and make love to her the way he always used to. 'You're right,' she said, 'I probably don't.' Then, needing to change the subject, she said, 'How is Betty? Has she left yet?'

'This morning. Back next Sunday, so I'm what you would call home alone for the next week. Still, I've survived in the past, so I've no reason not to expect to again. Now, what about Rousseau's *Discourse*? Apart from everything else, did it yield up the message you were expecting?'

Carla shook her head slowly. 'I'm not sure,' she answered. Then with a dry laugh, 'It's definitely not an easy read. At least not for me. Have you read it?'

'Oh, a long time ago. Probably when I was a student. Are you quite certain that it's supposed to have a meaning that's relevant to you two?'

'You know Richard,' she smiled. 'He wouldn't have chosen it at random. He'll be trying to tell me something, and revelling in all the intellectual somersaults that go along with me working it out. In their way they keep me connected to him.'

'But for the moment you're stumped?'

She nodded. 'I thought I might find a clue in one of his letters, but when I went upstairs to look for them they weren't there. I expect Sonya will know where they are. She put everything away after Mum died. It could be they're in storage with my things from London, which reminds me, I'd better pay the bill or it's all going to be evicted. Anyway, moving on to our famous film star. Guess where he wants to go for our first programme?'

'Surprise me.'

'Zanzibar.'

'You succeeded,' he responded. 'How did that come about? I can't see you making the suggestion.'

'Actually, in a way I did,' she said, 'because I gave him the Zanzibar file, without realizing, and wouldn't you just know it, it's come out top of his list. Needless to say I can't think of anywhere I less want to go. In fact, just the thought of it makes me break out in a sweat. Can you imagine? Following in their footsteps like that? Oh God, no,' she shuddered, clasping her hands to her face. 'I just wish I knew how the hell to get out of it.'

'When would it be? I mean, if you don't get out of it,' he asked.

'Probably January. Maybe, if I've seen Richard by then . . .' She picked up her drink, and took a sip. 'You know, I still find it hard to make myself accept that he's with Chrissie,' she said. 'It just doesn't seem to make any sense. They seem so wrong for each other.'

'Children always make things so much more complicated,' he said.

'As if they're not complicated enough, dealing with someone like Richard,' she muttered.

146

'Would you have it any other way?'

Carla looked surprised.

He smiled. 'I only mean that nothing was ever straight-forward with Richard, and there was a time when you thrived on his complexity.'

'It's true,' she conceded. 'But given the choice I'd definitely have Chrissie out of the picture.'

'But not the baby?'

'The baby's innocent. She didn't choose this. Chrissie did.'

'So let Chrissie pay?'

'Why not? Yes! Let her pay.'

Graham's eyes moved to his drink in a way that unsettled her, for it wasn't like him to withdraw at the height of an exchange, and as she watched him she wondered if maybe her tone had been too strident, too suggestive of the violence she'd once threatened. But she hadn't been in her right mind before, she'd said all kinds of things then that she hadn't really meant. Graham knew that, he'd even been the one to assure her that such feelings were normal in her situation. But he was troubled, she could sense it, and since the situation between her and Richard had now altered from when they'd first broken up, she thought that maybe she should be more careful about what she said, and the way she said it, even to Graham. The last thing she wanted was anyone thinking she was some kind of crazy who was vengefully plotting the downfall of the woman who'd stolen her man.

Chapter 9

The following day, fearing that her neighbours would be unable to leave John Rossmore alone if they went to the Coach and Horses, Carla got Avril to waylay him about a mile before the village and steer him in the direction of the George at Norton St Philip, where she'd already reserved a table. Of course everyone was going to recognize him there too, but as none of them knew Carla they probably wouldn't feel quite so free to interrupt – at least that was her theory. And in the event she was almost right, though it was clear from the minute they arrived at the oldest inn in England, with its magnificent original Tudor frontage, cobblestone courtyard, tiny leaded windows and low wooden doorways, that there was going to be no escaping the adulation and autographs. However, Avril and Lionel, John Rossmore's publicist, were well used to these scenes, as was the man himself, so the first ten minutes after their arrival were spent signing and chatting, until a very firm but friendly Lionel eased the star attraction out of the crowd and off into the dining room where Carla was already being shown to a table.

Watching how pleasantly and skilfully he dealt with everyone, from Lionel, to Avril, to his adoring public, had been quite fascinating, she'd found, though mainly because she in no way failed to recognize it for the cleverly disguised manipulation it actually was. In fact, with those eyes and that smile, he probably didn't need to be famous to work his magic, for his physical gifts alone were quite sufficient to enslave the masses. How extraordinary, and sad, that people could be so sucked in by a bit of charm, a few good looks and a sizeable helping of fame. Even Richard, it seemed, from the

148

email she'd received this morning, was affected, for though he'd gone into some wonderful and erotic detail of how their shared experience had been for him last night, he'd ended with a playful warning to her not to be too drawn in by the legendary Rossmore charm. The caution had surprised her, and gone quite a long way towards pleasing her too.

As John joined her at the table, where she sat with her back to the view of the valley, where the rain-washed hamlet of Littleton Barrow glinted like a silver tea set on a vast green and yellow cloth, she noticed two minders closing in behind him. Their purpose, she imagined, was to ensure that John Rossmore was able to eat his lunch and conduct a meeting with no further interruptions.

'Do you always have to go through this?' she asked him, as Lionel and Avril joined them. 'It didn't happen when we met at the hotel.'

He shrugged and pulled out the chair facing hers. 'Heathrow's a pretty anonymous place,' he answered. 'At least those hotels are. Places like this . . . Well, they've got a much more personal feel, and the way I see it, if I'm coming on to their territory I should at least say hello. Trouble is, I could spend the next two hours saying hello, and that's not what we're here for.' He smiled, and, turning to the others as he rubbed his hands together, said, 'Right, what are we all having to drink?'

Carla ordered a shandy, then made a pretence of going through her notes, while he passed their order on to one of his minders. He looked like a cat burglar, she thought, the way he was dressed in tight black jeans and black polo-neck sweater. It would have been embarrassing if she'd worn the same, because she almost had, but in the end she'd decided on an old pair of 501s and a cream-coloured fleece. She hadn't spent much time fussing about with her hair either; after all, they were only going to a pub, and she didn't want anyone thinking she'd got herself all dolled up just because she was meeting a famous actor.

'Hey, we've forgotten the dog,' he cried. 'What's his name, by the way?'

'Eddie,' Carla answered, looking down at Eddie's attentive little face and feeling her heart flood with love.

149

'So, Eddie, is water OK for you?' he asked.

Eddie's head tilted curiously to one side, then he looked up at Carla. Good boy, Carla mentally transmitted, you're not taken in either, but he obviously thinks he can use you to soften me up, so stay with it, buddy. 'Water'll be fine, won't it?' she said, fussing his ears. Then to John, 'He's a bit shy of strangers. But he'll be OK once he gets to know you.'

John held out a hand and Eddie, the treacherous beast, trotted happily over to lick it.

'I'll bet you're a wow with children and old people too,' Carla remarked.

'I've had my moments,' he confessed, his dark eyes simmering with laughter.

Carla tore her own away and looked at his publicist, Lionel, whose resemblance to Bart Simpson was so striking that she'd almost laughed when they were first introduced. Avril could have warned her! 'I got your fax this morning,' she told him. 'The interview schedule's looking extremely good, but unless I've misread something, on one of the days you seem to have John in Newcastle and London at the same time.'

Lionel was leafing swiftly through his paperwork.

'I can answer that,' Avril piped up. 'The Newcastle interview's for radio, and is being done down-the-line from the BBC, just prior to a recording for some afternoon show at Broadcasting House.'

'I see,' Carla responded, looking at the fax again, and when their drinks arrived some five minutes later she was still putting Lionel through his paces with all the points she wanted clarified.

Then Avril took over, and Carla watched John's handsome features settling into a scowl of concentration as Avril talked him through the three-page document she'd just handed him. Most of the details had been provided by Carla, and consisted of everything from how the first series had been devised to anecdotal material on the six locations they'd featured. On a scale of need-to-know it was probably way over the top, but better that than leave him with egg on his face over something that could have been avoided.

As they progressed she listened to his several questions, most of which were points of clarification, though some, she

150

realized, were just to tease Avril, whose responses were, well . . . To put it kindly, Avril and John Rossmore seemed to have quite a rapport going, and Carla was just hazarding a guess as to how long it might be before the connection became physical, when she was brought up sharp by an extremely important point that she had failed to cover.

'What do I say,' he was asking, 'if someone wants to know why the series is only going out now, when it was shot a year to eighteen months ago?'

Carla floundered, as all the real reasons rushed in to fudge up her excuses. How could she have overlooked this? It was unforgivable.

Avril, being the great publicist she was, came sailing right in with, 'You simply tell them that there was a bidding war for transmission rights, and that by the time it was resolved the season had been missed. But everything's been updated to reflect next season's rates.'

Carla was impressed. A gross inflation of the truth, but certainly one she could live with.

John was noting it down.

Lionel said, 'Do we need to go over the locations you're featuring for the next series at this point?'

'No,' John answered. 'Carla and I still have to discuss that, and I don't know about anyone else, but I'm starving, so why don't we make the menu our next point of focus?'

As they spent some time trying to decide between celery and Stilton soup, braised lamb shanks, roast beef and Yorkshire pudding, or tiger prawns in garlic, Carla idly fondled Eddie's ears while noting John Rossmore's apparent oblivion to the attention he was still attracting. And it was plenty, for all the other tables in the large oak-panelled room were now full to overflowing, as was the snug bar that was adjacent, leading her to suspect that word had gone out for miles around that John Rossmore was at the George. Though not a bit convinced by his oblivious act, she had once again to hand it to him, for she'd yet to detect any trace of vanity, nor had she managed a glimpse of the infamous ego. Of course, the man was a gifted actor, everyone knew that, which was what made her so mistrustful of him. And what she was witnessing now, albeit in subtle ways, she realized, was his

151

innate skill for taking charge, which, in less silky terms, was a presumption that everyone would always fall in with what he wanted just because of who he was.

Still, it would be downright childish of her not to order just because he'd suggested they should, so after choosing the lamb shanks, and a packet of pork scratchings for Eddie, she was about to move on to the next point on the agenda when he and Avril suddenly took off on a voyage of discovery, wondering who they might know in common, while trying to recall the odd occasions they'd met before, and showing Carla once again that she was not calling the shots here. Which was precisely why she hadn't wanted him on board, because a power struggle with celebrity was worse than an exercise in total futility, since the entire world was so damned impressed by fame that mere mortals such as she were completely trampled in the rush to the glory.

When she repeated this to Avril, in the car on the way back, it was quite some time before Avril could stop laughing.

In the end, such mirth started to get on Carla's nerves. 'It wasn't that funny,' she snapped. 'In fact, it wasn't meant to be funny at all.'

'I know,' Avril responded. 'That's what makes it so funny.'

Carla turned to glare out of the window.

'You don't get it, do you?' Avril said. 'You just don't get that it's your own ego that's having such a problem here. His is in check, but yours . . . Well, yours is like some pantomime dame trying to steal every show.'

Carla's lips pursed with annoyance, for there was a chance Avril had a point, and if she did, it definitely wasn't one Carla liked.

'What does it matter who the boss is, as long as your goals are the same?' Avril said, steering the Porsche onto the minor road that wound for several rural miles through to Cannock Martin.

Carla chose not to answer.

Avril glanced at her, then, still smiling, she said, 'So you're off to Zanzibar.'

Carla's eyes closed and she inhaled deeply, as though to suppress what she really wanted to say. 'Something else he's managed to get his way on,' she retorted.

'But it's a damned good idea. And if he can get Phoebe Marsh to play the black woman . . .' She allowed a few seconds to pass, then said, 'Look, I know Zanzibar's going to be a tough call for you, so I've got to tell you, I really admire the way you're handling it.'

Carla looked at her in surprise.

'Well, no-one at that table would ever have guessed you had any kind of issue wrapped up in the place,' Avril told her. 'And I have to confess, if I'd been consulted first, I'd have predicted you'd fight it all the way.'

'I wanted to,' Carla grudgingly admitted, 'but he's such a smooth operator he had me agreeing before I could even get my tongue round no.'

For some reason Avril seemed to find that funny too.

'You know,' Carla said, trying not to sound peevish, 'no-one would ever behave the way they do towards him if he weren't famous and so damned good-looking. If he was just your regular Joe, as you Americans say, no-one would take any notice of him at all.'

'Well, he wouldn't be much good to us then, would he?' Avril retorted.

Even Carla had to raise a smile at that. 'So,' she said, once again looking at the passing hedgerows and glimpses of open fields beyond, 'you seem pretty interested in him. Is it something you might pursue?'

Avril's eyebrows went up. 'You never know,' she responded, and brought the car to a stop in front of the cottage. 'And now I can hardly wait to get down to the nitty-gritty of the weirdo ménage à trois you had last night with the focus of your universe and Jean-Jacques Rousseau.'

Carla opened the door for Eddie to jump out. 'You consider yourself such a wag, don't you?' she commented dryly.

Avril grinned and got out too. 'Think I'll stay the night then drive up to London tomorrow,' she said, as Carla let them in the front door. 'I'm sick of staying in that hotel, and the agent's not exactly outperforming herself on the flat-search front. But we'll get there. Tea?'

'Love some,' Carla answered. 'I'll just check if there are any messages.'

There was only one, from Sonya, who still wasn't over the

153

fact that a bric-à-brac stall at the school fête had kept her away from a lunch with John Rossmore. 'Call me the minute you get in, you two,' she said, 'I want every detail. And next time, don't you bother putting yourselves out, I'll see him on your behalf and you can go and freeze your tits off in a field.'

Laughing, Carla went to relay the message to Avril, but when they tried Sonya she'd obviously gone out again.

'She'll call us,' Avril said, curling up in her favourite chair as Carla got the bellows to restart the fire. 'So now, come on, what was the Rousseau thing all about last night?' she demanded.

Carla smiled and picked up her tea as Eddie joined her on the sofa. 'Actually,' she said, 'I don't think it was as much about Rousseau's *Discourse*, as it's about Rousseau himself.'

Avril wrinkled her nose. 'In that?' she encouraged.

'Well, Rousseau believed that man is born good, you know, by nature, but that as he grows up he's corrupted by society.'

Avril waited, then realizing that was it, she threw out her hands and said, 'Oh well, that explains everything! I can't imagine how I managed to miss the point.'

Carla looked at her.

Avril gave an ingenuous smile. 'What the fuck are you talking about?' she said.

'What Richard's saying, as far as I can make out,' Carla replied, 'is that though he strives to be a good man, and believes himself at heart to be one, he is, of course, only human, and therefore susceptible to human weaknesses and society's corruptions. In other words it's a variation on the same theme as his email. In both cases he's asking me to understand that though he gave in to Chrissie, and then followed the path dictated by society in marrying her, it hasn't changed the way he feels about me.'

Again Avril was screwing up her face. 'My God,' she murmured. 'Either your powers of deduction are as convoluted as his messages, or I'm coming at life from the back of a cereal box.'

Carla laughed.

'Well, I suppose you've got to think like him if you're ever going to understand him,' Avril said, still looking as though her eyes might cross. 'So, where do you go from here?'

'I sent him an email telling him how I felt while I was reading the book, knowing he was reading it too . . . Believe it or not, it was quite a sexual experience . . . All right, we'll move on past that, because I can see something rich is about to erupt from your plebeian soul again. I had a message from him this morning, which I answered, and now, well, I suppose I just wait for him to email me back again.'

'God, it's all so fraught with excitement, isn't it? I don't know how you stand it.'

Carla's eyes narrowed.

'Well, don't you want to see him?' Avril asked incredulously.

'Of course I do. I'm practically going off my head wanting to see him . . . But . . .' She paused for a moment, wondering if she should confess how strange she found it that he hadn't picked up the phone to call her, or had yet to express any desire to see her, but getting into that with Avril probably wasn't going to be helpful. Nor did she want to tell her how sometimes she got the feeling she wasn't alone in the house, especially when Richard had yet to say if it was his car Betty had seen outside. It was nonsense, of course, because no-one could get past Eddie, and anyway, why would Richard come in and then hide? He wouldn't. But there was still the occasional sensation of another presence around her, and the only explanation she could come up with was that it was either her mother, or grandmother, which wasn't an answer she was happy with at all.

'But?' Avril prompted.

Carla looked up. 'Of course I want to see him,' she said, 'but it's kind of working this way too. At least for now it is. I mean, obviously it's not perfect, but if we were to see each other, well, everything would take on a pace that we might not be able to control, and to be honest, after everything that's happened there's a lot to repair, and it suits me not to have to deal with it all right now. It's enough to be in touch with him, to be able to communicate, and tell him things the way I used to. And having him in my life again, well, I just can't tell you what a difference it makes.'

'It's no wonder I never go in for all this love shit,' Avril grumbled. 'I'd never hack it.'

'You'd be surprised. Besides, every relationship's different, and I don't expect you'd go for the Richards of this world.'

'Richards? Plural? Darling, he's a one-off, and coming at it from the simplicity of my cornflakes mentality, all I can say is he must have been one hell of a shag to keep you hanging on like this.'

Carla couldn't help but laugh. 'Actually,' she said, 'he is.'

Avril immediately made herself more comfortable. 'Now you're talking my language,' she said. 'So, hit the gas.'

Carla was confused.

'What makes him so fantastic?' Avril cried. 'Which notes does he hit on the way to the Hallelujah Chorus?'

Carla was grinning. 'I'm not telling you that,' she said.

'Yes you bloody well are.'

Laughing, Carla said, 'OK. Well, let me see. I suppose, to begin with, he's tender and passionate. He's always considerate. Very considerate. He's got a way of making you respond to things . . . This is embarrassing.'

'What? You haven't even got to the bit where you take your clothes off yet.'

'You are insufferable,' Carla laughed. Then, after a pause, 'OK, what else can I tell you? Well, he's got this way of touching you, yet not touching you . . . It's hard to explain, but it can drive you nuts, believe me. And then there are times when seeing the way he's turned on is . . . well, mind-blowing in itself. He's so *there* when he's making love. So with the whole experience . . .'

'Listen,' Avril interrupted, 'I'm a picture person, OK? All this cerebral, spiritual stuff – that's not me. Give me position, duration, size, technique, you know the sort of thing.'

Carla's face was aglow with mirth.

'Start with size,' Avril said helpfully. 'What is he? A tonsil-pusher or a toothpick?'

Carla exploded into laughter.

'Does it touch the sides when he goes in, or do you have to start whirling your butt about like a Magimix?'

'Stop!' Carla cried, gripping her sides. 'You're outrageous.'

'Come on. There's got to be something that sets him apart,' Avril urged.

'All right, all right,' Carla finally managed. 'His *thing* is being tied up, hands and feet, and having you . . . Having you massage his body with yours, using these oils he gets in the Middle East.'

Avril's eyebrows went up as the corners of her mouth went down. 'Mmm, not bad,' she said. 'Bit essence of esprit for us more earthy types, but I could live with it. And that telephone call is almost certainly going to be from my cousin, whose lousy timing is on a par with coitus interruptus.'

'Hello?' Carla said into the receiver.

'Hi. It's John Rossmore.'

'Oh. John,' she said, looking at Avril.

Avril swooned. 'Speak of sex and Priapus himself rings up,' she murmured.

'What can I do for you?' Carla said, smothering a laugh.

'Actually it's Avril I need to speak to,' he told her.

Carla passed the phone over, then left them to it while she went to check on the email.

As she waited to go online she could hear Avril chatting and laughing in the next room, and considering how sobered she now felt after describing her sex life with Richard, she could only feel envious of Avril's amazing gift for not taking herself, or life, too seriously. Certainly Avril wouldn't be here, doing this, Carla reflected sadly to herself, when she saw that there was no message from Richard. However, they'd already set a time and date for their next shared hours together, which, he'd insisted, should end in a climax for them both, and not just for him, as it had last night, so maybe, for now, there was no more to say. It wasn't enough though, damn it, for despite his consideration she'd still be alone when it happened, and though they'd shared sex like this countless times in the past, when he'd been away on location, this time around it wasn't leaving her feeling quite so good.

By the time she returned to the sitting room Avril had finished her call with John, and was now speaking to Sonya, assuring her that yes, as the programme's chief administrator, researcher, organizer, accountant and dog-walker, she certainly would meet John Rossmore in the flesh, but as for anything more than that, she could just get in line, because

Avril and a few hundred thousand others were in front of her. 'And now,' she finished, 'I shall hand you over to our very own Olive Oyl.'

Cuffing her, Carla took the phone and went back to the sofa. 'Hi,' she said. 'Without getting into why, do you know where all my letters are from Richard?'

'In your personal box upstairs,' Sonya answered. 'Why?'

'Did I say let's not get into why?' Carla cried. 'Anyway, they're not there.'

'They're not?' Sonya said, surprised. 'I'm sure that's where I put them. In fact I even tied a little ribbon round them, you know, like you see in the movies.'

Carla appreciated that. 'Thank you,' she said. 'But I promise you, they're not there.'

'Did you try the other boxes, just in case I slipped them into the wrong one?'

'Yep.'

'What about under the stairs? I put a few things there, I seem to remember.'

'No. I haven't looked there. But I will.'

'Failing that, they can only be with your other things, in storage. Which reminds me, you . . .'

'. . . need to pay the bill. I know. Don't remind me. Are you coming over in the morning?'

'When have I ever let you down?'

'Actually, never. But we're getting too deep now and there's a tone on the line telling me someone's trying to get through. Can I go?'

'Gone,' Sonya said, and rang off.

'Hello?' Carla said picking up the next call.

'Ah! You're back!' Graham said. 'Did you have a good lunch?'

Carla grinned. 'Graham, you old groupie!' she teased.

'Less of the old. Anyway, I've got something to celebrate,' he said, 'and since I'm home alone, I wondered if you and Avril would do the honours?'

'I'm sure we would. What are they?'

'Come and drink some champagne?'

'Too much of a hardship. But for you we can manage it. What are we celebrating?'

'Actually, my sixtieth birthday, but I only fess up to fifty-three.'

'Oh no!' Carla cried. 'Why didn't you say something earlier? Of course we'll be there. In fact, by the time you open the door we'll be on the threshold. Oh God, how could I have forgotten?'

'Well, you've had a lot . . .'

'No, don't let me off the hook, it'll only make it worse. We'll be there in less time than it takes to stop at Teddy Best's to get a couple more bottles,' and putting the phone down, she stuffed Avril's purse into Avril's hand, attached Eddie to his lead and marched them all out of the house into the twilight, taking just a few minutes longer than usual to lock up, as she got used to her new keys.

Chapter 10

The next two weeks flashed by so fast that even Avril, who was used to working at speed, was starting to get punchy with fatigue and excitement by the end of them. For this period of build-up the show was all hers, so, having lectured Carla harshly on matters of delegation and trust – in order to force her hands off the reins – she'd then ensured Carla's non-interference by setting her a task she was in no position to refuse. Only then were Avril and Lionel really free to mastermind the launch of the series.

'I want you to find me a small but smart office somewhere in the West End that will be suitable for my London base,' Avril declared. 'No, hear me out,' she protested when Carla tried to interrupt. 'This is something I've been meaning to get round to for a year or so, and now I'm here I might as well put it in motion. After all, I can't go on squatting in other people's offices and working out of hotels every time I'm in town. Which reminds me, we still need somewhere to live in London, so you can take that on too. Now, here's your budget. The figure on the right is for the office, not the apartment, OK, just in case you were getting any ideas of evicting the Queen. Keep everything central, I'm not into group travel. Let me see, what else? Oh yes, you and John will need to start talking to potential investors for the next series any time now, so I need a copy of your spiel just in case anything crops up during the promotional period, which it will. Then there's . . .'

'Stop! I absolutely insist on speaking,' Carla cried.

Avril waited.

Carla looked at her.

'Fascinating,' Avril commented, knowing very well that Carla was trying to tell her how nervous she was about going to London. But Avril didn't intend to give that the time of day. London was a city Carla knew well, was home to her previous success and was also where her future lay. Once she was there, immersed in the whirl and challenge of it all, it would soon be as though she'd never left. So when the time came Avril simply handed Eddie over to Sonya, put Carla and a small suitcase into the Porsche and zoomed off up the motorway straight to an appointment with the estate agent. Not that the flat and office search was all that Carla had on her agenda for the next two weeks: there were several meetings with possible investors, also with a couple of international distributors, and plenty of deals to start getting under way with the show's lifeblood organizations such as tour operators and airlines. Then there were the snatched get-togethers with John, who, despite being up to his eyes in the crazy publicity schedule, was still eager to start talking about staffing and casting the news series.

And then suddenly, there they were, three days before transmission, swanning round the West End in a chauffeured Mercedes, poring over all the print coverage the programme was getting, while stopping off every now and then to view the places Carla had shortlisted for Avril's office and apartment. And not a whimper had Avril heard from Carla in the entire two weeks she'd been there about being unable to cope, wanting to go home, or about her painful proximity to Richard. Of course, she was accessing the email regularly through Avril's laptop, and though Avril was no more approving of this peculiar affair than before, she had to concede that, for the moment at least, it seemed to be doing no harm. Carla's mood was generally up, and her dedication to getting it all back together was totally energized and effective. She was also totally torn apart with nerves, as promised funds failed to show up, throwing them all into panic, until suddenly a call came from the bank saying the accounts were now flush, and before they knew it the next lot of funding was going through its little heart-stopping routine of no-show, then show. Added to that was the mounting anxiety of transmission, though in Avril's opinion Carla

161

would have to be some kind of manic-depressive not to feel anything other than delighted with the amount of coverage it was getting, and at how brilliantly John Rossmore was handling it all.

'He's on *The Quinn Wylie Show* tonight,' Avril said, clicking off her mobile and opening her agenda. 'And apparently there's a big piece going into the Saturday *Express* tomorrow that Lionel's just told me about. He also wants to meet with you, or at least talk to you, before you go back to Cannock Martin for the weekend.'

'Who? Lionel or John?'

'John. He's on his way back from Leeds. He's going to call us at the hotel when he gets in. Where are we?' she said, looking out of the car window at the grand terraced houses that lined both sides of the street they were passing through.

'Somewhere between Chelsea and Victoria,' Carla answered, glancing at her watch. 'Kind of Pimlico. The agent's meeting us there in . . . we're already late,' she declared, picking up her mobile as it rang. 'Carla Craig.' Her heart skipped several beats as a voice at the other end informed her that yet another major tour operator didn't want to commit to anything until after the first transmission. 'OK, then I'll be on the phone to you first thing next Tuesday morning,' she told the executive, and rang off. 'Oh God, I don't know how much more of this I can take,' she muttered, but her eyes were bright and her cheeks flushed with the sheer adrenalin of it all.

'Is this office or flat we're about to see?' Avril asked.

Carla was sitting forward, talking to the driver. 'It's just along there, the last one after the tree. That's it, the one on the corner with the black door.' She turned to Avril with a smile that took Avril by surprise with its mischievousness. 'I've saved this one till last,' she declared, 'because this is really something. I just wanted you to see what else was on offer first, then you'll probably have a better understanding of why . . .' Her grin widened. 'Well, come and see for yourself.'

Though the mid-afternoon air was damp, and the sky overhead was grey, it wasn't particularly cold as they stepped out onto the wide leafy street that Avril knew for a fact belonged to the infinitely more exclusive Belgravia, rather

162

than Pimlico. Not that she had a problem with that – home or office, addresses didn't come any smarter than those owned by the Grosvenor Estates. She looked up at the four-storey, double-fronted house that had obviously once been a seriously fancy single residence to somebody famous, though who the chap was, mentioned on the blue circular plaque over the front door, she didn't have the faintest idea. She'd put money on it, though, that he hadn't been responsible for the massive plate-glass windows that turned the entire first floor into a veritable fish tank. Apart from that, the house was like any other on the street, all white stucco and wrought-iron balconies, shiny black railings with gold fleur-de-lys tips and the traditional casement windows. Very upmarket. Suicidally expensive.

'Ah, Carla,' the agent puffed, trotting along from her car where she'd been waiting. 'And Avril. Shall we go in?'

The look that Carla tossed Avril was one of such childlike intrigue that Avril decided to ask nothing, and just let this be the surprise Carla obviously intended.

And boy, what a surprise it was!

'My God!' Avril murmured, as they stepped over the threshold into an entrance hall that spread the entire width of the double-fronted house, and swelled out to the back wall in a perfect half-moon shape. It was so unexpected, and unusual, that it, and everything around it, was hard to take in.

'Start up there,' Carla advised, pointing to the Italianate ceiling that was two storeys above them and boasted the kind of fresco a Renaissance master must have inspired. Avril saw now the reason for the massive windows across the front of the house, to shed light not only on the fresco, but on the extremely spacious hall they were standing in.

'Now the balcony,' Carla said.

Obediently Avril stared at the gently curving gantry that ran along the wall opposite the large windows and overlooked the hall. It was reached by a cantilever staircase with its exquisite filigree banisters that rose from either end of the hall to form a perfect, flat-topped arch over it. She could see that two doors opened off the balcony, and three more opened off the hall, right in front of them.

She looked at Carla. Words were failing her. Behind Carla,

163

Jeannie, the estate agent, with her scruffy little bun and Aquascutum raincoat, was beaming encouragement.

'Words fail me,' Avril said, stating her case.

Carla laughed. 'The same happened to me the first time I saw it,' she said. 'But wait,' and taking off across the black and white tiled hall she opened the middle of the three doors. 'Right,' she said, turning back. 'Now, imagine this. Here, in the hall, we have enough room for eight, possibly ten, desks. OK? And in here,' she continued, throwing an arm through the open door behind her, 'we have a kitchen. And here,' she was now indicating the door to the right of her, 'we have what used to be known as a boot room, but is now a cloakroom complete with toilet and shower. And on the other side we have a meeting-cum-viewing room.'

Avril was blinking.

Carla moved into the centre of the hall, grabbed Avril's arm and pulled her up to the balcony. 'In here,' she said, throwing open the first door, 'we have the master bedroom and en suite bathroom. As you can see it's huge, and the carpets are practically new. The room next door is a bit smaller, but has its own bathroom too.'

Avril was blinking faster. 'I'm not getting this,' she said. 'Desks, kitchen, boot room, bedrooms.'

Carla's eyes were dancing. 'It's going to mean living over the shop,' she said, 'but I thought . . . No, listen . . . I thought we could use downstairs as an office, and up here as two independent studio flats. You could have this one, which is the biggest, and Eddie and I can have the one next door. And guess what! There's a small garden off the kitchen, which can also be for Eddie.'

'Oh, thank goodness for that,' Avril cried faintly, 'I thought for one awful minute you'd forgotten him.'

Carla laughed. 'Don't you think it's fantastic!' she cried.

Avril's eyes were round. 'Fantastic? I've never seen anywhere more fan-fucking-tastic in my life. I take it you've already signed the lease.'

Carla grimaced. 'Ah, well. There's the rub. It's a bit, um, expensive. *But!*'

'I'm listening,' Avril assured her.

'I thought this was something we could do together.

164

Jeannie's already checked with the landlords to see if it's all right for us to use it as a twin-purpose premises, and they've agreed in principle, but they want more details on exactly who we are and what we intend to do.'

In the hall below Jeannie was nodding vigorously.

'So, what I was thinking was that you could run your London operations from here, and I can start up a production office, and when we're in town we've always got somewhere to stay. We can put locks on each of the bedroom doors, to make them entirely independent, and . . .'

'It works!' Avril cut in. 'You don't have to sell it to me any further. I just want to know how much.'

Carla put up her hands defensively. 'It's a lot,' she warned. 'But, great news, British Airways have actually bought the series now, for their in-flight systems, thanks to you, and there are a couple of international deals that are looking really positive. Plus, once we get some real financing going for the next series . . . Well, I can pay my way. Not yet, maybe. But soon. And we can just add up how much I owe you and when I'm in a position . . .'

Avril was walking away. 'Do I speak to the Duke of Westminster himself?' she said to Jeannie. 'Do you have his number? I want to get this in the bag now.'

'Oh yes, yes, yes, yes!' Carla cried, with a twirl of triumph. 'I knew you'd love it. I knew it was going to work.'

'What about furniture?' Avril said, taking out her mobile phone.

'I can get mine out of storage,' Carla answered. 'And we can go shopping for yours.'

'What about the desks etc?'

' I've still got the stuff from Soho, and the rest we could rent . . .'

'Leave it to me,' Avril said, punching in a number. The connection was made quickly, and she was put straight through to Lyle Coates, her business manager, who was based in Studio City, Los Angeles. 'Lyle?' she said, starting to grin. 'We're movin' and a-groovin', so I want you over here as soon as you can make it. Call Hans and have him come too. That's right, we're about to make our official expansion into Europe. What? Sure, I know it's about time, which is why I want you over here . . . OK, just let me know when to expect you.' She rang off, then turned to Jeannie: 'The Duke?'

'Well, it's not actually His Grace himself one speaks to,' she responded. 'And I think I'd better talk to his agents first . . .'

'Do what you have to,' Avril replied looking up at the ceiling. 'What's above?'

'Two more flats,' Carla answered.

'Access?'

Carla looked at Jeannie.

'Around the side,' Jeannie told them. 'Doesn't interfere with this part of the house at all.'

'Right,' Avril said. 'Will someone please now tell me how much the rent on this place is?'

Carla squirmed.

Jeannie turned pale.

'Oh, that much,' Avril said. Then prompting, 'Fifteen thousand a month?'

Carla shook her head.

'Twenty?'

'No. No. Less.'

'Eighteen.'

'No, less than fifteen.'

'Twelve?'

Carla nodded. 'And five hundred,' she added.

'Eleven's our top dollar,' Avril told Jeannie. 'So offer ten.'

'I'm afraid we're talking about pounds,' Jeannie said.

'Just coining a phrase,' Avril explained. 'So, when can we move in?'

Jeannie was still reeling from the speed at which all this was happening.

Carla answered for her. 'Once we've agreed terms, straight away,' she said.

'OK,' Avril decided. 'Seems we're about done here, then. Jeannie knows where to get hold of us, and I think we've got a man to go and watch on TV.'

Ten minutes later they were back in the Mercedes, making slow progress through the early evening traffic. Like Jeannie, Carla was still feeling the after-effects of Avril's lightning decision, whereas Avril was already on the phone to somebody else, discussing something else entirely, as though it, and only it, was of significance in the world. She was amazing, an absolute powerhouse of energy, with a quickness and acuity of mind that was like a whirlwind sweeping through the caution and procrastination of the mere mortals around her. It was no wonder she was so successful for she wasn't only gifted in her field, she was also blessed with the kind of courage most other people only ever dreamed of possessing. In fact, Carla probably hadn't realized just how successful she actually was until she'd seen her in action these past two weeks, and watching the way people sat up when she walked in a room, took notice whenever she spoke and virtually fell over themselves to please her, had been an extremely eye-opening experience. And now, because of Avril, there probably wasn't a person in the country who didn't know that a 'brand new travel programme with a difference' called *There and Beyond*, was being aired at eight o'clock on Monday night. How, Carla wondered, would she ever have done it without her?

After taking several calls herself, she turned to look out of the window. The temperature had dropped like a stone in the last half an hour, and the way the early evening commuters were hunched into their scarves and coats as they scurried around Sloane Square towards the tube almost made her shiver. She watched the leaves, scudding about the gutters, then looked up at all the familiar buildings as they turned into Sloane Street and began heading towards Knightsbridge. Not for the first time in the past two weeks she felt her heartbeat quicken as she wondered where, in this sprawling metropolis, Richard and Chrissie might now live. Though she and Richard were in touch virtually every day, she still hadn't asked, nor would she, for she never knew when the temptation to see him might overwhelm her.

Watching the exclusive streets and houses, garden squares and expensive boutiques pass by, she felt the stirring inside her that told her he was probably thinking about her right now, and trying to imagine where she was too. Her heart turned over, with sadness, happiness and not a little unease, for the strange reality of what was happening between them was in essence no reality at all. What did he really want from her, she wondered. Where did he think this was going? Was he really trying to find a way through for them, or was it all just a cruel and manipulative mind game? But no, she had only to think of his email that morning to know that wasn't the case. 'Nothing is as strong,' he had said, 'or matters as much, as the connection between us. It makes our lives as they are now, mere deviations from a far bigger journey, and proves that time, in its prosaic concept, is unable to separate two halves of the same spirit.'

'Silly bastard,' Avril declared, snapping off her phone and bringing Carla back to earth with a bump. 'Are we there yet?' she demanded, peering out of the window.

'Almost,' Carla answered. 'What time is it?'

Before Avril could reply her phone rang. 'Avril Hayden,' she trilled. 'Oh, it's you. How goes it down there in those rural parts, ooh arrr?'

Guessing it was Sonya, Carla laughed, then reached out for the phone as Avril said, 'Yep, she's right here, I'll pass you over, me ol' babby.'

'I do *not* speak like that!' Sonya was protesting, as Carla put the phone to her ear.

'We all do,' Carla told her, 'to one degree or another, even the fake Yank here. So, what's new?'

'I've emailed all your messages,' Sonya answered. 'Couple of urgent ones from Hayes and Jarvis and NatWest. We're still on a cliff edge, I'm afraid, about to plunge into the black beyond, unless this first programme's a wow! But don't worry, at least the NatWest thing isn't your personal account, which is empty again by the way, it's from their business section. I think they're caving in a bit over the loan terms.'

'Brilliant.'

'Everything's in order for the party on Monday. Maudie Taylor's coming, so Faith says, and the Reverend wants to know if he can bring his nephew who's just getting over the mumps. I told him yes. The nephew's thirty-two, by the way, and, according to Faith, a very good friend of Robin's, our illustrious helicopter pilot who called to say he'll be there, and can he bring his latest boyfriend? Again I said yes. I could go on, but the real reason I'm calling is to find out where the heck you've put the storage bill. They rang me up earlier and threatened to jettison all your stuff if we don't pay by the end of next week.'

'I left it on the desk,' Carla answered. 'In the pending tray.'

'Not there.'

'What about the file?'

'The file's not there either, so obviously one of us has taken it out and put it back in the wrong place. That one of us is probably you. Anyway, you didn't take the bill with you, intending to pay it, then forgot?'

'No.'

'So I'll get them to fax me a copy. Oh, and before you go, what time shall I expect you tomorrow?'

'About lunch time. I'll get the train because Avril's not coming until Sunday. Can you meet me with Eddie?'

'OK. Got to go now, because I want to be home in time to watch *The Quinn Wylie Show*. John's on tonight, isn't he?'

Carla grinned, knowing how thrilled Sonya was to be on first-name terms with her heart-throb. Not that they'd actually met yet, but in her capacity as Carla's office manager and personal assistant, there had been plenty of reasons for Sonya to speak to the great man on the phone this past couple of weeks.

As Carla rang off she was thinking about the missing file, and feeling oddly disturbed by its disappearance. It was only a file, and as Sonya had said, she could easily get a copy of the bill, so where was the problem? Of course there wouldn't be one, were it not for her peculiar feelings of sometimes not being alone in the house, though why anyone, ghostly or otherwise, would be interested in her storage file was beyond her. So Sonya had to be right, somehow it had been put back in the wrong place, and would no doubt surface in the fullness of time.

The car was now pulling up outside the Dorchester – a hotel Carla had never set foot inside, never mind stayed at, until Avril had re-entered her life. Even Richard had been impressed when she'd told him, and in describing the incredible grandeur and opulence she had made it sound as though they were experiencing everything from the expert cuisine, to the marble bathroom, to the enormous silk-canopied bed, together. Maybe not as good as the real thing, but rather arousing and even satisfying in its own incorporeal way.

When they got to their suite Avril headed off to the shower, leaving Carla to retrieve her messages from the email. She saw straight away that two were from Richard, but despite the excitement that sped up her heart, she dealt with her other messages first. Then, after helping herself to a drink from the minibar, she returned to the computer and read both messages through slowly and deliberately, so that she could lose herself totally in every word he had written, every nuance he conjured and all the emotions he aroused.

The first one began, 'Darling, I want you to know how hard this is for me too, knowing that you are so close, feeling you even closer still, and yet being unable to see you. But I do see you, in my mind, in my heart and always, always in my dreams. I am with you, with every fibre of my soul, every yearning of my body. When you lie down on that beautiful bed you describe, I want you to think of me, lying behind you, feel my arms reaching for you, hear my breath as I pull you against me. Let everything that is in your heart flow into mine, as I shall release all that is in mine to yours. Sleep with me, breathe with me, love with me, cry with me. Be always a part of me.'

A knot gathered in Carla's throat as she read the message again and again, and felt his longing and pain sinking deeper and deeper into her heart.

Then finally she moved on to the next.

'Darling, I haven't heard from you since this morning. I've been thinking about you all day, imagining you and everything you've been doing. Knowing where you are at every minute, who you're with and your purpose there, enables me to feel a part of your life, and to be the support to you I always strive to be. You are such a beautiful, courageous woman that my heart sings with the joy of belonging to you. There will be a time for us to reunite physically, for our bodies to share the intimacy of our minds. How I wish that time was now. "We all have the strength to endure the troubles of others," said La Rochefoucauld. Remember that, my darling. Remember it for me, as I shall remember it for you.'

Carla sat back in her chair and took a deep, steadying breath. He never complained about his life, never mentioned Chrissie at all, or the baby very often. She understood why: they weren't a part of this, they were another reality, another existence that had him anchored in a place that he could only escape through expressing his thoughts and sharing his dreams with her. Yet she knew, from little things he said, the odd nuance or allusion, that the burden he was carrying was not only heavy, but deeply painful and worrying. Sometimes she sensed his despair of ever finding the answers: the quote from La Rochefoucauld had conveyed that this evening. But she never pried, never asked for details that she had no desire to know, and would be too painful to hear.

Knowing he would want to hear from her tonight, she clicked open a blank message screen and started to type. 'My darling, I don't need to lie on a bed to feel you near me, or to hear you breathe and know how deeply you love me. You are with me all the time, wherever I am, whatever I am doing. I speak to you in my mind, and know the answers you will give, because I know you are me as I am you. I remember the first time you quoted La Rochefoucauld's words on having the strength to endure others' troubles, and we smiled then, because we felt we had no troubles, but knew that if we did, we would be each other's strength. Know that I am yours now, as you are mine. I will be with you, as arranged, at ten tonight, and already I can feel my desire mounting. Think of my lips and let me feel your own kissing them. Think of my breasts and let me feel your hands caressing them. And later, as I lie with my legs open to receive you, I'll know your desire is filling me in ways that will bring me a brief release from my undying need. *A bientôt, mon cher.*'

By the time Avril emerged from the bathroom the computer was off, and Carla was lounging in front of the TV wearing a thick terry robe and oversized slippers bearing the hotel's gold emblem.

'So, any messages from the great electronic lover?' Avril asked.

Carla smiled. 'Of course.'

'Saying?'

Carla's eyebrows went up.

171

Avril stifled her annoyance and concern, and flopped down on the sofa beside her. It was beyond bizarre, this email-fucking, and though Avril was always interested in sex, in whatever shape or form, this wasn't just sex. This was unscrupulous and controlling, and was leading Carla to a place that Avril was afraid she might be unable to escape from. But what the hell could she do to stop it? Every relationship had its own nuts in the chocolate and Carla was a grown woman, with a mind of her own. Except Avril was convinced Carla knew it wasn't right, though so far she'd shown no signs of breaking it off. Quite the reverse in fact, for she claimed she needed it. It made her feel whole and worthwhile again, she said, and if Avril knew what it was like not to feel those things, she'd understand why this contact now was so vital.

Being in no mood to argue it out, Avril plonked her feet up on the coffee table next to Carla's, and said, 'OK, let's get on to what's really important around here, which is what time the great love of *my* life is coming on the telly.'

'The programme's already started,' Carla told her. 'We're on a commercial break. Incidentally, he called while you were in the shower to say he was going to Kensington Place for dinner, if you want to join him. Apparently there're going to be a few people there you know.'

'Great. What time?'

'Eight thirty.' Then with a grin, 'Shall I expect you back?'

Avril frowned. 'What do you mean, you're coming too, aren't you?'

Carla shook her head. 'I've got an arrangement with Richard.'

Avril's lips tightened.

'So? Shall I expect you back?' Carla prompted.

Avril cast her a look, then deciding to let the Richard issue go again, with her usual drollery she said, 'This is hard for me, but I have this rule, never to screw the client. And right now, thanks to you, John Rossmore is a client. But I'm working on firing him, just as soon as I've got you all launched.'

Carla laughed. 'I thought you preferred strangers,' she said. 'No promises, no strings, no breakfast, is that how it goes?'

'Something like that. Great philosophy. You should try it. Anyway, here's our man.'

Carla turned to look at the screen where John Rossmore was entering the set to wild applause, which he saluted repeatedly, and waved his arms to increase. He then drew a fast sharp line for silence, which everyone obeyed, and laughed at.

Quinn Wylie, a rotund little man in his late fifties, was waiting to greet him, which he did warmly, making it clear that this wasn't the first time they'd met. 'So how are you?' Wylie said, as they both sat down on the grey box-like easy chairs.

'Great,' John answered. 'And who wouldn't be, after a welcome like that?'

A few people started clapping again.

'No! No! Please!' he cried. 'It's already gone to my head. In fact, even I'm beginning to find me insufferable.' He grinned at Wylie. 'And I'm definitely not the first.'

Wylie laughed. 'So what's happening with the bad-boy image?' he asked. 'We haven't heard anything disgusting or reprehensible about you in a while.'

'Hey, we can soon put that to rights,' John said, springing to his feet. And descending into Wylie's lap he attempted to engage him in a passionate embrace.

The audience went crazy.

John returned to his seat and straightened himself up. Wylie was still flushed, and laughing.

'Headlines tomorrow,' John stated, '"Rossmore comes out of the closet with Wylie." Or: "Randy Rossmore at it again."' He stretched his legs out, and bunched his hands in front of him. 'So? Got any drugs?'

This time the audience erupted into near hysteria, since there had recently been an exclusive in a Sunday tabloid accusing Wylie of hosting marijuana parties at his Oxfordshire estate.

John made a show of not knowing what all the fuss was about, then after a quick high five with Wylie, he settled back into his seat.

'This new travel show,' Wylie said.

'With a difference,' John added.

173

'Yes, what is the difference?'

'You mean apart from it being great, compulsive viewing, which alone sets it apart from all the other travel programmes on our screens?'

'I've got to tell you,' Wylie said to the audience, 'I've seen the first episode of this series, and it really is something different. So now,' he said to John, 'over to you for what makes it different.'

'OK. Well, it's not just taking you to a holiday destination, and telling you why you should go there,' he said. 'It goes beyond that, by dramatizing something of the country's culture or history in a ten- or fifteen-minute sketch that might depict anything from a love story between a conquistador and a native Indian girl in Mexico, to a pirate attack on board an East India ship off the Philippines, to a naked fertility dance in Uganda.'

Wylie said, 'So does that mean we could be seeing you naked in the next series?'

The female section of the audience whooped their approval.

John was laughing. 'I know, it's a heady prospect,' he admitted, 'but I'm afraid it's not on the agenda, *yet*. However, I'm working on the executive producer, because you all know how I'm never happy unless I've got my kit off.'

More laughter and applause, as everyone had heard the frequent criticism that he never took a film or TV part unless it called for him to be in the buff at least half a dozen times, for whatever reason.

'Actually,' he said, when he was able, 'there are no plans for me to appear in the new series at all. My role is to direct it, and I should tell you that once you've seen the first couple of episodes you'll understand why I begged Carla Craig, the exec. producer, to let me do it.'

'Did you really have to beg? I can't believe that.'

'Almost,' he laughed. 'She certainly wasn't keen.'

'Would that have anything to do with the rumours that no-one wants to take the risk of having you in their movie any more?'

John frowned. 'I don't know,' he answered pensively. 'Could be. She never mentioned it, but I guess it could be giving her a few problems. But I'm such a great guy really. I never lose my cool – unless provoked, and all those stories about women and drugs and boozing and gambling – I mean, look at me, do I look like the kind of guy who'd be into such a good time?'

A great cheer rose up out of the audience, who clearly adored his bad-boy image and were no doubt hoping he'd do something outrageous now, right in front of their eyes, that they'd be able to read about in the papers tomorrow.

'So has directing always been an ambition?' Wylie asked.

'It has. I've enjoyed being an actor, and I'm not saying I'll never do it again, but I'm ready to make a change and who wouldn't want to be involved in a programme that takes you all over the world and pays you for going? Not that I'm getting paid, you understand. I'm doing this for the love of it – and of the exec. producer,' he added with a wink. 'Gorgeous.' He drew an air picture of an hourglass figure.

Carla's mouth and eyes were wide open as she turned to Avril. 'I don't believe this,' she murmured.

Avril was laughing. 'Don't take it personally. Just look at them, they love it. God, he really knows how to play them.'

'So who will we see on our screens, fronting the new series?' Wylie asked. Then to the audience, 'I should explain that one half of this programme is much like the travel programmes we're used to, with a reporter talking you through the location and prices etc.' To John, 'So who's presenting the new series?'

'We'll be starting auditions sometime in the next couple of weeks,' he answered. 'But we've still got plenty of money to raise yet, which is why we want everyone to watch this first series, so the advertisers will look at the ratings and say hey, I want to stick my Bounty bar in there, or my Mercedes Benz, or my extra-strong mints.'

Avril said to Carla, 'Have you thought about asking John to present it himself?'

Carla nodded. 'Actually yes, it has crossed my mind,' she answered.

'You're just afraid it'll give him too much control.'

Carla's eyes remained on the screen.

Avril sighed. 'You control freaks,' she lamented.

175

Still Carla didn't respond. She was happy just to sit here and watch the rest of the programme, and wonder what Richard was making of the fact that John Rossmore had described her as gorgeous. Knowing Richard, he'd probably found it as amusing as everyone else, but if it had caused him a moment's concern, or even a frisson of something akin to jealousy, well, she had to confess, that was all right by her. After all, in the real world, she was living night and day with the concern about Chrissie, who shared his house, his bed, his name and even his baby. And that, by anyone's reckoning, was a hell of a lot harder to deal with than the throwaway comment of a man who meant no more to her than what he could do for her programme.

Chrissie was lying in bed, propped up by pillows. The room was in darkness, except for the grey, bobbing light from the TV, and the hazy glow of a street lamp shining through the blue velvet curtains. Richard was lying next to her, on top of the covers, the baby asleep on one shoulder, a clean nappy on the other.

The Quinn Wylie Show had finished two hours ago, but neither of them had mentioned it, they'd simply gone on lying here, quietly watching the three programmes that had followed. She thought that maybe Richard had dropped off too, for his breathing was deep and rhythmic, and he hadn't moved since he'd gone to get the baby. He often came to lie here with her, now that she didn't get up any more. The rest of the time he spent at his computer, or out interviewing people about the book he was writing. She didn't know who the people were, he rarely mentioned them, and she never asked. His professional world was where he went to escape her, so she didn't try to follow, she just released him, and envied him, because she had nowhere to go to get away from herself.

Tears rolled from the corners of her eyes, trickled down past her ears and into her neck. Watching John Rossmore earlier had been like watching life go on after she was dead. She was somewhere else now, part of another existence, and those who were left never mentioned her name. What was it going to be like when the programme itself went out, she wondered. Didn't anyone want to know where she was now, or what she was doing?

More tears welled and rolled.

Even if they did, how could she tell them, when the answer was that she was in hell, bleeding? She didn't want anyone to know that. She wanted them all to think that she was the wife Richard deserved, and the mother Ryan needed.

She'd made Richard cry the other day, when she'd refused to see a doctor. But she was afraid of doctors. They might take her away and never allow her to see Richard or Ryan again. Richard said that was nonsense, but he didn't know. Nobody knew, except her, because she'd already been there, in a place where they'd kept her locked up and under guard, and no-one had ever come to see her. She'd rather die than go there again.

Maybe that was the answer. To kill herself – and Ryan. She'd been thinking that a lot lately. Richard would be free then. Free to go back to Carla.

It was where he wanted to be. Chrissie knew that, because he'd never stopped loving Carla, nor would he. She didn't ask him any more, because she couldn't bear to hear him say that he loved them both, but in different ways. She didn't want him to love Carla, but there was nothing she could do to stop it. So if she killed herself and the baby, none of it would matter any more.

She'd thought of several different ways to do it, but the energy it took, and the courage, was defeating her. The most she'd managed these past few days was to get herself to the bathroom. She wasn't eating much either, but she tried, because it seemed to matter to Richard. She didn't know why, because, in the end, nothing mattered really, they were all going to die, it was just a question of when, and how. And what did that matter once it had happened? Death was final, irreversible and eventually everyone was forgotten anyway.

Maybe if Carla was dead, Richard would forget her. Maybe then Chrissie could start living again. They could make it as though Carla had never existed, in much the same way as Carla had made it for Chrissie. And after a while Carla's ghost, which seemed to dominate their lives, could be exorcized, and Richard would be set free.

These were the silent, desperate ravings of a mind that had lost its way. She knew that, but she seemed unable to rescue it. She only went on planning, and crying, and wishing it were different, for Richard's and Ryan's sakes, if not for her own.

Beside her Richard stirred. She closed her eyes, but opened them again when he turned her to face him.

'Hungry?' he whispered.

She nodded, but only because that was the answer he wanted.

'I'll go and make us something,' he said. Then taking a tighter grip on the baby, he swung his legs to the floor and got up.

Ryan started to whimper.

Chrissie turned away. She didn't want to hear the crying, it only reminded her of how useless she was.

Richard carried the baby over to the window and peered out at the darkness. 'It's raining again,' he said, then, dropping the curtain, he went downstairs to prepare some food.

If it was raining, maybe the man she kept seeing out there was getting wet. She pictured him with rain running through the greased grooves of his hair, dribbling down his roughened face then dripping into the collar of his dark brown overcoat. She'd talked to him for a while last week, after he'd stopped to admire Richard's silver BMW. She still wasn't sure what had made her go out there, but she was glad she had now. It had proved that she was still able to communicate with others, even if they were no more than strangers. Richard had asked who he was when she'd come back inside, so she'd told him, just a neighbour: a lonely middle-aged man with a small passion for cars, and enough time on his hands to listen to other people's chat.

It wasn't long after talking to the man that she'd felt a terrible lethargy creeping into her bones, weighting her with a stultifying sadness and exhaustion. So she'd come up here, to lie down, and now she never wanted to get up again.

Chapter 11

The countryside around Cannock Martin was emerging drably through the morning mist as Avril's Porsche roared along the narrow winding road towards the village. When she got there she screeched to a halt in front of Carla's cottage, just as Carla pulled open the front door.

'Are you all right?' Avril demanded, leaping out. 'Stupid question. Of course you're not all right.'

'I've certainly been better,' Carla responded, her pale face glancing anxiously around to see if anyone was watching. No-one appeared to be, but it wasn't always easy to tell.

The kitchen smelled of freshly brewed coffee and toast. The table was laden with Sunday papers, the culprit, Avril noticed, lying open on top of the pile.

'Coffee?' Carla offered, sounding shaky.

As she went to pour Avril shrugged off her coat and tugged at her gloves with her teeth. 'I don't suppose you had any warning,' she said, knowing the answer already.

'What do you think?' Carla retorted. 'Did you?'

'None.' Avril took her coffee over to the Aga where she shivered and stamped her feet. 'I'd like to get my hands on whoever's responsible for this,' she commented tartly.

'That makes two of us,' Carla responded.

'Someone sold them the story,' Avril stated. 'That much is clear. I'd just like to know who.'

Carla went back to where she'd been sitting at the table, and picked up her coffee. She was still wearing the thick woollen scarf and grey tracksuit she'd jogged up to the shop in, and her face was still showing signs of the shock she had received when she'd opened one of the tabloids.

179

'Don't worry, you're not on my list of suspects,' she told Avril.

Avril was relieved to hear that, though she hadn't really expected to be. However, she was one of the few who knew the ins and outs of what had happened between Carla and Chrissie, which formed the basis of the article, though Chrissie's current depression was as much news to Avril as it was to anyone else. 'Trying to put a positive spin on this,' she said, sitting down too, 'it'll probably get everyone watching the programme.'

Carla's eyebrows went up. 'Well, that's good,' she said dryly.

Though Carla had given her the gist of the story on the phone, Avril had yet to read it, so reaching across the table she dragged over the paper that contained the damning piece. Flicking it open to the centre pages, she looked at the pictures of Carla, Chrissie and Richard as they'd been a year or more ago – and then at the one of Chrissie as she was now. She looked so awful it was hard to tell it was her, but the caption said it was, so she supposed she had to believe it. The headline read: 'Chrissie Banished from *Beyond*'. The accompanying story was written with usual tabloid sensationalism, telling why Chrissie Fields, the 'sexy presenter' of the 'much-hyped *There and Beyond*', had been banned by executive producer Carla Craig from taking part in any of the run-up publicity.

'"Craig's fury,"' she read, '"stems from being rejected by her one-time lover, foreign correspondent Richard Mere, in favour of the lovely Chrissie. Chrissie, who is now married to Mere, is said to be devastated by Craig's decision to drop her, not only from the publicity, but also from the next series, which is to be directed by actor John Rossmore. Apparently it is the rift between the former friends that is behind the programme's late transmission, which was originally due on screens at the beginning of the year. We are also told that relations between the two women were severed completely following the birth of Richard and Chrissie's daughter Ryan, now five months old. The childless Craig is said to still be extremely bitter over the break-up of her relationship with Mere."'

180

Reading those words to herself had been bad enough, hearing them spoken aloud turned Carla's insides weak with humiliation and anger. 'Funny, isn't it,' she said tersely, 'how those small inaccuracies can really piss you off? I mean, there were no relations between me and Chrissie from the day I found out. And as for being bitter . . .' Her face tightened. 'Well, I'm sure as hell bitter now!' she spat, then her eyes closed as the fear of what Richard might be thinking caught in her chest.

Returning to the page, Avril continued. ' "A source close to both women claims that it is Craig's brutal treatment of Chrissie that has set Chrissie back several years in her battle against depression . . ." Just who the hell is this source?' Avril demanded.

Carla shook her head.

Avril went on: ' "Chrissie is said to have been willing to promote the programme in the hope of repairing relations with Craig. However Craig, who was unavailable for comment, spurned all Chrissie's offers and when asked by a friend how she felt about Chrissie's depression, is quoted as saying 'After what she did to me, I hope she rots in hell.' " ' Avril's head came up. 'Just when did you say that?' she demanded angrily. 'And to whom, may I ask?' Then, shoving the paper away, 'What am I getting so het up about? I know what they're like. They'll put quote marks on anything. Actually, I'll tell you what I'm so bloody angry about . . . I should have known something like this would happen. I should have been ready for it, and I damned well wasn't.'

'We both should have been,' Carla retorted. 'Though how the hell we were supposed to know Chrissie's in a depression . . .'

'It's my job to know. But it's bullshit. I mean, most of the rest of it is, so why shouldn't that be?'

Carla said, 'It would account for why Richard's unwilling to see me, right now.'

Avril stared at her hard. 'Do you think there's any chance he could be the source of all this crap?' she demanded.

Carla's head jerked back in amazement. 'No!' she cried. 'My God, what's going on in your mind? He'd never do anything like that. Chrissie's got a history of depression, everyone knows that, so anyone could be behind this story.'

Avril was still watching her closely. 'Well, it's obviously someone who's known her a long time,' she pointed out. 'With all the detail they're going into on her past, the suicide attempts, and everything . . .' She went back to the paper, and continued reading.

'Don't!' Carla said, pressing her hands to her face. 'I already know what it says, so please, just read it to yourself.' But though Avril read quietly there was no escaping the worst parts that Carla knew were now imprinted on her mind for ever.

'. . . Craig is said to run an exclusive show, with her own ego as the star, and any actors or crew who she feels might threaten her position are immediately blacklisted . . .' She'd never had anything like a blacklist, nor would she, so who had fed them these lies? Then there was the claim that had shaken her most of all. 'Mere has taken a sabbatical from the job that has seen him reporting from all over the world, in order to write a book and spend more time with his wife and daughter.' Such a picture of cosiness and containment was almost suffocating in its horror. It wasn't at all how she'd imagined them. In fact, she'd had no idea until now that he was no longer travelling, because he'd never mentioned a sabbatical, or a book. But with everything else being lies, maybe she could assume that was too.

'This is obviously someone who knows both you and Chrissie pretty well,' Avril observed. 'Someone who doesn't like you very much either, considering the slant of the story. Does anyone come to mind?'

Carla shook her head.

Avril looked at her with uncompromising eyes. It might be nice to think you had no enemies, but most people did. 'There is one person,' she stated finally.

Carla looked back at her, then, dashing a hand through her hair, she said, 'I know who you're thinking of, and OK, it's the only answer I can come up with too.'

Avril glanced at the paper again, then said, 'It's a damned effective way of getting back at you for blocking her out the way you have.'

'She's got Richard,' Carla said through her teeth. 'Did she really need any more?'

'Some wouldn't have thought so,' Avril replied. 'Are there any emails from him?'

'There weren't an hour ago,' Carla answered. Getting sharply to her feet, she went to stand at the window and gaze out at the misty fields. Inside she was boiling with so much hate and anger and crippling humiliation she could barely think straight, though uppermost in her mind was the fear that Richard would call a halt to their contact now. 'It has to be Chrissie,' she suddenly seethed. 'The timing's too perfect for it not to be. Right on the eve of transmission . . .'

Avril nodded her agreement. 'And given her history of mental stress, or whatever they're calling it, this could be just the kind of thing she'd do, with no regard for herself or how she might come out of it. Her only purpose was to get back at you, which just goes to show how threatened she still feels by you, and which would be why she made sure to get in all that stuff about Richard spending more time with his family. Considering what's going on between you and him these days, her insecurity is justified, but that's her problem. Ours is deciding how we're going to handle the negative effect on your standing. I turned my phone off on the way down here, but it's not going to be long before someone tracks us down.'

'What do you suggest?' Carla asked.

Avril pulled a face. 'Well, first up, do you want to give any interviews?'

'Are you out of your mind?' Carla exploded.

Avril remained calm. 'I thought you might not,' she said. 'So I'll have to do the talking for you. Personally I'd like to attack back, and make it crystal clear that the bitch was screwing Richard for God knows how long while he was living with you, and that she chose the day your mother . . . No, it's OK,' she said when Carla's eyes grew even wider. 'I won't go that route, I'm just saying I'd like to. I guess what we need to do is take the line of surprise. In that this was all over a long time ago and Chrissie's remarks, as well as her depression, have come right out of the blue.'

'What about the fact that *you*, under my instructions, asked reporters to stay away from her? Doesn't that add to her case?'

'I played it right down when I did that,' Avril replied. She'd never told Carla about the conversation she'd had with Chrissie personally, and didn't see that there was any reason to now. 'More than asking them to steer clear of Chrissie, I asked them to concentrate on John. So I think we could shift the blame for Chrissie's exclusion onto my shoulders, because I thought John would get us more airtime and print space. Which he has.'

Carla's tension relaxed a little. 'Do you mind doing that?' she said.

Avril shrugged. 'Why would I? It's a damn sight closer to the truth than most of that bullshit can claim to be. Is that Eddie barking?'

Carla was already at the door. 'I hope to God it's not reporters,' she muttered.

But it wasn't. To her surprise it was Detective Inspector Fellowes, who'd been waylaid going into Graham's by Maudie Taylor, asking him to come and check out Gilbert's cottage again.

'That woman's turning into a royal pain in the neck about this place,' the detective grumbled from an upstairs window. 'There's not a sign of anyone having been here . . . There never is. Still, I don't suppose you heard anything in the night?'

'Not a peep,' Carla answered. Which was true, she hadn't, and Maudie's constant paranoia was starting to get on her nerves.

'She says she heard singing, or something,' Fellowes informed her.

'Well, that could easily have been coming from my place,' Carla told him. 'I had an opera playing on the CD.'

'Oh, then that'll be it,' he declared. Then with a sigh, 'I suppose I'm going to have to try convincing her of that now.'

Carla managed a smile. 'Good luck,' she said, and taking Eddie back inside she closed the door on a quickening wind.

By the middle of the afternoon Carla, though still smarting and worried, had calmed down considerably, and Avril, an excellent troubleshooter, was confident she'd dealt with as many calls as they were going to get, both on her mobile and on Carla's office line. Precisely how effective she'd been in buffing up Carla's tarnished reputation wouldn't be clear until the next day's papers came out, but it was unlikely that many of the dailies would follow up on this kind of Sunday story with much more than a few lines. Some of what was said would almost certainly be damning of Carla, for the simple reason they'd be unable to resist it while Carla was poised for success.

'Well, that's something I'll just have to live with,' Carla responded when Avril warned her.

'And keep in mind that none of this is likely to hurt the viewing figures,' Avril added. 'Which, in the end, is all that matters.'

A light of humour returned to Carla's eyes. 'You're so American,' she teased.

Avril laughed. 'OK, your image counts too,' she conceded, 'but only to you and those of us who love you. And since we know the truth, there's no real harm done.' As she spoke she was reaching for the phone on Carla's desk. 'Avril Hayden,' she said into the receiver.

'I've been trying to get hold of you for hours,' John Rossmore told her. 'Actually, that's a lie. It's Carla I'm after.'

Avril held out the phone. 'It's John,' she said.

Carla froze, then waved a hand to say she wasn't there.

Avril looked at her in amazement. Then cupping a hand over the receiver she said, 'What's wrong? I can't tell him you're not here now. He'll know I'm lying.'

'I don't want to discuss it with him,' Carla whispered.

Avril's eyes flashed. 'In case you'd forgotten,' she said tersely, 'he's working on the next series, which is probably what he's calling about.'

Suitably chastened, Carla took the phone, and to cover her chagrin affected a cheery tone as she said, 'John! How are you?'

'Great. How are you?'

'OK. What can I do for you?'

'Actually, I've got a favour to ask. Well, I'm not sure it's a favour, it's probably more of an intrusion.'

Avril said, 'I'm going upstairs to take a bath.'

Carla waved her on.

John was still talking. 'Avril tells me there's a party at your local tomorrow night for the programme's launch,' he was saying, 'and, I guess, this is me trying to cadge an invite.'

Carla took a breath, then held it.

'I know it's supposed to be a private thing,' he continued, 'but I was hoping you might consider me worthy . . .'

'No. I mean, yes. Of course,' she blurted. 'Please come.' What else could she say? Certainly not what she wanted to say, which was a categoric no. This was her territory, her friends, her family, he had no business here . . .

'Great,' he responded. 'What time?'

'It starts around seven.'

'OK, see you then,' and he ended the call.

Grudgingly grateful for his failure to mention that day's story, she replaced the receiver and wondered how long it would take him to bring it up the following evening. He was almost bound to, considering he was the one who'd been out there, spinning the tall tale on why the programme was being transmitted almost a year later than it should have been. He was probably, and understandably, a bit pissed off that she hadn't trusted him with the truth from the outset, especially if he'd been bombarded by his own set of calls from the press today, wanting to know what he knew about the rift between Carla Craig and Chrissie Fields. Actually, it hadn't occurred to her until now that he might be in the firing line too, so instead of going to her computer, which was where she was heading, she went out into the hall and ran upstairs.

'Of course he'll have been getting calls,' Avril confirmed, swishing her bathwater to create more bubbles. 'But don't worry, I spoke to Lionel on the way here, and we decided that John's script would be "nothing to do with me, before my time".'

Carla was content with that. 'OK,' she said, less interested in John Rossmore now than she was in the enormous breasts Avril had just freed from a D-cup bra. 'What do they feel like?' she asked, peering at them through the steam that was wafting up from the taps. 'I mean, do you still have the same, you know, sensation and everything?'

Avril cupped them with pride. 'Of course,' she replied. 'They're just firmer in the middle. And bigger, obviously. Actually, they're probably not as big as yours, it's just that you're taller and I'm such a titch, so they look bigger on me.'

'Do men notice the difference?' Carla wanted to know.

'Depends how familiar they are with implants. Some don't have a clue.'

'But they still feel like yours?'

Avril squeezed and rotated them. 'Yes, they definitely feel like mine,' she confirmed. 'Why, are you thinking of getting some?'

Carla laughed. 'I'd be more likely to go the other way and have a reduction,' she answered. 'Though, come to think of it, Richard was always extremely fond of my boobs.'

'And that's all that counts,' Avril responded smoothly.

Slanting her a look, Carla trotted back down the stairs and with a renewed onslaught of nerves turned on her computer. This time a message was waiting, but it was several minutes before she could pluck up the courage to open it. When she did, it was hard to stop her eyes skimming through it in search of the reassurance she needed, but finally she managed to steel herself and start at the beginning.

'Oh my darling,' he began, 'after trying to protect you from the way Chrissie is, to keep her condition a secret from the world, I now find it exposed in the most brutal fashion with you as its cause. But of course it is I who am to blame, not you. Strangely, she seems brighter today, though she hasn't seen the paper, so has no idea that her failing state of mind is being discussed by all who care to discuss it. I am trying to persuade her to see a doctor, but so far she is resisting me.

'But those are my problems, and shouldn't be allowed in any way to be a burden to you. I am wondering, now that reality has impinged on us this way, if, for the sake of others, we should cease this beautiful, oh so painful, discourse we have. *L'homme est né libre, et partout il est dans les fers.* Man was born free, and everywhere he is in chains. Maybe our love is binding you in chains, and I should be strong enough, honourable enough, because I love you, to set you free. Perhaps you are the only part of me that can be free. The rest of me is bound in the prison of my guilt, and only in a future existence can we be allowed to join again as one.'

Carla didn't give herself a moment to think, before her fingers hit the keyboard with an impassioned reply. 'You know we cannot be so easily separated, so I beg you, don't try. Let's allow these events to run their course, and know that I am here, enduring your troubles with a strength that is made all the greater by its connection with you. There will be a way through this, we just have to be patient and understand that freedom and chains, guilt and innocence, belong to a relative world, as do our bodies and minds. But our spirits, our souls, will always be one.'

Avril's eyes boggled when she read that. 'Blimey,' she said, raising a leg from the soapy water to rest it on the edge of the bath, 'very Jean-Paul Sartre.'

Carla's smile was wry.

'Well,' Avril said, handing back the printouts, 'you know me, I don't really buy all this existential stuff, but if it works for you . . . Hand me a towel, will you? If it works for you, then who am I to say come on Carla, get a life?'

Carla's eyes darkened.

Avril laughed. 'Now don't start getting pissy with me,' she said. 'I'm having a hard enough time getting my head round all this . . . Who was the French bloke this time, by the way?'

'Rousseau.'

'Oh, him again. Anyway, I don't know what you want me to do here. The story's in the paper, Chrissie's revealed her colours, and you and Richard are still soaring about in a celestial cuckoo land. Sounds to me like all's right with your little world.'

'Not quite the way I'd have put it,' Carla said, with irony.

'I daresay not,' Avril intoned. 'Now, go and get us some wine, so we've got something to sustain us through the evening as we start planning our new offices and apartments. Oh, just one other thing,' she said, as Carla started to leave, 'what did John want?'

'John?' Carla frowned. 'Oh, John Rossmore. To come to the party tomorrow.'

'And you said yes.'

'I said yes,' Carla confirmed.

'Good. Now, summon your earthly presence and trot it along to the wine shop while I dry myself off here.'

Laughing, Carla went to fetch her coat, and a minute later, hearing the front door close, Avril was on the point of braving the chill air of the landing to go and get her clothes, when she suddenly stopped and turned to look over her shoulder.

It was the weirdest thing, but she could have sworn she'd just heard someone sigh. Her heartbeat quickened, and her skin started to prickle. Never, in all the years she'd been coming here, had she felt scared in this house, nor had she ever sensed any kind of presence beyond those she could see. She wasn't sure she sensed anything now, but she was damned sure she'd heard that sigh, and apart from her there was no-one else there to heave it.

In the end, deciding to put it down to the plumbing, she opened the bathroom door and almost fell over Eddie who was lying on the floor right outside.

'Oh, it was you!' she laughed, stooping to tousle him. 'You gave me the fright of my life.'

Never one to refuse attention, Eddie rolled on to his back and crooked his paws either side of his face.

'Let me get dressed first,' Avril told him, starting to shiver, and pulling the towel more tightly around her she hurried into the warmth of the guest bedroom, where she unpacked the Vuitton holdall she'd brought with her, dressed quickly, then opened the wardrobe to hang up the rest of her clothes. To her surprise, the memory boxes that took up most of the space were in some disarray, though she quickly realized, as she started tidying them, that it was only Valerie's thesis that was creating the mess. Careful to make sure it was all there, she gathered it up and slipped it back into the envelope. She gave a fleeting thought to the letter Carla had found rucked in the bottom, and wondered if she'd ever found the rest of it. Avril imagined not, or she'd have mentioned it, and since it was most likely that Richard had it, there wasn't much chance they'd ever get to know what it had said.

A few minutes later she found herself recalling Richard's mysterious visit to the cottage while she and Carla had been in Monaco, as though there might be some connection between that and the thesis being out of its envelope. But surely not, for why on earth would he be looking for the missing page to a letter that had been written well over a year ago, and whose contents had been rendered benign almost as soon as they were penned? So no, she was just putting two

189

and two together and coming up with intrigue for intrigue's sake here, which was what happened to a person after they'd been in Hollywood for a while. However, she didn't trust Richard, and wasn't at all impressed by the fact that he'd never actually admitted to receiving the letter. Or indeed to being at the cottage. It was weird, that, the way he was proving so reticent about details that, on the surface at least, didn't seem to matter much. There was obviously a reason for it, which was why, at some point, she was going to make Carla sit down and discuss what was happening, if for no other reason than to be sure that Carla was aware that something wasn't right. However, after the nasty shock Carla had been dealt today, now probably wouldn't be a good time. So, closing the wardrobe door, Avril turned the key and went down to the kitchen where Carla was searching out the corkscrew while speaking to her brother on the phone.

'OK, fairy godmother,' Carla said to Avril the following evening, 'you've organized the ball, so how about changing Eddie into a nice new dress for the night?'

Laughing, Avril said, 'You should have thought about that a week ago, because that's how long it takes to kick-start my wand.'

Carla looked down at Eddie, who was gazing raptly up at her. 'Even you've got something new to wear to the party,' she said, straightening up the smart black bow tie Sonya's kids had given him earlier. Then, wafting back into her bedroom, she opened the wardrobe again and, grimacing, pulled out the trusty black cashmere dress that she'd bought at huge expense some three years ago, and laid it out on the bed. It would have to do, and she could always liven it up with the diamond pendant Richard had once surprised her with on one of his own birthdays. She couldn't help wishing he could be there tonight, though he'd sent a message earlier assuring her that in spirit he would be, and that she should spare him many thoughts throughout the evening, and speak to him in her mind, so that he could speak back to her and share it all with her. He'd sent two messages today, and hadn't mentioned Chrissie or the newspaper article in either. She knew why:

190

he didn't want anything to spoil this special time for her – but how wrong it all seemed to be doing it without him, in fact without either of them.

Going over to the dressing table, she sat down to continue her make-up. Considering the significance of tonight's party, she was surprisingly calm, though she didn't mind admitting that she'd be glad when the programme was transmitted, the reviews published, and that spiteful attack in yesterday's paper well on its way to history. It was hard coming to terms with the fact that she was in the paper at all, never mind being referred to as 'Craig', as though 'Craig' were some kind of unmentionable disease, or a hard-nosed killer on the run from a life sentence. And having so many lies and injustices printed about her was so horrible and enraging that she could hardly get them out of her mind.

However, for this evening, at least, she had to try, since her neighbours had gone to a lot of trouble to make this party special, which Faith had been at pains to let her know when she'd delivered the post that morning.

'. . . and course, we all knows that was just a load of ol' rubbish in the paper about you, yesterday,' she'd assured Carla. 'And that's why we all wants to make tonight a real good do for you, to make up for it, like. Everyone's going to be there, and we got a couple of surprises which I'm not going tell you about, or it'll spoil 'em.'

There was a good chance, had Avril not virtually lassoed her off down the garden path at that point, that Faith's secrets would have burst their seams, but for the moment they remained securely stitched in.

Now, as Carla dusted a tawny blusher lightly on to her cheeks, she realized how easily she could become emotional over all the kindness that had gone into this evening. None of them had been a part of making the programme, didn't even really know what it took to get one on the air, but because it mattered to her, it mattered to them too, and she could only feel glad that she'd decided to share its official launch with them.

By ten to seven she was downstairs, settling back the fire and getting her big winter coat from the hall cupboard. Which reminded her, Sonya had looked in here for Richard's letters

191

and hadn't found them. So she'd look herself tomorrow. Failing that, they had to be in storage, which she'd find out soon enough, since everything was due to be delivered to the Belgravia *ménage*, as Avril was calling it, at the end of the week. Just thinking about that caused Carla's heart to judder, for having committed to it, she now had to pay for it, and if tonight's programme wasn't well received . . .

'Are you going to get that?' Avril shouted, as someone banged on the front door.

By the time Carla got there Avril was already halfway down the stairs.

'*Mesdemoiselles*,' John Rossmore declared with a swooping bow, when Carla opened the door. 'Your carriage awaits.'

Slightly thrown, Carla looked back at Avril.

'Well, for God's sake let him in,' Avril cried. 'Can't you see it's raining?'

'Sorry,' Carla said, standing back to make room.

Avril swept up behind her, then laughed delightedly as John scooped her up to his height to kiss her.

'You look magnificent,' he told her.

Which was certainly one way of describing it, Carla thought wryly, though exactly what her neighbours would make of Avril's totally transparent black net dress, with its few lavishly embroidered red roses covering her modesty . . . Well, it was going to be interesting to find out.

'And so do you,' John said, turning his smile on Carla.

'Thank you,' she replied, and turned to Avril in order to escape the humorous warmth of his eyes, as well as his oppressive proximity in the dark, cramped hallway.

'I thought,' he explained, looking at Avril too, 'that as it was raining, I'd come and get you.'

'Does that mean you've already been to the pub?' Avril said, wrapping herself in a blood-red pashmina.

'And met half the village,' he confirmed. 'Lionel's here too, I hope that's OK.'

'Of course,' Avril assured him. 'But I'll tell you what, you can take Carla on ahead and come back for me. Or send Lionel. I need to call my office,' she explained, when Carla glared at her.

'I'll get my coat,' Carla said shortly.

Avril watched her disappear into the sitting room, then winked at John. 'She wants to be a producer when she grows up,' she said.

John was stooping to greet Eddie, who was staring at him from the bottom of the stairs. 'Well, look at you,' he said. 'I didn't know this was a black-tie affair.'

Eddie wagged his tail, then rolled onto his back and put his legs in the air.

'Funny, that's what I always feel like doing when you talk to me,' Avril remarked.

Carla was back. 'Maybe I should take an umbrella and walk,' she said to John. 'You won't want Eddie messing up your car.'

'I've got a better idea,' Avril said. 'Why don't you let John drive your car, because nothing can make that old heap any worse than it already is.'

Carla blushed, and tried not to notice the amusement in John Rossmore's eyes.

'Sounds like a plan to me,' he said. 'But my car's a Range Rover, so we can always put Eddie in the back.'

'He likes to sit with me,' Carla retorted.

'Then he can sit with you.'

Avril had to stop herself screaming. 'I don't believe how long this is taking,' she cried. 'Just get in a damned car, will you, and I'll meet you there.'

Five minutes later Carla arrived at the pub in John's Range Rover, with Eddie sitting at her feet in the foot well.

'Thank you,' she said, as John held an umbrella over the door to cover her while she got out. She wished she could be friendlier, but she was too angry at being forced to turn up here with him, as though he was her partner, to be able to put any warmth into her voice.

He said nothing, merely walked beside her as they dodged round the puddles in the car park to get to the pub. Then, as he opened the door for her to go in ahead of him, a rousing cheer of welcome finally brought a smile to her face. As she was pulled into the crowd she soon forgot about John Rossmore, who, Avril told her later, had had the good grace to turn up early so that her friends and neighbours could meet the celebrity guest before Carla's arrival. That way,

193

Carla's big entrance would in no way be upstaged by the idiocy, as he put it, of his fame.

'Bring her over here,' Sylvia was calling from behind the bar. 'That's it. Right over here. We've got the champagne all set out. What are you going to have, our Carla? A Buck's Fizz or a *coupe*, as they d'call it in France? That, for you peasants, means straight bubbly.'

'Either,' Carla laughed, gazing round at all the decorations and blinking lights. 'Just look at all this!' she cried in delight. 'It's amazing. I had no idea you were going to all this trouble.'

'We made the banner!' her niece and nephew shouted, jumping up and down in excitement.

'Hey, I didn't see you two there,' Carla gushed, sweeping them into her arms. 'And you made the banner. The one that says There and Beyond?'

They nodded eagerly. 'Daddy helped a bit,' Kitty admitted, looking up at Mark.

'It's the best banner I've ever seen,' Carla told them, hugging them again. Then she hugged her brother, whose eyes were shining with pride.

'Everyone here's seeing this as their triumph too,' he told her. 'Even Maudie. Wait till you see what she's got you.'

'Maudie?' Carla echoed.

'Over here! Make way! Make way!' Faith demanded, pushing open a path in the crowd.

To Carla's amazement Maudie, the old crosspatch, was standing in front of the food table, holding a magnificent cake in her arms, while scowling horribly at Carla.

'You made that?' Carla cried.

'Course she did,' Faith answered. 'Bloody brilliant, isn't it?'

'It certainly is,' Carla agreed, as genuinely touched by the gesture as she was impressed by the expert replica of a Boeing 747 with *Carla goes There and Beyond* piped in icing across the wings. 'Maudie, I don't know what to say . . .'

'I've got my camera,' Sonya shouted, pushing her way through. 'We've got to get a shot of this. Maudie, try smiling, will you?' She looked through the viewfinder. 'On second thoughts, Maudie, you look a bit scary when you do that.'

At that everyone exploded into laughter, even Maudie, and Sonya quickly captured an historical shot.

'John!' Sonya cried, turning round to find him. 'Come on! You've got to have your picture taken too. No, not with Carla, with me!' And thrusting the camera at Mark, she grabbed John's arm and smiled glowingly into the lens.

'He hasn't got a drink!' Robin Jessop called over the noise. 'Sylvia, pass one of the glasses, will you? And then it's my turn for the photo.' And mincing up to John's other side, he linked arms with the star and affected an outrageous pose, which John promptly mirrored, much to everyone's delight.

'Here, did you see the telly we've got in special?' Jack, the landlord, said to Carla.

Carla turned to where he was pointing, and actually gasped out loud. 'How did I miss that?' she laughed, unable to believe the size of the screen. 'Where on earth did you get it?'

'Fleur and Perry found it in a shop in Bath,' he informed her. 'So we rented it for the night. Not going to miss anything on this one, are we? Three foot by three foot, it is. Course, they do have them in their homes like that in 'Ollywood, so Avril says.'

'What do I say?' Avril demanded, coming in the door with Lionel. 'Let me through, will you? I need some champagne. And who the hell's in charge of the lights around here? Turn them down, for God's sake! It's supposed to look like a Roman bath, not a bloody swimming bath.'

'That'll be a great dress when it's finished,' Sonya shouted, as Avril discarded her pashmina to a chorus of bawdy whoops and whistles.

'She's got some nerve, coming in here like that,' Maudie grunted.

'Well at least she's got the figure for it,' Angie remarked, enviously.

'More women should dress like that,' Jack decided. 'It's feminine, is what it is.'

'Listen to him,' Sylvia jeered, 'he wouldn't know feminine if it got up and bit him on the bum.'

'I wouldn't need biting on the bum if you had a pair like that,' Jack countered.

'No, you'd need rescuing, is what you'd need,' Joe Locke told him, making everyone laugh.

Avril gave a shameless waggle of her shoulders, then took the glass John was passing her.

'More photos,' Sonya insisted, shoving her way back in.

Carla linked arms with Mark and after Sonya had snapped them she eased him to the edge of the crowd, making space for those jostling to have a picture taken with John.

'He seems like a really nice bloke,' Mark commented, his handsome face reddened on one side from where he'd been standing in front of the fire.

Carla shrugged. 'He's used to all this, remember. It happens to him all the time.'

'Yeah, but he doesn't have to be so good-natured about it.'

'He does if it's my friends and family,' Carla declared hotly. Then, smiling, she squeezed his arm and said, 'I'm so nervous about this transmission. I wish it was already over.'

'It will be soon enough,' he responded, 'then you'll be saying, *Oh, I wish it could happen all over again. It went too fast. I missed it.*'

Laughing, she said, 'Your gift for mimicry is almost as good as Avril's.'

'I don't know about that,' he replied, 'but I do know we were beginning to wonder if we'd ever see this day. You, with your very own programme going out on TV. Amazing! Who'd have thought it?'

'It's been a long journey,' Carla admitted, 'and looking back, it seems nothing short of miraculous that we ever got it going, never mind to this point now.'

'Well, it's certainly an ambitious project,' he agreed. 'But it'll all be worth it, you'll see.' He hesitated before continuing, and Carla knew instinctively that he was going to say something about Richard. Obviously Sonya would have told him about the renewed contact, even though she'd asked her not to, and the thought of trying to explain it to Mark was worse than trying to explain it to Avril. At least Avril was a woman, which gave her some empathy. As a man, and particularly his type of man, Mark was never going to understand the kind of bond that held her and Richard together, not when there was no physical contact to support it. All Mark would remember was how utterly devastated she had been when Richard had left her, and that being a married

196

man now Richard had no right to be messing around in Carla's life again.

To her relief, the door opened at that moment, and Graham stomped in from the rain. It fleetingly occurred to Carla to put him and Mark together so that Graham could try persuading her brother that he didn't need to worry, but it was hardly Graham's problem, so it would be unfair to ask.

'Graham!' she cried, going to greet him. 'I was beginning to wonder what had happened to you.'

He held up his hands. 'I had to take Betty to the station,' he said. 'Her sister's sprained her ankle, so she's gone to look after her for a couple of weeks.' He chuckled. 'All that walking in the Pennines and then poor old Daphne goes and slips on the kitchen floor at home.'

'Well, at least you're here,' Carla said, ushering him towards the bar. 'Come and get a drink. The programme's starting in ten minutes.'

Angie was in front of the champagne, and pushed one into Graham's hand as he said to Carla, 'So, do I get an introduction?'

Carla frowned. Then, realizing who he meant, rolled her eyes and said, 'Not you too. Come on,' and, turning round, she searched John out in the crowd and began pulling Graham through.

Sonya was at the ready with her camera and managed to capture the three of them laughing, as John shook Graham's hand and got in first with, 'I've always wanted to meet you.'

At that point Carla's empty glass was removed from her hand and replaced with a full one, then Avril joined them and began flirting with John, only to be outdone by Sonya, Sylvia, Angie, Fleur and the most gregarious of them all, Randy Robin, which was what the other men had dubbed him.

Graham looked at his watch. 'Not long now,' he said to Carla.

'Don't,' she responded with a shiver of nerves.

Grinning, he said, 'Come on, let's get ourselves some good seats, I've been looking forward to this for a long time, so I don't want to miss anything.'

'Oh no, please,' Carla groaned. 'Let's stay near the bar so I can get drunk. I've got a feeling I might need to.'

As she spoke, the large screen adjacent to the bar flickered into life, and not long after that Avril shouted for everyone to be quiet. The preceding commercials were playing. It was only a matter of minutes now before *There and Beyond* was aired to the nation.

An expectant hush hovered over the gathering as Jack lowered the lights and Sylvia turned up the sound. An advert for Andrex was showing.

'I feels so bloody nervous, reckon I could do with some of that meself,' Teddy Best commented, sending a titter round the room.

Carla looked at Graham and failed to raise a smile. Then John Rossmore came to stand the other side of her, and before she knew it the familiar soundtrack of the opening titles started to play – and her heart stopped beating.

'Catchy tune,' Lloyd Lamar commented.

'Sssh,' his wife hissed.

Carla was very still and very tense. She knew this programme inside out, was only too aware of how the magnificent opening shot, of the sun rising over the rolling plains of the Kruger Park, was soon going to give way to a big close-up of Chrissie, welcoming them all to South Africa.

As the transition happened, and Chrissie's lovely face filled the screen, Carla felt her insides turning to liquid. It had to be the size of the screen making her feel so peculiar, or perhaps it was a reaction to yesterday, and being confronted now with Chrissie's face and voice. There was an odd rushing sound in her head and she felt vaguely sick. Then dimly she was aware of a hand squeezing her shoulder, and the steadying reassurance that seemed to flow from it set her breathing again. A few seconds later she was able to glance at John Rossmore, whose gesture was reminding her that he was well acquainted not only with first nights, but with being maligned and misquoted by the press, so he knew how she was feeling.

He looked at her for only a moment, then, returning his eyes to the screen, he removed his hand. It was the right thing to do, for she'd only have felt awkward if he'd kept it there, and now the programme was really under way she found herself able to detach from its content and silently pray that everyone who was out there watching was going to love it.

After the introduction, and more stunning shots of the South African landscape, the programme moved on to the dramatized section, a comedic misunderstanding between two Zulus, whose communication through coloured beads had been read by one macho warrior as a request for a night of passion, when what the other was actually expressing was anger at a slight to his family. The players were genuine Zulus, whose performances, though obviously amateur, were still good, but having written it, rehearsed it, shot it and watched it a thousand times in the edit, Carla now knew it so well that she saw only its flaws, cringed at the dialogue and wanted to bury herself alive in the hideous pauses. How could Jed have allowed that? Why hadn't she seen earlier that the style was just too feature-film for a meagre little TV sketch? And then the midway break was upon them, and the Zulu story was only half over.

Of course that was the problem with a Channel 4 transmission. If it had been going out on the BBC, as originally planned, there would have been no break, and they wouldn't have to endure this ludicrous hiatus in a piece that wasn't good to begin with. She saw now how right John was when he'd suggested they should start with the dramatization, and come in with the contemporary insert later. That way it wouldn't matter which channel they transmitted on, there would be no pause in the drama.

No-one was saying anything, they were just looking around, waiting for someone else to speak first, then Teddy Best broke the terrible silence by asking for a drink.

Carla caught Avril's eye and smiled weakly when Avril gave her a thumbs up. Then she noticed that Mark, too, was beaming encouragement, and Sonya, who'd seen it all a hundred times anyway, was aglow with pride. But they were family. Of course they were going to like it. They probably didn't dare not to.

The second half rolled on to the screen, and everyone was once again making a great show of being riveted. Carla wasn't sure she could bear any more. What the hell had she been thinking, making a programme about places that were so exotic and expensive and out of most people's reach that condescending was the kindest word she could think of to describe her insufferable elitism and arrogance. In fact, the longer she watched, the less able she felt ever to face anyone again. But maybe the catastrophe had one saving grace, that of persuading the world that she'd been justified in dropping Chrissie. Not because Chrissie was no good, but because the public was generally unable to distinguish between a presenter's performance and a programme's weakness, so ultimately, in the audience's mind, Chrissie would take the blame for the programme's failure.

Finally the end credits appeared from the bottom of frame, and closing her eyes she braced herself for the bemusement, or worse, of her neighbours. It was a moment before she realized that the noise drowning the music was applause, and that accompanying that were cheers of bravo and more! But of course, they would do that; she was standing right there so they had to be polite.

'Best travel programme I've ever seen!' Teddy Best roundly declared.

'Fantastic. Absolutely marvellous,' Beanie Lamar added.

'Divine, darling. Simply divine,' Robin crooned.

'What I wouldn't give to go to a place like that,' Sylvia lamented.

'What about those couple of old buggers and their beads?' Jack chuckled.

'Great stuff,' Joe Locke agreed. 'Clever to stay away from the political thing. Just concentrate on the culture and landscape.'

Graham was grinning at Carla's surprise. 'A winner!' he declared. 'An absolute winner!'

Carla's face was starting to light up. They genuinely did seem to like it, and the sound of more corks popping, to the accompaniment of Cliff blasting across the sound system with 'Congratulations', started her laughing. Obviously someone had already cued that up, but it was no less welcome for that. And tomorrow's reviews, and audience ratings, would come soon enough, so why not just go with it now and have a good time?

'The rocket's launched! Let the party begin!' Avril cried, and, hoisting a full magnum of champagne in Carla's direction, she refilled her glass and whispered, 'You're on your way, baby. Today Cannock Martin, tomorrow the reviews.'

Carla's smile was wider than ever. 'Thanks for reminding me,' she cried over the noise. Then, biting her lips as emotion brinked, she added, 'I'll never forget what you've done, Avril . . .'

'Speech! Speech!' Teddy Best shouted.

'Yes! Speech!' the others started to echo.

So Carla got up on a chair, made everyone gasp and laugh by almost losing her balance, then somehow managed to get through a short and slushy thank-you for the party, the support, the friendship and 'The cake!' she ended, raising her glass to Maudie.

John Rossmore was standing with Graham, listening and applauding along with the others, then laughing when she collapsed into the arms of her brother and sister-in-law. Reaching for a bottle to top up his and Graham's glasses, he said, 'She has every right to feel proud tonight.'

Graham was beaming with pride. 'An unusual approach to an innovative idea,' he commented. 'And having you on board for the next series is about the best validation she could hope for.'

John looked surprised. 'Modesty prevails here,' he responded. 'But I thank you for that. And I don't mind telling you that I really do believe in this programme. And in Carla. She knows what she's doing and she's not afraid to take chances.'

Graham was still watching her as she grabbed Avril and started to dance. 'She's a remarkable young woman,' he said, 'and this past year has been far from easy.'

'Avril told me about her mother,' John said. 'Amazing the way the papers manage to skip over the most crucial issues when it suits them.'

'Mmm,' Graham grunted. Then, after a moment's pause, 'She thinks Chrissie sold the story, but I'm not so sure.'

'Why would she think that?' John asked, frowning.

'Ah, now we're getting into the female psyche,' Graham grimaced, 'which, I have to confess, is territory I've never successfully charted. However, Carla, and the way her mind works, is certainly a fascinating study.'

John laughed. 'I was forgetting you're a writer,' he said, 'so I guess we're all subjects of study to you.'

'To one degree or another,' Graham acknowledged. 'And despite how many years I've been at it, I can tell you the human capacity for survival never ceases to amaze me. But of course that's my field, and as you know it gets considerably more complex, not to mention sinister, the further into it you go. Were I writing historical romances I'd no doubt have a very different view of the world.'

Like many of Graham's readers John was only too aware of the macabre trails the author followed to obtain his story. 'It must have an effect on you,' he said, 'dealing with all those depraved aspects of human nature.'

Graham's eyes danced merrily. 'I try to keep it in check,' he joked.

John smiled too, then, after taking a sip of his drink, he said, 'Going back to this newspaper thing. As a detective manqué, who do you think was behind it?'

Graham thoughtfully scratched his chin. 'Not knowing all the players in this particular scenario,' he said, 'it's hard for me to say. But I'll tell you why I don't think it was Chrissie.'

John waited.

'I don't think it was her,' Graham said, 'because based on the personal knowledge I have of Chrissie, I'd say that she's not the vindictive type. Self-destructive, maybe. But certainly not vindictive, which would therefore make it unlikely that she was behind that story.'

John's eyebrows were drawn together. 'But you're not hazarding a guess who might have been?'

'Impossible when, as I said, I don't know everyone involved. But I do know that it can often be the person you least suspect who turns out to be the culprit.'

John grinned. 'Something you've made an extremely good living out of,' he commented.

Graham cocked a humorous eyebrow. 'Thanks to my close association with the police force, most of what I write has its roots in truth,' he replied. 'Now, I think, if I want to remain on good terms with my neighbours, I should stop hogging your company.'

It was well after midnight before the party finally started to calm down, and those who'd danced and drank themselves senseless began staggering about in search of their coats. Carla, both exhausted and elated, disappeared into the ladies for a few minutes to communicate on a telepathic level with Richard, then came out again to have a last jig around with Sonya. Despite having had a fabulous evening, she'd hardly stopped being aware of the gap at her side that Richard, not John Rossmore, should have been filling. It wasn't that John had pushed his way in, in fact they'd only danced together once, and that without touching, it was simply that John's instant popularity with her neighbours had felt like an intrusion on a place that had always been Richard's. But the occasional quiet moments she had taken to connect with Richard had helped ease her over the resentment, and thankfully no-one but Graham had known anything about it. And the only reason she'd confided in him was so that she could speak Richard's name out loud. It was a way of bringing him right into the party, and Graham, she knew, would neither judge nor mock her need to do it.

Now, as Sonya spun her off towards the bar, she almost collided with Maudie, who was waiting for the Reverend to see her home.

'Ah!' Carla said, staggering to a halt. 'I'm glad to catch you. If you hear any singing tomorrow night, it'll be coming from my CD player.' She didn't add that this was a 'date' with Richard, to listen to one of their favourite operas.

Not quite sober, Maudie blinked a few times, then said, 'There's something going on in old Gilbert's house, you mark my words, and I'm going to speak to that detective friend of Graham's about it.'

Coming to join them, Avril said, 'You already did that.'

Maudie swayed from side to side. 'Did I?' she said. 'What did he find?'

'That Carla had her CD player on too loud.'

Maudie was shaking her head. 'Not that,' she said. 'I know it wasn't that.'

'So what was it?'

'Ah, there you are, Maudie,' the Reverend said, coming up behind her with her coat. 'Ready to go?'

After punching thin air a couple of times as she tried to

insert an arm in a sleeve Maudie finally managed to get into her coat, and after slurring a frosty goodbye, she followed the Reverend and his nephew out into the night.

'Silly old bag,' Avril commented, then, catching Carla's arm, she dragged her over to where Graham and John and several others were engaged in a one-upmanship contest as to who had seen or heard the weirdest things.

'Oh God, Maudie should still be here,' Carla laughed, sitting down between Gayle and Perry.

'Sssh,' Angie said, 'Fleur's telling us about the aliens she and Perry have been making contact with lately.'

'We haven't actually managed to speak to them yet,' Fleur insisted, 'but we will, soon. We've ordered all this high-tech equipment from the States that'll help us communicate better. It should be here any time. But we can definitely hear them, can't we Perry?'

'So what are they saying?' Sylvia wanted to know.

Fleur's angelic face was earnestly sober. 'Hard to make it out,' she answered, 'but they're definitely talking about our planet.'

'So they speak English?' Teddy said, hiding a smirk.

Fleur nodded. 'The ones we've heard do.'

'So how do you know they're talking about Earth?' Angie asked.

'And where are they, exactly?' Faith demanded. 'Just in case I gets any letters for 'em,' she added, making everyone laugh.

'They're somewhere in their own craft,' Fleur answered, not in the least bit fazed. 'We haven't managed to locate it yet, but it can't be far away, and once we've got all our stuff from America set up . . .'

'Did you see that film, *Contact*?' Gayle said. 'You're going to be like the Jodie Foster character.'

'Hah!' her husband laughed. 'That's the one where they had Pensacola, Florida as paradise. Can't say I want to go there much, when my number's up.'

'I think Jodie Foster's wonderful,' Beanie swooned. 'Have you ever met her?' she asked John.

He shook his head. 'Avril probably has,' he offered.

'Not yet,' Avril confessed, 'but give me time.'

Teddy was eager to get back into the bizarre. 'Come on, Graham,' he said, 'you must be full of weird and wonderful stories. So what's the worst thing you've ever seen or heard?'

Graham pulled a face as he thought hard and stared down at his drink.

Everyone was agog, and Carla could see he was going to do his best not to disappoint them.

'Well,' he said finally, 'I suppose the worst thing I've ever seen has to be someone being murdered.'

Virtually everyone's jaw dropped. 'You've seen someone getting killed?' Sylvia breathed. 'How? I mean, what, were they chopped up, or strangled, or what?'

Graham lifted his glass, then said, 'I'm sorry. I shouldn't have brought it up.' He put his glass back on the table. 'It happened a long time ago, but it was very distressing, and I . . . Well, I never talk about it, and as I said, I shouldn't have brought it up.'

It was clear that everyone was dying to ask who it had been, where it had happened, how he'd come to be there, was it in one of his books now, and many other questions, but the pale, closed expression on his face made them hold back.

Stepping into the breach, Angie said, 'Come on, Pete, we should go home, we've got work tomorrow.'

'Bloody hell, don't remind me,' he grumbled.

Avril said to John, 'Where are you staying?'

'I've booked a hotel in Bath, so I should leave my car here and get a taxi.'

'Won't hear of it,' Graham told him. 'Plenty of room at my house, and it's walking distance. My wife's away, so we'll have to fend for ourselves, but I'm sure we can manage.'

'I was going to invite him to stay with me,' Avril protested.

'So was every other woman in the village,' Gayle added.

'Plenty of room at my place,' Robin chirped up.

Laughing, John held up his hands. 'I'll take the first offer, if it's OK,' he said to Graham. 'But I should see Eddie and his girls home first.'

'Oh, don't worry about us,' Carla said. 'We could do with the air.'

'The most gorgeous man on earth offers to see her home, and she wants air,' Avril complained.

It wasn't until they were walking back through the village, with John and Graham heading in the opposite direction, that it briefly occurred to Carla how little she knew about John Rossmore's private life. This was surprising, considering how often it must have been written about in the press. However, gossip had never held much appeal for her, so she only ever got the gist of what was going on, like how difficult he could be to work with, and how hard he partied. She'd yet to witness either, though it was still very early days and the way he'd thrown himself into this evening certainly proved he had no aversion to the good time. She presumed he was single, and straight, or Avril wouldn't be making such a play for him, though one could never tell with Avril, who wasn't the type to let such trivialities stand in her way. Carla toyed for a moment with asking, then decided against it. She didn't want Avril reading anything into her interest, which was only mild anyway, and could easily be satisfied by tapping into the Internet, if she was that keen to know. Which she wasn't. It was simply an idle curiosity, promptly dismissed, for, unlike many of her neighbours, she had no desire whatsoever to fall asleep thinking of John Rossmore.

Chapter 12

Moving into the Belgravia *ménage* turned out to be a riotous affair, thanks to Lyle and Hans, the two stand-up comics who, in true Hollywood fashion, were moonlighting as a team of first-rate business managers, currently working exclusively for Avril. Their outrageous approach to the world, and mind-boggling talent for making things happen, meant that any angst Carla might have suffered at this next big step in her life was immediately tossed in the air and blasted to smithereens by their scathing wit. Sonya and Avril were having a real trip with them, while Carla and John Rossmore attempted to discuss the programme, unpack boxes, put up shelves and dodge round removal men.

For the moment John had disappeared, and Carla was under a desk trying to plug in a computer and suppress the dread of Zanzibar that she'd woken up with that morning, and had little hope of shaking now that everything was going ahead.

'OK! What's going on out here?' Avril suddenly demanded, banging out of the kitchen in her fuchsia pink dungarees and blue spotted hairband.

'Ah, here she is, like a page out of *Vogue*,' Hans crooned.

'And I've never seen a woman more out of vogue,' Lyle added.

'Yes, very funny,' Avril responded. 'What's happened to John Rossmore? I hope he's not shirking . . .'

'I'm up here!' he shouted, from the balcony.

Avril turned to look up. 'Why?' she asked. 'Those are our private quarters.'

'Because someone threw a pile of bedding at me, and told me to bring it up here,' he answered reasonably.

'That was me,' Sonya owned up, appearing from behind a tall cupboard with a mobile phone pressed to her ear. 'I've got the delivery department from Harrods on the line,' she told Avril, swerving round a couple of removal men who were lugging in Carla's furniture from storage. 'They can bring the new bed and sofas for your flat today, but the rest of it won't be available until next week.'

'Whenever,' Avril responded, waving a dismissive hand. 'Is the plumber up there with you, John? One of the taps isn't working in the kitchen.'

Sonya was beetling after the removal company's foreman. 'I asked your boss for a printout of everything. Did he remember to give it to you?' she asked, grabbing his arm.

'Didn't give nothing to me,' the foreman grunted.

Sonya immediately got on the line to the storage company. As she waited to be put through Avril backed into her, dragging a heavy box. 'What time are you leaving to drive home?' Avril wanted to know.

'About four,' Sonya answered. 'That should get me back for seven at the very latest. Why? Oh, hang on. Yes, Mr Fox? Sonya Craig here. That's right, the printout. I need the total of everything we've paid over the last fifteen months, including the charges for today, to give to the accountant.' She paused as he spoke, and glanced at Avril. Then she was frowning. 'You gave it to who?' she said. 'But I didn't send anyone . . . No, I didn't ask for anything to be taken out of storage until today. Are you sure you've got the right account?'

Avril was looking at her curiously.

'Well, I don't know anything about that,' Sonya said. 'There must be some mistake. Anyway, could you put the printout in the post to me, please?'

'What was all that about?' Avril said, as she rang off.

Sonya shrugged. 'Got his wires crossed somewhere,' she answered. 'Says someone took some things out of storage last week and he gave them our statement. With any luck they'll pay it, whoever they are.'

'Didn't he say who it was?'

'No, just said "the gentleman" I sent. But believe me, I've been dealing with this company for over a year, and I've lost count of how many times I've received bills that weren't ours

208

and letters asking us for keys we never had. Now, where were we? Oh, yes, I'm leaving at four.'

'Great. Could you run Lyle out to the airport on your way, he's got a friend flying in from LA who he wants to meet.'

'No problem,' Sonya answered. 'Oh, crikey. Look at that. What are they doing with those filing cabinets?' and off she zoomed to carry on supervising the deliveries.

By late afternoon everything was finally in, and as the door closed behind the heavily-tipped removal team Avril conjured a magnum of Laurent Perrier from the fridge, which she got John to crack open so they could drink a toast – in hastily produced coffee mugs – to their excellent *ménage*.

'I've got to hand it to you two,' John said, looking up at the huge picture windows and exquisitely painted ceiling, 'this place is definitely unique.' He was standing at the centre of the room, dust from the shelves he'd put up smearing his face, sweat dampening his clothes, so that his T-shirt clung to his body in a way that made Avril glance at Carla with wicked eyes.

'Have you decided what's going where yet?' Hans asked, slumping into an executive swivel-chair and looking doubtfully at the utter disorganization of desks, filing cabinets, bookcases, framed prints, boxes of stationery, stacks of video cassettes and dozens of unlabelled boxes.

'My section's over there in front of the fireplace,' Avril answered, going to sit cross-legged on an unpacked box. 'I'm not going to need as big a staff as Carla, so her desks and stuff will take up about two-thirds of the space.'

'Which means I should be paying more rent,' Carla stated, from where she was perched on the top of a stepladder.

'In lieu of which I've taken a share in her company,' Avril announced. 'So let's drink to that too.'

Too tired to get up, they merely raised their glasses, then Sonya, noticing the time, dragged Lyle off to where she'd left her car, on a meter that had happily jammed.

Carla was watching John as he strolled over to the stairs and sat down on the bottom step. Catching her eye he winked and instead of smiling she looked quickly away, which was a stupid reaction, when she should have just come right out with what she was thinking, and thanked him for helping

209

today. After all, he probably had a thousand other things to do and places to be, but in choosing to come here and muck in with everyone else he'd shown where his priorities were. Besides, it wasn't everyone who could lay claim to having John Rossmore put up their shelves and shift around their bedroom furniture, which alone deserved a word of acknowledgement.

'I'm knackered,' Avril yawned. 'And starving. Who's for pizza?'

'Definitely,' Hans replied.

'Me too,' Carla added.

John drained his glass. 'I'm afraid you'll have to count me out,' he said, glancing at his watch. 'I should leave here in half an hour, so make use of me while you can.'

Avril looked him up and down. 'Now there's an offer,' she responded seductively.

Carla laughed, then coloured slightly as she looked at John, whose eyes were dancing. He was obviously well used to women like Avril, and not for the first time Carla found herself wishing that she too could occasionally be a little more laid-back.

'But you've still got all sorts of trust issues going on,' Avril reminded her, when Carla brought the subject up later, as they wearily climbed the stairs to their studio flats, 'which is bound to make you a bit nervy around men. And besides, it's just not in your character to be as brazen as me. Your attributes, oh long-legged, tousle-haired beauty that you are, are elsewhere placed. Now, what do you say we bunk up together tonight, because I don't think I've got enough energy left to make up more than one bed?'

'Fine by me, but we should make it mine, because Eddie'll want to crash out with us and all your bedding's brand new. Which reminds me, we'd better trot him round the block before we turn in.'

'You're on your own,' Avril muttered. Then, looking down at the madness below, she groaned out loud and sent up an impassioned plea for Mary Poppins to swoop in and rescue them.

However, somehow, over the next two days, a semblance of order was culled from the chaos, as telephones were connected, computers were installed and the great unpacking began to look marginally less like a scene from *Twister*. With so much organizing and arranging to be done, there wasn't much time for Carla to dwell on some of the terrible reviews the programme had received the morning after transmission, or how utterly terrified she'd felt by them, though there were plenty of moments when they stole up on her anyway, and left her feeling almost physically sick. Three critics had absolutely torn it to shreds, calling it pompous, non-directional, out of touch and, in one particularly nasty case, a patronizing and xenophobic attempt to disguise utter twaddle as cultural enlightenment.

The rest of the reviews had been glowing, calling it fresh, imaginative, funny, and a cut above the more mundane approach to this type of programme. Maddening, how the praise never seemed to soften the blows of censure and ridicule. It was like a tender caress after a sharp, painful slap – welcome, but not very effective. Not even the high viewing figures had been much of a balm either, since they were attributed to the promotional build-up, rather than audience approval. However, the second programme, set in Mexico, had now gone out, and the ratings, to Carla's surprise, and relief, had held steady. Had they dropped, she honestly didn't think she'd be taking the risk of moving into the *ménage*, but that small boost to her confidence, combined with John's unshakable belief in the programme, and Avril's refusal to countenance failure, had refuelled her determination to make this show work. So now there was never any discussion about her misgivings for the future, only about how they were going to continue raising enough money to finance it, which was an exercise that she and John were throwing themselves into with praiseworthy zeal.

Virtually every day over the following few weeks was taken up by meetings with bankers, businessmen, industry financiers and sponsorship brokers. That they could produce such impressive viewing figures was certainly holding some sway, though Carla was very aware that John's involvement, and charm, were responsible for many of the positive decisions, especially now that he had agreed to appear in the programme.

'Sure, I understand why you're asking,' he'd said when she first approached him on the matter, 'and all modesty aside, I think it's the right move. I just wanted it to come from you, rather than me.'

Carla's eyebrows went up. 'I thought all modesty was aside,' she teased.

Laughing, he sat back in his chair and signalled for a waiter to bring the bill. They usually lunched together now, since most days found them somewhere in the City or West End, in between meetings and with a need to eat – or even sometimes to celebrate, when a potential backer became a committed investor.

'I think the way to go,' he said, 'would be for me to alternate between presenting and acting. The weeks I'm not presenting we can call on a guest celebrity to front the show, that way we'll add more variety and keep it looking fresh. Incidentally, did my agent call you about my contract yet?'

Carla nodded, and felt a flutter of unease as the prospect of Zanzibar moved one step closer. 'It's with the lawyer, and should be ready for our signatures by the end of the week,' she told him.

He grinned. 'So then we'll be officially attached.'

Feeling a slight colour rise in her cheeks, she mumbled, 'Something like that,' and picked up the bill.

She knew he enjoyed teasing her, and on the whole she didn't mind, for it had been a long time since a man had flirted with her in such a harmless, yet flattering way. With Richard everything was on a level that was much more soulful and intense, and even frightening since he'd begun suggesting they meet. She wanted to, of course, indeed the very thought of it filled her with such excitement and anticipation it was often what carried her so blithely through the day, but in the evenings, when she was alone and playing out the erotic instructions he'd given her, she invariably ended up feeling almost sick with embarrassment to think of herself writhing naked on the bed, as though she were some remotely controlled sex object. It was no way to be living, making love to herself and pretending he was there, so why was she continuing to do it? Why couldn't she just say no, it's over now, and move on? Or even yes, and agree to see him?

212

Why was she allowing this to happen? Because she loved him, of course, and because she was afraid of losing what little of him she now had. But what about when she was in Zanzibar? The very thought of it, masturbating in a place where he and Chrissie had made love, turned her skin hot and cold with loathing. Dear God, just being on the same island was going to be bad enough; to think of humiliating herself like that made her want to tear herself to pieces rather than even consider it. She so desperately didn't want to go, but there was no backing out now, the plans were already under way, and John was so looking forward to it that she didn't have the heart even to suggest she might not be.

Avril sensed how reluctant she was, Carla knew, but Avril clearly had no intention of indulging her by discussing it, at least not in any depth, for she was too busy becoming fully operational in her London base. Mainly thanks to Lyle and Hans, who'd stayed for three weeks setting everything up, she now had an executive vice-president, Jeffrey Calder, two account managers, Felicia and Leo, and a vacancy for a personal assistant. On Carla's side great progress had been made too, though the staffing of the programme was a joint effort between her and John, and so far they'd recruited the previous series' production manager, Frazer Jackson; a researcher, also from last time, Verna Pope; and John's choice of lighting cameraman, Kit Kingsley. The assistant director John had approached was tied up on a film for the next few months, so he was currently scouting around for another. As Carla also required an assistant it was decided that she and Avril would share, since Avril wouldn't have need of anyone on a full-time basis.

'Sonya would be perfect, of course,' Avril declared one evening, as they made themselves comfortable in the glowing warmth of Carla's candle-lit studio. 'Can't we get her to move up here?'

'You might get *her* to, but I don't think Mark would,' Carla answered, patting the sofa for Eddie to jump up.

'Have you asked him?'

'No. Nor will I, because Sonya's got two kids, which means she can only commit part-time anyway, and to cover both of us we need someone full-time.'

'Can't she get a nanny?'

Carla laughed. 'Drop it,' she said. 'Sonya can't do it, and we've got to concentrate on finding someone who can. Shame Davey, who did the last series, has gone back to Oz. He'd have been perfect. Bit of a slave to his libido, but a great assistant.'

'Has John come up with any ideas?' Avril wanted to know. 'Where is he, by the way?'

Carla shrugged. 'God knows. It's past eight o'clock, he's generally out of here by six thirty, seven at the latest.'

'He is? I hadn't noticed. Where does he go?'

'I don't *know*,' Carla cried, laughing. 'Home, I expect. Or out somewhere. If the amount of calls he gets are anything to go by, then he's got such an active social life I'm amazed he manages to get up in the morning, never mind drag himself over here for a full day's work.'

'But you're getting along well with him?'

'Of course.'

Avril looked pleased. 'So you haven't given him the slip in favour of Richard again?' she said.

Carla's annoyance showed. 'Richard and John are two entirely separate issues in my life,' she responded, 'so the question of giving one the slip in favour of the other doesn't come into it.'

'It did the night after the party, when John cooked a meal at Graham's, and you couldn't make it because you were listening to an opera, supposedly with Richard, but actually *on your own.*'

Carla's expression was tight. 'I'm not getting into that again,' she retorted. 'I told you at the time, what I do, and when and how I do it, is my business. I don't get on your case over the male escorts you choose to go out with, so don't get on mine over how Richard and I choose to spend our time.'

Avril looked at her hard.

Carla refused to justify herself further.

With no preamble Avril said, 'When was the last time you had sex?'

Carla blinked. 'What?'

'You heard me.'

'What's that got to do with anything?'

'You know damned well what it's got to do with anything. All that e-masturbation and cyber-screwing, it's not real, Carla . . .'

'It's not like that, now let's leave it, shall we?'

Avril continued to look at her, then finally moved her eyes around the room, which was cosily furnished with a deep beige sofa and matching armchair, queen-sized brass bed, Oriental rugs and cabinets, loaded bookshelves and lushly draped windows. 'Anything in here that didn't come from your and Richard's flat?' she asked lightly.

'I'm not in a position to go out and buy everything new, the way you did,' Carla reminded her tersely.

'No, of course not. Sorry.'

A few more tense moments passed, then Carla's expression softened. 'No, I'm sorry,' she said. 'I guess I'm tired, and anxious about tomorrow . . .'

'What's tomorrow?'

'John and I start casting for the Zanzibar programme.'

'Oh, right. Have you told Richard you're going?'

'Not yet.'

'But you're still in touch with him? Every day?'

'More or less.'

'Does he ever say how Chrissie is?'

'No.'

'The baby?'

'No. Look, let's get off the subject, or we'll end up falling out.'

'OK. But just answer me this. Has he asked to see you at all, now he knows you're in London?'

Carla's answer was to look down at Eddie's face, resting on her lap.

'Well, thanks to the papers we now know he's in Knightsbridge,' Avril pointed out. 'A hop and a skip from here.'

Still Carla said nothing.

'Don't you think it's odd, that he hasn't asked . . .'

'He has, OK?' Carla snapped. 'In fact, if you must know, he's suggested it several times and I'm the one who's holding back.'

Avril couldn't have looked more surprised. 'Why?' she demanded.

215

'I don't know. I suppose because I'm just too afraid of being hurt again.'

'Well, I can understand that,' Avril responded. 'But it's not really healthy, is it, going on the way you are?'

'So you think I *should* see him?'

'As a matter of fact I do, because it's probably the only way to lay the ghost.'

Carla shifted restlessly. Even discussing this was hard, especially in terms of breaking it off. 'If I do see him,' she said, 'it won't end there. We both know that . . .'

'And where do you think it's going to lead, considering the commitments he now has?'

Carla threw out her hands. 'I don't know,' she cried, irritably. 'I haven't got the faintest idea. Now let's get off the subject. Tell me how long you're going to be in LA. Will you be back for Christmas?'

Sighing and stretching, Avril said, 'I'm not sure. I've already been away longer than I should have. But I'm considering coming back for the Zanzibar trip. It's OK, I'll pay my own way, *and* handle the publicity, so how's that for an offer? When is it, by the way?'

'John's going in about three weeks, to recce and cast locally,' Carla answered. 'The actual shoot's due to happen in January.'

'You're not going with him on the recce?'

'There's no need for me to, so there's no point adding to the expense. When are you leaving, by the way?'

'Sunday,' Avril answered, looking at her watch. 'Shall we go out to eat, or shall we see what we can rummage up in the kitchen downstairs?'

Half an hour later Avril was heaping piles of steaming hot pasta and spicy tomato sauce into a couple of bowls, while Carla set a fresh bottle of wine on the big pine table then reached up to get some glasses from one of the shiny oak cabinets over the sink. Though the kitchen was slightly beaten, and old-fashioned, it was homely and functional, and during the day offered a sunny view on to the disastrously untidy patio-garden. By now the conversation had moved on to the current state of financing for the next series of *There and Beyond*.

216

'We've probably got four programmes covered,' Carla was saying, as she filled the glasses, 'and there are still plenty of possibles who haven't come back to us yet. The fact that the ratings have increased is working wonders, and all the positive press you're managing to get us is definitely making a difference.'

'Which other locations are you planning to feature?' Avril asked, pulling up one of the Victorian-style stickback chairs.

'Argentina, India, Bali, and the others are still up for discussion. John's quite keen on Greece, which I've already done part of a script for.'

'Mm, interesting choices,' Avril commented. Then, going to get the pepper mill from next to the hob, she said, 'Has it occurred to you that John might have a bit of thing for you?'

Carla immediately stopped eating. 'I can't believe you said that,' she finally responded. 'He's never done anything to give even the slightest impression he's interested in me, and by suggesting it you're going to make it uncomfortable for me when I see him again.'

Avril laughed. 'It's OK,' she said, sitting down again. 'I don't think he's about to leap on you. Though a spot of leaping about with John Rossmore would probably do you the power of good. Release some of that tension you've got building up over there. And you can't tell me you don't find him attractive.'

'Actually, I don't,' Carla lied. It certainly wasn't a huge attraction, but considering how charismatic, not to mention good-looking and physical, he was, it was hard not to imagine what he might be like in bed. But she had no intention of telling Avril that, for there was every chance Avril would pass it on to John, and she'd rather hang upside down naked in a public place than be numbered amongst the millions who were all dying to know what John Rossmore was like in the sack. 'Anyway,' she said, 'I thought you had designs in that direction.'

'Me!' Avril laughed. 'I'd like to shag him every night for a month, but I value our new friendship too highly to jeopardize it for the sake of mere fleshly fulfilment.'

'Well, the same goes here. Not that I want to shag him, as you so eloquently put it, but I wouldn't want to jeopardize the working relationship we already have.'

217

'Glad to hear it, because God knows it would be the easiest thing in the world to find yourself taken in by all that wit and charm. Regardless of whether or not he's got the hots for you, I can tell you this: all women are, to men like John Rossmore, is a reason to change the sheets. And being tossed out with the laundry once is enough for any woman.'

Carla was looking perturbed, as, cutting herself a slice of olive bread, she said, 'You know, I hope his womanizing isn't going to prove a problem while we're shooting, because the last thing we need is him causing havoc amongst the female members of the cast and crew.'

'Well, you're going to be in some wickedly hot climates, and you know what heat does to the libido,' Avril warned. 'But he's behaved like a professional thus far, and I for one am pretty convinced by how committed he seems to the programme's success.'

'Mm,' Carla responded dubiously. In fact, were it not for Sonya faxing her the occasional article that popped up in the diary and gossip columns, placing John Rossmore at various hot spots around town, she might not have been even half so concerned. After all, the way he'd conducted himself with her these past few weeks hardly suggested a tempestuous, hard-drinking egomaniac with an incurable passion for women and gambling. However, the papers were nothing if not consistent in their portrayal of his bad-boy image, frequently commenting on how he was rarely seen with the same girl twice, and how, just last week, he'd been involved in a scuffle with the police after they'd been called to deal with some 'threatening behaviour' at a Mayfair casino.

Being ever mindful of how she had failed to detect any signs of Richard's duplicity, Carla was doubly unnerved by this apparent split personality in John. Still, at least in this case she knew about the aberration beforehand, so she didn't have to be afraid of it coming out of nowhere the way it had last time.

'Do you think what we read about him in the papers is true?' she said to Avril.

Avril shrugged, and, finishing a mouthful of food, said, 'Probably. At least a lot of it will be, but all you have to concern yourself with is the fact that he didn't get where he is today without talent and tenacity, or without a killer knowledge of how to play the press to his own ends when it suits him.'

Carla carried on eating. Avril was right, of course, she didn't need to concern herself with anything about John other than what he was bringing to the programme. As that amounted to just about everything, including the go-position they were now rapidly sliding into, she reminded herself of how fortunate she was to have him on board, then turned her thoughts to Richard and the ever-increasing dilemma of what, if anything, she should do about seeing him.

Chrissie was pushing Ryan's stroller through the crowded food department in Harrods. The overhead lights were dazzling, the various smells and noises were a bouquet and cacophony that felt joltingly at odds with her own reality, much like the towering pre-Christmas displays and seasonal music were out of place so early in November.

People kept stopping to admire her beautiful baby, so Chrissie smiled and thanked them, but never looked at Ryan herself for fear of starting her screaming. But so far Ryan had been an angel, and since Chrissie had been taking the medication Richard had insisted on, she'd felt better too. At least now she had the energy to get out of bed, she even cooked on occasion and went out for walks with Richard and Ryan. She'd only agreed to take the Prozac because Richard had looked so anguished when he'd tried to persuade her that she'd been afraid of what he might do if she didn't. Though he'd sworn he'd never let anyone take her away, she didn't believe him, because she'd heard the doctor telling him that in the end it might be the only solution. She hadn't seen the doctor herself, not even when he came to the house, she'd just listened from the top of the stairs as he told Richard about psychoses and depressions and an urgent need for intense psychotherapy.

So she took the medication, and life did seem a little brighter now, so much so that she'd even chatted on the phone with some of her friends. No-one ever mentioned that horrible spread in the paper, nor did she and Richard any more. It had been awful at the time, so hard for them to deal

219

with that in the end they'd made a pact to try and forget it. But before the pact they'd tried to work out who might have been behind the story. Richard had suspected the man with the grey hair who was so often outside the house. Certainly they hadn't seen him since, but Chrissie knew she hadn't told him anything about Richard, or Carla, or even herself to the degree it was in the paper. Of course there was the new nanny, but she simply hadn't known them long enough to give so much detail on Chrissie's past. That left only one other person, but Chrissie hadn't mentioned that person to Richard, because if she was right, she didn't want anyone to know the shame she felt for having led someone to avenge themselves on Carla for something Carla hadn't even done.

But she didn't need to worry about Carla now. The programme was in its fourth week of transmission, the ratings were fantastic, and whatever damage the article might have inflicted had no doubt been obliterated by the heady swell of success. And she knew how that felt, because people were recognizing her and congratulating her all the time, now that she was coming out more, and seeing the reaction for herself. Carla might have snatched away her power, but there was nothing she could do to steal her glory.

Stopping at the chocolate counter, she helped herself to one of the truffles a girl was handing out, found it delicious and bought a box for Richard. Moving on, she came across another promotion, this time for punch, and giggled with the woman as she downed three straight off. The cheese counter was one of her favourites, and as usual there were plenty of varieties chopped into cubes for tasting. She thought about what to get for dinner, but wasn't sure if Richard would be back in time. He'd gone to see someone he'd been trying to get a meeting with for ages, someone to do with Middle East intelligence, he'd said.

An hour later she found herself being tempted by the exotic fragrances of the perfumery department. She was laden with parcels by now, though with no real recollection of what was in them, or even of buying them. It wasn't the first time she'd mentally blanked like this, but such lapses happened to everyone, and everyone had an inbuilt autopilot that steered them about when they had lots on their mind, like when she'd taken the car last week and driven out to the cemetery where her father was buried. She couldn't remember anything about getting there, not even taking the decision to go, but she'd known exactly where she was when she'd arrived, and had then found her way back again without Richard even knowing she was gone. It wasn't the first time she'd gone off like that, and he didn't know about the other times either.

The house was empty when she got home. She put her parcels on the kitchen table, then sat down to wait. Her breathing was unsteady, and fear was billowing through her heart in huge, terrifying waves. She wasn't entirely sure when she'd first realized Ryan and the stroller had gone; maybe it was only a few minutes ago, when she'd come in the door and realized everything was so quiet. She thought of ringing Harrods to see if anyone had found her, but she was too afraid of discovering that nobody had.

'Oh my God!' she suddenly sobbed. 'I'm sorry. I'm so, so sorry.'

A long time later Richard came home and found her cuddling Ryan on the sofa, making such a fuss of her, and looking so happy and relaxed with her beautiful daughter, that his surprise made Chrissie laugh.

'How did it go?' she asked, as he kissed her, then Ryan. 'Did you see the man?'

'Yes,' he answered. 'How are you? You look wonderful.'

She laughed again. 'I feel it,' she said. 'I went shopping and spent all your money. Then I came back here and gave Ryan her tea and a bath, and she didn't cry once, did you, you little sweetheart?'

She wouldn't tell him that Ryan's screaming earlier was what had alerted her to the fact that she'd left the pushchair outside in the cold. It wasn't something he needed to know, it would only worry him, and seeing how pleased and happy he was to find her and Ryan together like this was so heartening that she really shouldn't do anything to spoil it.

221

Chapter 13

'OK, you two,' Carla called up the stairs to her niece and nephew, 'last one down is a silly fat frog.'

She was barely back in the kitchen when the thunder of four small feet pounding down the stairs startled Eddie from his breakfast, and very possibly registered somewhere on a Richter scale.

'I'm first and you're a silly fat frog,' Kitty sang, bursting into the kitchen with her sweater inside out and her leggings back to front.

'*You* are,' Courtenay said, giving her a shove. 'Toasted soldiers for me,' he told Carla, 'and can I have three eggs, please?'

'Three?' Carla cried, making him laugh with her shock.

'I want thirty-three,' Kitty declared, her big blue eyes simmering with mischief.

'I want ten thousand,' Courtenay boasted. 'I can eat ten thousand.'

Carla looked at Kitty. 'I think he's a bit of a banana, don't you?'

'I'm not a banana!' he cried, waving his spoon and fork in the air. 'You're a banana, and an apple.'

Carla rolled her eyes in horror. 'He called me an apple,' she gasped. 'What shall we do with him?'

'Put him in the rubbish and throw him out,' Kitty shouted. 'Because he's rubbish.'

'You're rubbish,' he told her, trying to hit her.

'All right, enough!' Carla barked. 'Two eggs each and lots of toasted soldiers coming up. Then we'll take Eddie for a walk. Did you remember to bring your wellies?'

'Yes,' they chorused.

'And can we go and see the baby sheep in the farm?' Kitty asked.

Courtenay creased his cute, freckly face into a puking expression, then howled in protest when Carla squeezed his cheeks and pushed his head back to give him a kiss.

'Auntie Carla,' Kitty said, when Carla finally sat down to join them. 'Who was that lady outside last night?'

Carla frowned, and handed her a piece of kitchen-roll. 'Wipe the egg off your nose,' she told her. 'What lady?'

'The one who was outside last night,' Kitty repeated.

'I don't know what you mean, darling,' Carla said. 'There wasn't anyone outside last night.'

'There *was*,' Courtenay declared. 'We saw her, didn't we, Kitty? She was down by the tree, and Eddie was barking.'

Carla was confused, and not a little alarmed, though Eddie often barked in the night if a fox or a badger, or some other nocturnal creature ventured into the garden, so it wasn't so unusual. However, with the uneasy feelings she'd been having these past few months, of either being watched, or not exactly being alone, this was not something she wanted to hear.

Realizing she was in danger of scaring the children too, she rolled her eyes and said, 'Oh, I expect it was Beanie looking for Dumbbell.' Which it could have been, though she'd never spotted Beanie down by the tree searching for Dumbbell before, but what other explanation could there be, if she wanted to keep this rational? And even if she didn't, she wasn't about to start believing in Maudie's ghosts or squatters, or whatever they were supposed to be, next door, or anywhere else. 'What did she look like?' she asked.

Kitty looked at her older brother. 'Um,' he said, 'she was about this big,' his hand was as high as he could reach, which was about four feet off the ground, 'and she had, um, hair, and . . .'

'And she was wearing a coat,' Kitty finished.

'Oh, then that'll definitely have been Beanie,' Carla said decisively.

'Phone!' Kitty suddenly yelled.

'You don't say,' Carla responded, tilting her chair back to

223

pick up the one on the dresser. 'Hello, Carla, Kitty, Courtenay,' she announced rapidly, presuming it was Sonya, and making the children grin with the alliteration they found so amusing.

'I see. Does that mean you've got company, or have you taken to announcing all your names when you answer the phone?'

Carla laughed. 'Good morning, John,' she said. 'I was expecting my sister-in-law.'

'I am not she,' he confessed.

'That you are not,' she agreed. 'So, what can I do for you at nine o'clock on a Sunday morning?'

'You can tell me where you've put the first-draft script for Zanzibar,' he answered. 'I'm at the office, and I don't like to go snooping around your desk, in case of what I might find.'

'You're at the office!' she cried in surprise. 'Don't you have a life?'

'You don't know the half of it,' he sighed. 'I've been out auditioning starlets all night, and I've cast so many parts we might have to rethink the entire piece.'

Carla's eyes were shining. 'I thought we were casting the harem locally in Zanzibar,' she said, 'not in London nightclubs.'

'Ah, but you should see these girls,' he groaned. 'And if I've got to be playing the Sultan, I should have a say in who my babes are, shouldn't I?'

'Absolutely,' she agreed, knowing very well that he was sending them both up. 'So, why the first-draft script?'

'Because there was something in it that doesn't seem to have found its way into the second draft, and I think it should have.'

'OK. It's in the middle filing cabinet, bottom drawer, under Zanzibar. The keys are in the clay pot on the bookcase next to my desk.'

'I see it,' he said. 'And now I'll leave you in peace. Enjoy the day,' and he rang off.

It wasn't until a few minutes later, as she helped Kitty to straighten out her clothes, that it occurred to Carla that Avril must be at the *ménage* too . . . So the reason John was there so early on a Sunday morning was very possibly because he'd

224

spent the night there, with Avril, who wasn't flying back to LA until late afternoon. For one surprising, and unpleasant, moment Carla felt much as she did with Richard and Chrissie, as though she was on the outside of a relationship, being almost deliberately excluded. Obviously, it wasn't quite the same with John and Avril, but she still wasn't thrilled by the idea that they might be getting involved. However, if they were, she wanted to know.

'You are *so* nosy,' Avril laughed, when Carla called and asked point-blank if John had spent the night there. 'And what's it to you if he did, may I ask?'

'Nothing,' Carla assured her. 'I was just wondering, that's all.'

'Well, wonder away, because I'm not telling.'

'Is he still there?' Carla asked.

'Yep.'

'Dressed?'

Avril chuckled.

Carla had to laugh too.

'If you must know,' Avril said, 'we went out last night, a whole gang of us, and yes, John did end up staying here, but he slept on the sofa. OK? Happy?'

Carla was dying. Obviously he'd just heard every word Avril had said, and she didn't even want to think about the conclusions he might be drawing. 'I'll kill you for that,' she muttered. Then blithely added, 'You must be losing your touch if you didn't manage to get him off the sofa.'

'Maybe I am,' Avril agreed.

Carla could hear John's voice in the background, though she couldn't make out what he was saying. Then, to her dismay, Avril burst out laughing.

'Do I want to know what he just said?' Carla asked her.

'Probably not,' Avril answered. 'But don't worry, it wasn't about you.'

Once again Carla cringed. 'I'm going,' she said.

'No, wait,' Avril cried. 'I need to talk to you about the speaking globe thing. Jeffrey's been in touch with the manufacturer, and they want to know how many you need.'

'Two,' Carla answered. 'They're the runner-up prizes. I think Abercrombie and Kent are going to spring for first prize with a safari. I'm seeing them on Wednesday. It could be a good idea for Felicia and Leo to come with me, since they're devising the competition.'

'OK. You can work that out with them. But make sure they keep me informed.'

'I will.' Carla turned to where Kitty and Courtenay, only half in their coats and wellies, were tearing open the back door to run outside and collect conkers. It reminded her of what they'd said about seeing a woman last night, so, changing the subject, she repeated it to Avril. 'Who do you think it could have been?' she said.

'God knows. What time was it?'

'I don't know. The kids didn't go to bed until late, so I suppose it must have been after eleven.'

'And you don't have any ideas yourself?'

'I told the children it was probably Beanie looking for her dog, which I guess it could have been . . .'

'Strange,' Avril commented. 'Maybe you should ask Maudie if she saw anyone, because not much gets past her.'

'I don't think I could bear to set her off again,' Carla groaned. 'Maybe it was just a shadow they saw. You know, some kind of trick of the moonlight. Anyway, I'm going, before they break their necks climbing the tree. Call me when you get to LA.'

'Will do. Oh, hang on.'

John was talking again.

'Sorry, I thought he was giving me a message for you,' Avril said, 'but he's thinking about his stomach and reminding me that we've arranged to meet everyone for breakfast. So, bye. Speak to you late tomorrow,' and she was gone.

By six o'clock that evening the children had gone home, and Carla had not only finished the work she'd brought with her, she'd also composed a long email to Richard, and carried out yet another search for his letters. Since they hadn't turned up with everything from storage, they surely had to be in the house somewhere, but once again she'd failed to find them. She could now only presume that they had somehow been thrown out by mistake, which was a prospect she found almost as upsetting as the fact that she hadn't heard from him at all in the past three days. Her heart gave a small, panicked beat as she thought of what that might mean, and could she bear it if he abandoned her again? With nothing material to bind them together, or acknowledge them as a part of each other, this unexpected silence had left her drifting in a fog of frustration and doubt. But maybe he'd gone off on assignment to a place where it was difficult to connect his computer. She'd never asked him about the sabbatical that had been mentioned in the paper, mainly because if she found out it was true, she would only start tormenting herself with the reasons behind his decision.

Sighing heavily, she turned off the light in the study and went to stoke up the fire in the sitting room. She wasn't at all proud of the way she kept skirting round questions that really ought to be asked, or of how she hadn't insisted on answers to those that she had managed to pose. Her only excuse was that her sense of self-preservation was so strong now that she couldn't even get a need for the truth past it, because the truth might bring pain, and pain was something she'd had more than enough of. However, ignorance was no state to be in, nor was this awful feeling of being so cut off, unable to call him, and so totally disconnected from the real events of his life. Avril was right, it wasn't healthy, carrying on this way, so maybe she should summon the courage and agree to see him. It could even be that his silence these past three days was a deliberate ruse to bring her to this very conclusion. Her heart fluttered as she wondered when the best time would be, but there was no good time for something like this. Whenever it happened, it would be disruptive in the extreme, and she not only owed it to herself to be focused and together at all stages of the upcoming production, she owed it to John and the others too.

Looking at the clock, she considered going back to London tonight. Graham was taking her and Eddie to the station in the morning, but maybe he wouldn't mind taking them now, instead. But what was she going to do when she got there? Sit around her studio with nothing to do, and nowhere to go? At least here she could pop along to the pub. The trouble was, she didn't feel like going to the pub. She wanted to go out and have some of the fun Avril always managed to have. Frankly, she wouldn't mind some of the sex too, because God knew how long it had been ... Long enough for her fantasies to have become confused, that was for sure, because just lately she'd started thinking about John in that way, and some of the thoughts were so unbelievably erotic that she could only thank God he had no way of reading her mind.

Since talking to him this morning images of him making love to Avril had flashed in her mind all day, and though she knew it probably hadn't happened, the idea of him naked and aroused, and her own body in place of Avril's, was really stressing her out. Of course, it could as easily be Jeffrey, Avril's VP, she was fantasizing about, or Frazer, her own production manager, because lust wasn't particularly discriminating, so the fact that John had become its focus was simply because he was there, and the occasional attention he paid her was mildly agreeable. And if she weren't always working, or sharing telepathic time with Richard, she might not be getting into this state! She'd be out there with Avril, and everyone else, partying and going to shows and dancing ... Her heart turned over, and she wanted to scream at the frustration of feeling so restless in her body and uncontrolled in her longings.

'Tonight?' Graham said into the phone. 'You want me to take you to the station tonight?'

'Only if it's convenient,' Carla assured him.

'Oh dear. You see, Betty's just got back and we're about to sit down and have dinner.'

'Then, please, forget it,' Carla insisted. 'I'll call Teddy, or Angie. Or maybe I'll just stay with my plan to go back early in the morning.'

Ringing off, she returned to the sitting room and stared down at the fire. Maybe she'd just take a long hot bath and find something to read that she could later discuss with Richard. Or maybe she should send him an email demanding to know why he hadn't been in touch!

The bath helped soothe her a little, but curling up in front of the fire with Rousseau's *Discourse* failed to engage her thoughts the way it had before, when she'd been searching for Richard's hidden message. Nor could she find anything to which she could allude herself, in an effort to get him guessing

228

what she might be trying to tell him. Her mind just wasn't there. It was flitting about all over the place, from John, to the programme, to Avril, to Graham, back to John, and not until Eddie started barking did her thoughts jar on the recollection of the woman the children had seen down by the tree.

'What is it?' she said, her heart starting to pound as, still barking, he ran into the kitchen then back to the sitting room. His little face was so earnest as he looked at her, still barking away, that it wasn't hard to work out that he wanted her to follow him.

'No. You're not going out there chasing foxes at this time of night,' she told him, trying to calm herself with a sharpness of tone.

He ran back into the kitchen, still barking.

Carla's heart was thudding even harder as she pulled her dressing gown more tightly around her, and got up from the sofa. The curtains were drawn, so she couldn't see out, nor, she acknowledged with some relief, could anyone see in.

'Eddie! Stop it!' she cried, as he raced back in. 'What's the matter? There's no-one out there.'

But Eddie clearly thought there was.

'Oh God,' she muttered. 'Eddie! Please, stop barking. I'm not going out there, and nor are you.' Then she almost leapt out of her skin as the telephone suddenly rang. 'Hello?' she gasped, grabbing it up.

'Carla? Is everything all right? Why's Eddie barking?'

'I don't know,' she answered. Then, puzzled, she added, 'You can hear him, at the other end of the village?'

Graham laughed. 'I can hear him down the phone,' he reminded her.

Carla smiled, and put a hand to her head. 'Of course,' she said. 'He's just been going so berserk . . . Probably just a fox, but he's spooked me a bit. The children said they . . .'

'Hang on,' he interrupted.

She heard his hand go over the mouthpiece, the sound of muffled voices, then he was back on the line.

'Sorry,' he said. 'Betty's just come in. She forgot to take her key. Anyway, I was calling to find out if you'd gone back to London, or if you still need a lift in the morning. I take it you do.'

'Yes, please. That would be wonderful,' she said. 'Can we leave at six thirty? Is that too early?'

'Not at all. Six thirty it is. Now, is everything all right? Eddie seems to have calmed down a bit.'

Carla looked at him, slumped on the floor as though nothing had happened. 'He's a menace,' she scolded, 'but he's fine now. I was just feeling a bit edgy I suppose, and irritable because I haven't heard from Richard . . . Tell me, do you think I should see him?'

'Mmm,' Graham responded, pondering the question. 'I suppose it'll have to happen sooner or later. Do you feel ready for it?'

'I don't know,' she sighed. Then, to her dismay, she embarked on a lengthy account of the dilemma and doubts she'd been putting herself through for weeks.

Though Graham listened with his usual understanding and patience, and offered some heartening suggestions, she was no more settled in her mind by the time she went to bed than she'd been before.

Scooting Eddie over so she could uncover the spot he'd just warmed up, she slipped in between the sheets, then reached across him to turn out the light. Her mind was racing, but it wasn't very long before she was completely tangled up in a dream that was about Richard, who became John, who then turned into Graham, before moving on to Betty hanging from the horse chestnut tree, though she wasn't dead, and then Richard was there with Chrissie and it was Chrissie hanging from the tree, where Richard had put her. However, Carla's most vivid recollection the next morning was of the powerfully erotic sex she'd had with John, up against the bookshelves next to her desk, which then became a public place, where her orgasm was so immense that it drew a crowd, and finally shook her out of the dream.

Chapter 14

It had to be fifteen months or more since Carla felt this good. In fact, her old energy was flooding back with such gusto that she was having trouble keeping the emotion from her voice and euphoria from her words as she stood in front of the small cast she and John had chosen, and the production team that was going to enable the new series to happen, briefing them on what it was all going to be about. They were in the *ménage*'s spacious back room, which, for the next few weeks, was going to double as a rehearsal and viewing room. Standing here, in a brand new plum wool dress, the first she'd bought in over a year, and an expensive pair of black suede boots, addressing her new team as their executive producer, was saying more clearly than anything that she really had pulled through the worst of the bad times, and was now heading right back to the top – and beyond.

'The funding we've managed to raise so far, for the new series, has surpassed even my wild expectations,' she told them. 'Last time around we set some very high standards, which we now aim to exceed, and, thanks to the increase in budget, as well as the bonus of having John Rossmore on board – with an exceptionally talented group of actors and crew behind him – I've no doubt we will.' She didn't look at John, who was sitting in a chair to her right, legs stretched out in front of him, thumbs hooked into the belt loops of his jeans, though she could almost feel his irony, and was hard put not to smile herself. 'The last programme in the current series is due to air next Monday at eight, then the entire series will be repeated starting in February, on Tuesday nights at ten. This is a major bonus I wasn't expecting, and is confirmation indeed that we are as good as everyone says we are, with the notable exception of a few confused TV critics.'

After the amusement had passed Frazer, the production manager, said, 'Any dates for the new series' transmission yet?'

'Probably the same time next year,' Carla answered, 'with a repeat showing again in the spring. Everything's really taking off, but we'd be fools if we believed ourselves invincible, so let's understand right now that there's one heck of a lot of hard work coming up, for everyone, and I want you all to remember that no one person is more important than another, because that's not the way we work. We're a team, so we all pull together, which means you can feel free to share your complaints, concerns and especially ideas with either John or me, and give us any kind of input you think might be valuable.'

At that moment the door opened and Kit Kingsley, the giant bear of a lighting cameraman, came in with a fresh cup of coffee in one hand, a heavy holdall in the other, and a genuinely apologetic look on his face. 'Sorry,' he said, grimacing, 'nothing I could do. The flight was delayed . . .'

'It's OK,' Carla told him. 'We got your message.' She looked around the room. 'I guess most of you know Kit,' she said, 'if only by reputation.'

John was on his feet greeting the cameraman, who then sat down next to him on one of the assortment of second-hand chairs that were positioned around the edges of the room, with only the odd coffee table, rug, script and ashtray taking up the space in the middle. Carla was the only one standing, with her shoulders and one foot pressed up against a wall, everyone else was either perched on a window-sill or sitting on the chairs. Since Kit was the most senior member of the team, Carla began going through the introductions again, starting with Phoebe Marsh, the stunningly beautiful black actress who was going to be starring in the dramatic sketch on Zanzibar, then the various members of costume, make-up and production, and finishing with Rosa Gingell, whom John had cast as the slave trader's wife.

Rosa treated Kit to her most winning smile, then, without looking at Carla, returned her eyes to the script she had resting on her lap. Carla's eyes lingered on her for a moment. Rosa's coldness towards her had been marked from the moment she'd arrived that morning, and though Carla had no idea why, she could only wish that she'd remembered sooner how resistant Chrissie had always been to casting her. Rosa was too much of a gossip and troublemaker to make it worth having her around, Chrissie had always claimed. It was the reason she hardly ever worked, her reputation went before her. But though Carla had certainly baulked when John had first suggested her, it had been for reasons more to do with Rosa becoming a two-way grapevine between her and Chrissie and Richard, than with Rosa's spiky personality. Now, only able to imagine that Rosa's frostiness was part of some bizarre stand on Chrissie's behalf, Carla just hoped she understood that cold-shouldering the executive producer on day one was definitely not a good start, nor was sucking up to the director, who had only cast her because Yale Winfield – a good friend of Rosa's who was playing the slave trader – had made it part of his deal. So Rosa hadn't been John's choice either, and if Carla knew anything about John Rossmore by now, it was that his laid-back manner and ready sense of humour in no way blunted his ability to sum up a situation, or a person, in less time than it took most to get past hello.

'OK,' Carla said, the introductions over, 'I'm going to talk now about our plans for the upcoming series, starting with your particular episode, which is going to be shot in Zanzibar. For those of you who haven't yet familiarized yourselves with the island, it's off the east coast of Tanzania, which is on the east coast of Africa, south of Kenya and north of Mozambique.'

Frazer was on his feet, in front of an enormous map of the world that covered one entire wall. Locating Zanzibar, he pointed it out, though it was a bit like a pinprick on an elephant's back.

'I'm sure you'll agree,' Carla continued, 'that the name alone evokes all kinds of exotic images, and believe me, its history and culture outclass even the most vivid of imaginations. Its architecture has a strong Islamic influence, thanks to the long reign of the Sultans of Oman, but it also has several British customs left over from the days of the

Protectorate. It was one of the world's most prominent centres for trade between East and West during the seventeenth and eighteenth centuries, dealing in ivory from Africa, silks from India, porcelain from China, as well as all kinds of opiates, weaponry, coffee, tea and many of the spices that are still exported today, like cloves, vanilla, cinnamon, cardamom, you name it . . . But, as I'm sure you know, its major trading was done in the slave market, where men, women and children who'd been hunted down and captured on mainland Africa were herded, branded, whipped and a whole lot worse, before being sold to the highest bidders. An extremely emotive subject, but not one that we'll go into now.

'One of the island's most famous visitors was David Livingstone, as in "Dr Livingstone, I presume." He was there in the mid-eighteen hundreds, and the house where he stayed is now the Zanzibar Tourist Commission. Actually there are plenty of significant people and events that make up the cocktail of the island's history, most of which you'll find in the guidebooks that are outside in the office, and in the few pages I've written myself that are with the books. But please bear in mind that I haven't visited the place yet, so my information is culled from the guides, and from the initial research trip that was done a year or so ago.'

At this point she was deliberately not looking at Rosa, since Rosa would know that she was avoiding mentioning Chrissie's name.

'John, Kit, Hugo, Russell, Frazer and Verna will be going to recce the island in about three weeks,' she continued. 'I should mention at this point that those of you who aren't up to date on your vaccines should talk to Marjie, my temporary assistant, who'll tell you what you need and where to go. Marjie, by the way, probably knows more about television production than the rest of us put together, so be nice to her, because I'm doing my level best to turn her temporary status into a permanent one, and if any of you can discover her temptation of choice, I might be happy to indulge yours too, depending on what it is.'

As their attentive faces relaxed into laughter, Carla leaned down to John and said, 'I'm about done here, shall we break for coffee before you take over?'

234

'Good idea,' he answered. Then added, 'Did anyone ever tell you you're a hard act to follow?'

'All the time,' she answered without missing a beat, then, after announcing a fifteen-minute interval, she headed for the door.

In the office outside Marjie, who looked like everyone's favourite aunt with her grey wavy hair, gentle blue eyes and bosomy front, was in conference with Felicia and Leo, Avril's account managers, while Jeffrey, Avril's exec. VP, was at his desk over by the fireplace, talking on the phone and tapping into his computer. Eddie, who'd been banished from the meeting, leapt out of his sulk the instant Carla reappeared, and was soon quite delirious at being surrounded by so much cooing and fondling again.

After grabbing a coffee Carla returned to her desk, and the pile of messages Marjie had taken over the past couple of hours. Flipping through them, she sat down to start returning the most urgent, while John and his first assistant, Hugo, perched on the edge of John's desk opposite, and began discussing the various technical requirements. Kit and Russell, the designer, soon joined them, leaving the cast sitting around the table in the kitchen, either gossiping, looking through the script, or reading the notes and guidebooks Carla had mentioned.

By the time the coffee break was over Carla had only managed to get through two lengthy, but necessary calls, and though the urgency attached to the others was growing, John and the cast were about to embark on a read-through of the script, and as the writer, she had to be there. So abandoning the build-up of work to Marjie, who was so unflappable she could make a dead man look manic, she seized her own copy of the script and headed back to the meeting room.

John began by outlining the story. Naturally they'd all read it, but this was his first chance to give them some idea of how he, as the director, saw it. In less than five minutes everyone, including Carla, was aching with laughter. Though the story of a beautiful black slave girl was essentially a tragedy, it was John's take on his own role, as the dashingly handsome Sultan, that was making them all laugh, mainly because he was making it sound so utterly beyond belief that he, the

235

putative womanizer, gambler and rampant user of illegal substances, could ever have been cast in such a role.

'Rampant, of course, is a word that sums up this sultan chap to a T,' he said. 'I mean, what else can you call a man who's got two dozen wives and at least as many mistresses?'

'A dreamer?' Carla suggested.

John's head went back as he and everyone else laughed.

Carla crooked an eyebrow and glanced at Rosa, who'd failed to find the joke funny.

'OK,' John went on, 'whilst the evil slave trader and his harridan of a wife are doing double deals all over town for the exquisite beauty, I, being the dashing hero that I am, ride to the rescue on my sturdy white steed and carry her to the safety of my harem.'

'Which is a bit like taking her from the proverbial pan and dumping her straight in the fire,' Phoebe commented.

As everyone laughed, Carla looked at Phoebe's lovely face, then at John's, and felt a small flutter inside at how easy she found it to imagine them together, not only because of their matching good looks, but because of the chemistry that was already starting to flow. Swallowing her dismay, Carla tried to assure herself that John would be professional at all times, and respect the fact that Phoebe was married. She supposed she had to hope that Phoebe would respect it too.

'So, where were we?' John was saying. 'OK. I've got this fabulous creature hiding in my palace, when in burst the evil slaver and his wife to snatch her back. In this they succeed, and promptly sell the hapless beauty to the wicked pirate who buys her for his lascivious crew. Just a minute,' he said, looking at Carla, 'I thought I was the rampant one.'

'We're not dealing in reality,' she reminded him. 'In this, you're the good guy who happens to respect a lovely young girl's innocence.'

He frowned. 'Doesn't sound very sultan-ish to me,' he said.

'It's the way it happened,' she assured him, reminding them all that this was based, very loosely, on an actual story.

'OK, well, after that what can I say,' John continued, 'except you must have gathered by now that I want to play most of it tongue in cheek, but the seriousness of the undertone shouldn't in any way be lost. It's there in the writing, so it needs to come out in the acting. Today, we're just going to read through, then we'll have an informal chat about characters and costumes and that sort of thing. Next week we've got two rehearsals scheduled, a third just before I go to Zanzibar, then two more in the week running up to the shoot. Any questions? Frazer, you wanted to say something?'

'Just that the publicists have arranged a photoshoot for December ninth,' he said, with an habitual blush. 'If anyone can't make it, would you let me know so we can try to fit you in another time.'

'Will you be wanting them in costume for the photoshoot?' Jackie, the wardrobe mistress, asked.

Frazer looked at John, who looked at Carla. They both nodded. 'Where's it going to be happening?' John asked.

'At a studio over in Ladbroke Grove,' Frazer answered. 'Felicia's got all the details, I'll make sure I get them before everyone leaves today.'

'OK,' John said, rubbing his hands. 'Let's start reading, why not? Is anyone going to put a watch on it?'

Carla held up her hand. 'I'll time it,' she said.

Half an hour later, having clocked up a rough duration of twenty minutes, Carla returned to her desk feeling more than satisfied with the way it had read. The dialogue worked, the humour was subtle, and the undercurrent of menace was at just the right level. That wasn't to say no polishing was called for, because it was, and no doubt the rehearsals would throw up all manner of changes between now and when they left. On the whole, however, the rather fantastic love story was looking as though it would provide the perfect vehicle to take them not only into Zanzibar's colourful past, but all around its impossibly romantic present.

Actually, it was the romance of the island's tropical splendour, with its white sandy beaches and aquamarine sea, that had given her the most problems while she was writing, because it was impossible not to think of Richard and Chrissie experiencing it all and creating, no doubt, some of the most precious memories they now shared. Though she tried not to let herself dwell on it, it still hurt almost beyond endurance, but with everything moving ahead at its own rapid pace, there was simply no way of avoiding it now.

It was close to eight that evening by the time Frazer, the last one to leave, took his blushing face out of the door, having just had his offer to walk Eddie politely turned down by Carla, because she needed the air. In fact, she ended up staying out much longer than she might have, mainly because it was a bright, moonlit night that was almost warm, considering the time of year, and the air, the trees, the large white houses, exclusive restaurants and traffic were so magically London that she was absorbing it like an elixir. What an incredible first day of production, with everything going so well she was almost afraid of tomorrow, for she couldn't imagine it getting any better. But there was still tonight to get through, which was going to be her first alone at the *ménage*, and though she wasn't exactly nervous, she was a little apprehensive, mainly because of the loneliness she could sense waiting to claim her. Of course there were any number of old friends she could call and arrange to see, but not at this short notice, and with her schedule being so hectic now it was hard to make any firm arrangements for the future. Besides, there was too strong a chance that someone would start talking about Richard, and since things had changed in ways none of them could know about, she had no desire to hear what they might have to say.

Letting herself back in the front door, she closed and locked it behind her, then took Eddie into the kitchen to get him some supper. She should probably eat something herself, but she didn't feel like much, so, contenting herself with a glass of wine and a dish of nuts, she returned to her computer, linked up with the Internet and printed out the latest email from Richard. That done, she checked everything was turned off, then went upstairs to her studio, where she put on some music, lit candles under the pots of fragrant oils, and settled down on the sofa with Eddie to read the message.

It was long, slightly repetitive, and by an author she didn't recognize at all, though she presumed it was one of the French classicists, probably from the Age of Reason, as opposed to the later Romantic Movement. Until now he'd always quoted authors they'd discussed, and even read together, but this was a piece that seemed to have no place in her memory, and without his letters to guide her she wasn't even sure where to start looking.

Letting her head fall onto the back of the sofa, she picked up her wine and took a sip. Then she ate some nuts, giving a couple to Eddie, and before she knew it she was mulling over everything she had to do tomorrow, from the meeting at eight with the company accountant, to the lunch she'd been pressed into by a particularly aggressive agent, to the script changes for Zanzibar and story developments for Greece and India. But that wasn't even the half of it, and she could only thank God she'd managed to persuade Marjie to come and help out, otherwise there was no knowing what kind of mess she'd end up in.

Her thoughts drifted on, taking her to Christmas, which she'd no doubt spend with her family, then to New Year, which Avril would hopefully be around for, and finally to Zanzibar. Though her heart contracted, she was soon smiling as she recalled the way John had handled the read-through this morning, and if this first experience of him in production was anything to go by, then she had much less to fear from his rumoured ego and tantrums than she had from the wayward inclinations of her own mind. Even now, as she sat here thinking about how she'd addressed the meeting, in her fantasy scenario there was no-one in the room but her and John, in the exact same positions they'd been in this morning, though now his hand was moving under her dress, up over her thighs . . . Snapping the thought off, she took another sip of wine and ruffled Eddie's ears.

'Maybe I should get Avril to give me the number of her escort service,' she sighed wearily. Then, grimacing, she turned back to the email and began puzzling over it again.

'Oh God,' she groaned, after a while, 'what am I doing, sitting here trying to work out a message from one man, while fantasizing about having sex with another, with no real hope of ever achieving either? Why aren't I having a life, like everyone else?'

For one intensely awful moment she almost picked up the phone to call John, on the pretext of wanting to discuss the script, when what she really wanted was him to flirt with her again.

'How pathetic am I going to get?' she murmured to Eddie. 'And it's not only me he flirts with, it's all women, like Phoebe, Verna, Marjie, definitely Avril . . . I wonder who he's really sleeping with. You've got to pity her, whoever she is, because it must be hell living with a man who practically every woman alive wants to get into bed.'

Looking down at the email in her lap her heart gave a long and painful wrench as she came back to earth. What was she talking about? She didn't want John Rossmore, any more than she wanted dear freckly-faced Frazer . . . The only one she wanted was Richard, and she wanted him so badly that the wires between her mind and body were getting so confused by lust, that, if she wasn't careful, she'd end up doing something she'd bitterly regret.

'Darling,' she wrote, back at her computer, 'though I haven't yet worked out the significance of your last message, I just wanted you to know that I'm sitting here thinking about you, and feeling the need to see you so fiercely that I'm wondering if the time has come for me to let go of my caution and allow myself to return completely to your heart, where I belong. My day-to-day life is so full of the programme now that I'm afraid of it coming between us, though I know that in truth nothing can. I feel so confused about where we are going, how we can be together and not hurt other people, though of course I only mean your daughter, because I still find it so hard to forgive Chrissie for stealing you away. I ask myself so often, why, oh why, did you go? The answer, whatever it is, probably means nothing now, as time has moved on and I must accept that mistakes are possible, even between those who love each other as much as we do.

'The success I'm enjoying now is so heady that at times I feel more attached to it than I do my own heart. But that is only because it's here, at my fingertips, and you are . . . Where are you? I wonder that all the time, as I look around, expecting to see you, or feel you, or hear you. What does your last message mean? Where can I find the answers? Even as I ask I hear you telling me to look inside my heart, then I will know what you are saying to me, which has nothing to do with who wrote the words, only with what you are using them to convey. Good night, dream of me, as I shall dream of you.'

His message the next morning said: 'The words are Machiavelli's, the message is from my tortured soul. You remember we read *The Prince*, together, in the gardens of the Pitti Palace? Read it again, my darling, and understand its sense as well as its cunning. Hear what I am telling you, listen with your heart, and feel with your mind. Immerse yourself in the success of your everyday world, and know that whenever you look around, I am there, in my spirit, that is joined to yours.'

Carla's shock was almost palpable. Machiavelli! How could he have used words from a man whose detachment from moral values was almost frightening to contemplate when given in this context? What sense? What cunning? Was he saying that his behaviour was based on some convoluted sixteenth-century philosophy? If he was, then didn't that make her little more than an intellectual experiment, the human equivalent of a laboratory rat being tested by the unethical workings of a brilliant mind?

She was so upset, and bewildered, by the message that she forwarded it immediately to Graham, then picked up the phone to let him know it was there. He rang back, a few minutes later, having read the message and weighed it against her reaction.

'I think I can understand why you're upset,' he said ruminatively, 'but it's probably because you're seeing Machiavelli only as an unprincipled manipulator, and forgetting the skilled politician he actually was.'

'Which takes us where?' Carla said, a little calmer now, and willing to listen to a less hysterical viewpoint than her own.

'What about starting with Florence?' he suggested.

Carla frowned. 'Because that's where we read the book together?'

'It's just a thought.'

She was quiet for a moment, staring at Eddie, but not actually seeing him as she thought about Florence, and those magical hours they'd spent in the gardens of the Pitti Palace. Then she recalled how she had ended her own message with '. . . nothing to do with who wrote the words, only with what you are using them to convey.' 'I think I've got an idea what this is about now,' she said, finally, and started to smile. 'The

241

three days we spent in Florence were nothing short of perfect, but boy, what he had to go through to get the time off . . . It was in the middle of the Bosnian crisis, and in order not to jeopardize his assignment, but to spend his birthday with me . . . Well, you don't need to know all the favours he had to ask, and promises he had to make, and even lies he had to tell . . . I probably don't even know the half of it myself, but I think what he's saying is that sometimes you have to detach emotionally from one situation in order to attend to another.'

'Interesting,' Graham responded.

Carla smiled. 'In other words,' she said, 'the reason he wasn't in touch with me for a few days was because there was something going on at home that had to be dealt with. And it's likely to happen again, but that doesn't change anything about us, we're still a single spirit that, just like a single individual, often has more than one task, as well as more than one loyalty. Does that make sense to you?'

'Put like that it does,' he answered.

Carla grinned. 'Great,' she said, and after thanking him she hung up, closed her laptop and ran downstairs to where the office was already coming alive for the day. The fact that Richard hadn't responded to her veiled suggestion that they should meet was OK, because she still wasn't sure about it either. However, she had to confess that nor was she thrilled by the idea that it was now him holding back, rather than her, since the reversal could have adverse effects on the strength she had been drawing from being the wanted, rather than the wanter. Alarming, even frightening, how vulnerable, and unreliable, such strengths as resolve, self-esteem and confidence could be, when dealing with a difficult love.

There were two police cars outside, one in front of Richard's BMW, the other behind it. Only one had official insignia, the other was a dark red saloon that had brought a man in a smart black raincoat and a woman in a green eider-padded jacket. There were other cars there, but Chrissie wasn't sure who they belonged to, except the woman who'd got out of one, about fifteen minutes ago, had been carrying Ryan.

Who exactly had found her, in Kensington Gardens, Chrissie didn't know. She had no recollection of leaving her

242

there, she couldn't even remember taking her out. She only recalled being in the park, surrounded by trees and people and skaters and birds as she drifted weightlessly in another realm of consciousness where fear didn't exist, and inadequacy was never measured.

The call had come, only minutes after she'd returned home, telling her that Ryan had been found. Richard was in his study, so he'd had no idea, until the police turned up, that Ryan had even been missing. By then Chrissie had taken herself upstairs, into the bedroom, not wanting to see anyone, especially not Richard. Over the past fifteen minutes she'd heard snatches of the conversation below, so knew that if she wanted to avoid what they were planning she should go into the bathroom now, lock the door and never come out.

Though tears rolled down her face, all she knew was the fear that was riveting her to the landing, and the awful loneliness that seemed to be descending from the ceiling, closing in with the walls and rising up with the floor. Something terrible was happening to her, and she didn't know where to turn any more. She'd heard them explaining to Richard how the brain didn't always make a full recovery from substance abuse, and that even years later, the after-effects of hallucinogenics could distort the mind and incite paranoia. When combined with a clear case of post-natal depression, and the natural exhaustion of being a new mother – and one who wasn't quite so young any more – it must be understood that for her own sake, as well as her daughter's, she had to have professional help.

Richard was agreeing to everything, but was insistent that they didn't take her away.

Chrissie's heart swelled with love and pain. He was still protecting her, wanting to keep her where he knew she felt safe, and where he could help her through this himself. He just needed Dr Philbert to carry on advising him, as he had been these past few months, and he would make sure that she was never left alone with the baby again – at least not until everyone was certain she could handle it.

'I'm sorry to be so blunt,' a woman's voice said, 'but you should be made aware that there's a chance she'll get worse.

243

If that happens, she really will have to be hospitalized, you do understand that, don't you?'

'Let's deal with that *if* it happens,' Richard answered.

'Have you any idea when she stopped taking the medication?' another voice asked.

There was no answer, which suggested Richard had shaken his head.

'Mrs Crabbe, here, is from the social services,' the woman's voice said. 'She'll be calling on you regularly.'

'There's no need,' Richard assured her.

'I'm afraid you don't have a choice,' the woman told him. 'When something like this happens to a child, we have to follow up. I'm sure you understand.'

Again there was no answer.

Chrissie turned round and walked back into the bedroom.

A long time later she heard them leaving, the sounds of the car engines starting, and driving away. She was sitting on the edge of the bed, tight with the misery of her confusion, trying desperately to hold on to what little courage she had left. She had to tell him she'd see any doctor he wanted, she'd even go to the hospital if that would make him feel better.

When he came to stand in the doorway she couldn't look up. She was too ashamed of the pain she was causing him, and the terrible harm she might have done Ryan.

'Look at me,' he said after a while.

She shook her head, so he came forward and knelt in front of her.

'Do you remember leaving her?' he said, taking her hands.

For a moment she looked at his pale, stricken face, then, unable to bear it, she lowered her eyes.

'Please don't be afraid,' he implored. 'No-one wants to hurt you, or lock you away. We just want to help you.'

A huge knot of emotion was trying to choke her. She opened her mouth and a terrible sob mangled the words as she said, 'I know.'

Taking her in his arms, he pulled her gently from the bed and sat her on the floor with him. 'I keep telling you we'll get through this,' he said gruffly, stroking her hair, 'but sometimes you frighten me so much that I start to despair.' Holding her face between his hands he looked searchingly into her eyes. 'Where are you?' he whispered. 'Where's the woman I love?'

'I'm here,' she sobbed. 'I'm still here.'

'Then don't leave me. We need you. Me and Ryan. We love you.'

'I'm sorry,' she choked, hardly able to speak.

He pulled her back against him and rested her head on his shoulder. For a long time he merely rocked her and stroked her and whispered an occasional word of comfort. Then finally he said, 'Do you remember now, where you went in the car the other day?'

Sniffing, and wiping her eyes with the back of her hand, she shook her head. 'I only remember you coming to get me,' she said, haltingly.

'But you don't know where you'd been?'

'No. I think . . . I was in Chiswick.'

'That's where you were when you called me,' he told her. 'You don't remember where you were before that?'

She considered telling him she'd just been driving around, but didn't, because he'd know it wasn't true, and it would only worry him more if he thought she was starting to lie. The problem was, she had no recollection of how she'd ended up in Chiswick, or of how long she'd been gone.

'Did you see, or speak to anyone?' he asked.

'I don't think so.' She wondered why he was so concerned, when his life would surely be so much easier if she were just to get in the car and disappear for ever. Perhaps that was secretly what he wanted, and he was trying to find out now how likely it was to happen. In fact, she was able to read his thoughts so clearly he could almost be speaking them aloud, as he willed her to take the car and crash it head-on into a motorway bridge. He wouldn't have to worry about her then. She'd be dead, and he would be free. He probably had no idea that she could see through what he was doing, how he was making her think she was mad, pushing her to a point where she'd take her own life, rather than have to do it himself. The show he put on of loving her and wanting only to help was all very convincing, but she knew that what he really wanted was to get rid of her for good. And he was clever enough to trick them all into believing his act, even her. Or so he thought

. . . But she wasn't quite so stupid. She knew what was going on here, but if she let on that she'd worked out his plan, she'd be putting herself in even graver danger than she already was. So for the time being she'd continue the charade of believing he loved her, until she managed to think of a way to get herself and Ryan to a place of absolute safety.

Chapter 15

Carla was at her computer discussing the latest rewrites for Zanzibar, while John stood over her, watching her type them in, and making it hard for her to ignore the male scent of him, not to mention the omnipotence of his stance that was only inches away from a full embrace. In the end, feeling much more unsettled than she'd like to admit, she hit the save button and rolled her chair back so that he was forced to stand upright.

'You're a genius,' he told her, referring to her last suggestion. 'And if you want to be the one to tell Yale Winfield he's lost another half-dozen lines, don't let me stand in your way.'

Grinning, she said, 'Speaking of denting egos, have you told Rosa her two-hander scene with Phoebe has gone yet?'

His dark eyes started to dance. 'Actually, I have,' he answered. 'And she took it quite well, considering.'

Carla was immediately suspicious. 'Considering what?' she challenged. 'No, don't tell me. She thinks I made the cut. John Rossmore, you told her . . .'

'No! I swear I told her it was me who cut it, but she won't believe me. She's convinced it was you, and that I'm just trying to cover. And then I thought if one of us has to be the villain, it might as well be you, since you seem to fit the role so much better than I do.'

'Tell me about it!' Hugo piped up, his wide, boyish eyes and apple-round cheeks oozing indignation. 'She's just refused me a two per cent increase in budget, *two per cent!*, and Frazer tells me we're having to fly *economy*. I tried to resign, but she won't let me do that either. The woman's not a villain, she's a tyrant!'

247

Carla turned to John. 'He's your assistant, teach him some respect. And while you're at it, educate him in the use of loudhailers and vocal enhancement, they're cheaper than all the walkie-talkies and mobile phones he's asking for. Now, where's Marjie? Felicia!' she shouted across the office. 'Have you appropriated my assistant again?'

'She's on the phone to Avril, in the kitchen,' Felicia shouted back. 'Have you spoken to the photographer from *Maxim* yet?'

'Yes,' Carla answered, reaching for the phone. '*There and Beyond*,' she sang into the receiver.

A woman's voice said, 'Can I speak to John Rossmore? It's Karen.'

Carla put her on hold, and to John, who was now back at his desk opposite, she said, 'Another lady for you, Mr Irresistible. This one's called Karen.'

'Oh! Great!' he said, obviously pleased. 'Which line?'

'Three.'

'Carla!' Marjie called from the kitchen door. 'Avril wants to speak to you.'

'Put her through here,' Carla shouted over an eruption of laughter at something Hugo had just said. 'And pipe down, you lot! I can't hear myself think.'

'What's all the noise?' Avril wanted to know, when Carla picked up the line.

'God knows,' Carla responded. 'It's a madhouse here. Now tell me, did you get the amended copy of the Zanzibar schedule I attached to an email?'

'Yeah. And I can still make it, no problem.'

Carla's heart flooded with relief, for she didn't even want to think about making the trip without Avril. 'That's great,' she said. 'John and the others are off on the recce next week, you should speak to him before he goes. I'll pass you over when we've finished.'

'Sure. So everything's working out with you two? No clash of the titans, or wars of the roses?'

'Not even a small scuffle at mill,' Carla answered. 'And if this is you looking for material . . .'

'A falling-out between you and John Rossmore is not something I'd want to go public with,' Avril interrupted. 'However, if you want to fake it . . .'

Carla said to John, 'Avril's asking if we want to fake it.'

He grimaced, as he considered. 'Hard to fake the real thing,' he responded earnestly.

Startled out of a pithy response, Carla almost blushed as she said to Avril, 'Did you hear that?'

Avril was laughing. 'I most certainly did,' she answered. 'But is he talking about what we're talking about?'

Changing the subject, Carla said, 'Have you seen the new advertising budget for the repeat transmissions?'

'Yes, but before we get into that, what's all this I hear about an intruder at the cottage?'

Carla immediately went cold. 'What do you mean?' she said, her heartbeat slowing. 'What intruder?'

'I just spoke to Sonya,' Avril replied. 'She said someone was seen . . .'

'Why hasn't she told me?' Carla cried, only then spotting the Post-it telling her to call Sonya. 'Who was it, does she know?'

'I don't think so. She only told me that . . .'

'I need to call her,' Carla said. 'I'll get back to you about the budget.'

Hitting the connectors she picked up another line and dialled Sonya's number.

'Are you OK?' John asked.

She nodded, then realizing this might be a call she didn't want overheard, she quickly rang off and ran upstairs to her studio. Minutes later she was speaking to Sonya.

'It's OK, calm down,' Sonya was saying. 'Nothing's been damaged, nothing's missing, we don't even know if Maudie really did see anyone. You know what she's like.'

Carla did, only too well, though it didn't relax her too much. 'So what happened?' she demanded. 'You said you pulled up outside . . .'

'I pulled up outside just as Graham was letting himself out of the front door. Apparently Maudie went straight to him when she saw someone, and he went to check it out. We went back in together, but like I said, no damage has been done, and nothing's missing. In fact, if you ask me, Maudie's just stirring up trouble.'

'Did you talk to her? Did she say who it might have been?'

'She wasn't there, but Graham talked to her, obviously.' There was a pause, then Sonya said, 'I know you're probably thinking of Richard, but apparently Maudie thought it was a woman.'

Carla's heart turned inside out. Surely to God it wasn't a ghost Maudie had seen. Oh please no. She'd never believed in them before, but maybe that was only because she'd never seen one. She'd certainly felt something though, on more than one occasion, and now this.

'You know, I wouldn't worry too much,' Sonya advised. 'Maudie's always seeing and hearing things, we all know that, probably because she gets bored sitting behind those net curtains all day long, so she likes to create a little action for herself.'

Carla really wanted to believe that, and with someone calling out for her downstairs, and Eddie scratching at the door to be let in, she decided she had to, at least for now. So, ending the call, she went back downstairs, Eddie at her heels, as she tried comforting herself with how sensitive dogs were supposed to be to the supernatural, so surely what she was sensing when at the cottage couldn't be a ghost, or Eddie would have responded. And whatever Maudie had seen was probably nothing more sinister than someone delivering fliers or selling insurance.

By six that evening, after another hectic day of meetings and schedules, Carla came out of the viewing room where she'd been watching some of the competition's videos to find Phoebe perched on the edge of Marjie's desk while speaking to someone on her mobile phone. Marjie herself was arranging for a car to come and pick the actress up.

Carla linked fingers with Phoebe as she passed, then sat down at her computer to start going over the figures Frazer had entered. It was dark outside, and Hugo was putting on his coat while chatting to Leo and Felicia, who were also showing signs of leaving. Behind her, Carla heard Phoebe say, 'Fantastic! I'll ask him.' Then to John she said, 'Hey, do you want to come over to Holme House? There's a surprise party for Wes Powell. Starts at seven.'

'Sure,' John replied. 'What's it in aid of?'

'His birthday. I'm speaking to Tilly.'

'Tell her hi, and yes, I'll definitely be there, though maybe not as early as seven.' He was looking at his watch. 'Hell, it's already after six. What time's your car coming?'

'It'll be outside in less than a minute,' Marjie answered, putting the phone down.

'This woman's a magician,' Phoebe declared.

'Not a magician, merely fortunate enough to call just as someone was getting dropped off a few doors down,' Marjie responded. 'In fact, I think I'll cadge a lift myself, if you're going past a tube station.'

'Name it, we'll pass it,' John told her, putting on his leather jacket and tucking a scarf into the collar.

'Don't anyone mind me!' Carla cried. 'I can hold the fort.'

'Then watch out for those Indians,' John told her.

She slanted him a look, while hoping that nothing in her expression showed how much she'd like to be invited to the surprise party too. But it must have, for John said, 'Why don't you come? You can be my date for the evening.'

Carla's heart jolted.

'Now there's an offer that's never been refused,' Phoebe declared, winding herself seductively around John, while smiling her beautiful smile at Carla.

A thousand jumbled thoughts were racing through Carla's mind, like, could she go dressed as she was? How long would it take to get changed? What was his motive for asking? Who was Karen, who'd called earlier? What about leaving Eddie alone? And what about Richard? But what about him, for God's sake? Theirs was only a pseudo-relationship, which, when stripped of its metaphysical posturing and soul-journey gloss, was nothing more than something Zen-like and karmic to hold on to because neither of them wanted to let go. Well, it was about time she did.

'I'm sorry,' she heard herself saying, 'I've got a lot of work to finish up here, and I'm meeting a friend for dinner, later.' Why had she said that? It was a lie, she had no friend to meet, and she'd really love to go. But he might have asked out of pity, thinking she was going to spend yet another evening alone, and she loathed the very idea of being seen as a charity case. Such pride, and there she was, still smiling away, as though her empty social life belonged to someone else entirely.

251

'Oh well,' John said, 'old Fraze is still here to keep you company, so's Jeffrey.'

'Already gone,' Jeffrey announced, hefting his briefcase onto his desk and starting to pack up.

'Got a yoga class at seven,' Frazer informed them. 'Then I'm on my third date with the gorgeous Clarissa.'

Minutes later, in an exodus that almost caused a draught, everyone was gone and Carla was alone with Eddie. 'Well,' she said, looking down at him, the commotion of the day still echoing in her ears, 'he could have tried to persuade me.'

Eddie cocked his head to one side.

'On the other hand,' she said, 'I've got scripts to write for Greece and India, and while it's quiet like this, it would be just the time to get started.'

Eddie's head went to the other side.

'But first, we'll take you for a walk. As it's the only social life we have, we definitely don't want to miss out on it, do we?' And then, she added defiantly to herself, she was going to email Richard and tell him straight out that she wanted to see him.

'Carla's on the phone,' Betty said.

Graham looked up from the newspaper he was reading. Betty was standing in the sitting-room doorway, her small, sturdy frame cast in shadows from the darkened hall behind her, her solemn face glowing softly in the reflected firelight. 'Oh, good,' he said, smiling.

Betty waited for him to lift the receiver on the small table beside him, then returned to the kitchen to replace the phone there.

'Carla!' Graham said, pleasure deepening his voice.

'How are you?'

'Excellent. Where are you?'

'In London, but I'll be down at the weekend.'

'Then we'll make a date for Saturday evening at the pub,' he declared. 'Unless you've got other plans.'

'No. Saturday's fine,' she said. 'Sonya told me about Maudie, thanks for going to check the house over.'

'Not at all. There was nothing amiss. Not that I expected there to be, but you know Maudie, she probably wouldn't

252

have let up until someone reacted.'

'So you don't think there was anything to it?' Carla said.

'There didn't appear to be, but it would take a braver man than I to accuse Maudie Taylor of seeing things.'

The irony was audible in Carla's voice as she said, 'So it's safe to come home?'

'Oh, I think so,' he chuckled. 'Would you like me to pick you up at the station?'

'Wonderful. I'll call before to let you know which train we'll be on.' For a moment it seemed as though she might say more, but then she merely wished him goodnight and rang off.

After replacing the receiver Graham ambled through to the kitchen where Betty was taking a goulash from the oven. Hearing him come in, she said, 'What time do you want to eat?'

'As soon as you're ready,' he answered. Then, rubbing a hand thoughtfully over his chin, he said, 'I wonder if I should go and talk to Maudie again?'

Betty looked surprised. 'Do you think you need to?' she asked.

'I don't know,' he answered, shaking his head. 'Maybe not. Nothing to worry about, I'm sure.'

'Then leave it,' Betty advised. 'Best forgotten.'

Chapter 16

She'd slept for so long that the seasons had changed. That was how it felt, though it was only the wintry darkness inside her that was succumbing to a shadowy and tentative spring. Outside the streets were grey with cold, the trees barren and rigid with a frost that melted late in the day, sometimes to return in the morning. The pills were working a little like that, slowly dissolving the paranoia, clearing her vision and even easing her gingerly out of the black depths of despair. She didn't always feel so afraid now, though she was often nervous and querulous, but that would pass, they told her, and the periods of light were already getting longer. Ryan's crying still made her anxious, though, on the whole, she was dealing with it better now. Just the occasional burst of alarm, or flutter of dismay, but Richard was always there, watching her, encouraging her, never failing in his love as she struggled back from the terrifying abyss that had the power to suck her in like a clam.

Soon she would begin her sessions with a therapist, but not just yet. The medication needed more time to work, and everyone was warning her not to rush. Now she had agreed to accept help, the process would be slow, they told her, but much more effective if she learned to trust those around her, and take each day at a time. And despite the moments of utter bleakness, and spells of lethargy, she'd managed a Christmas-shopping trip with Richard and Ryan just yesterday, and today she had unpacked some of the boxes upstairs.

Now, she was sitting on the sofa next to Richard, feeling slightly bewildered, and remote, as she listened to Rosa gossiping about *There and Beyond*, while Jilly cooed and fussed over Ryan, who was now dressed in the cute little dungarees Jilly had just given her.

For her part Rosa was uncomfortably aware of Richard's eyes watching her across the sitting room of this smart Knightsbridge house, where half of his and Chrissie's belongings were still in boxes, and most of the upstairs rooms were so neglected they could almost be derelict. The way he fixed a person with that ruthlessly silent scrutiny, as though assessing them with that oh, so superior brain, was enough to make anyone squirm. But not her, because she had nothing to squirm about. She was just being honest about the way things were at *There and Beyond*, now that Chrissie wasn't part of it any more.

'There's just not the same atmosphere,' she complained, keeping her eyes on Chrissie, as though Richard didn't exist. 'You know, they don't have the kind of fun you used to have, and Carla's so full of herself it makes you want to vomit.'

Jilly looked up in surprise, but said nothing as Rosa lifted her wine glass and took a sip.

'Would you like some more?' Chrissie offered, suddenly sitting forward.

Rosa arched her eyebrows. 'I've barely had three sips,' she responded.

Chrissie sat back again, and glanced at Richard, who smiled and stretched an arm along the sofa behind her. Considering how terrible Chrissie looked Rosa couldn't help thinking it a miracle that Richard was still with her at all, never mind sitting so close. Her skin was puffy and grey, her hair looked dead, and her sweatshirt and jeans were so shapeless and masculine they had to be Richard's. Of course they'd caught her on the hop, popping in unannounced like this, but it was the way Richard had wanted it, or so he'd told Jilly when he'd called. 'Just say you were in the area,' he'd instructed, 'then come in and have a drink.' Exactly what his motives were for doing things this way was anyone's guess, because it would take some kind of genius to figure out the workings of a mind like his, but Rosa was pretty convinced that it was in some way linked to her role on *There and Beyond*, and an attempt to get the low-down on what was going on with Carla.

So, ever a one to oblige, she carried on with, 'You should see her, strutting about that place in Belgravia like she's the one who can afford it, when everyone knows Avril Hayden is funding it ... Honestly, she gets right up everyone's nose with her airs and graces, though obviously, with her being the exec. producer we all have to kowtow and pretend to like her. Except, you know me, I'm not afraid to let her know just what I think. And it bugs her like crazy that I won't suck up to her the way everyone else does. But I ask you, why should I, when we all know from past record that there's no way she'd have given me that part if it weren't for the fact that John Rossmore put his foot down and said she had to.'

Chrissie's smile was bland, as her eyelids blinked up and down.

Richard's expression remained as inscrutable as ever.

Chrissie said, 'How are you getting on with John Rossmore?'

'Oh, he's amazing!' Rosa enthused. 'You know, really easy-going, great sense of humour, really into the actors, which isn't surprising when he's one himself. That's what made you such a great director, when you were doing it, or so everyone said. Of course, if Carla hadn't blacklisted me, I'd have had first-hand experience of your talents, wouldn't I? You know, I'm so glad you told me about that, because I always wondered why you never gave me a part. I used to get really upset about it, didn't I, Jilly? Especially when there's not very much to the sketches. It just didn't seem right, not giving a part to your friend. Anyway, like I said, John Rossmore overruled her, so it doesn't look as though she's going to get all her own way this time around.'

'She never used to with me,' Chrissie said. 'Not on everything.'

'Maybe not, but you still know how overbearing and pigheaded she can be when she wants. Though, credit where it's due, she's really getting out there and selling the programme, and she seems to work all the hours God sends. If you ask me, that programme's the only life she has.'

Chrissie swallowed, and her head turned briefly towards Richard, before, steeling herself, she said, 'So she hasn't met anyone else yet?'

256

Rosa laughed nastily. 'Only Eddie, her bloody dog. She never goes anywhere without the damned thing, and we're all expected to make a fuss of him, and throw his flaming ball, and think he's as irresistible as she does. I'd like to hear what she had to say if one of us wanted to bring a dog to the office, and she was expected to drool all over it. I bet it'd be a different story then.'

'Eddie was her mum's dog,' Chrissie said, her eyes seeming very big.

Rosa shrugged. 'Well it's obviously hers now. She even sleeps with the bloody thing.'

Jilly's head came up. 'How do you know that?' she demanded.

'Everyone does.'

Jilly looked sceptical. 'And how do you know she doesn't have a boyfriend?' she asked.

Rosa rolled her eyes. 'Believe me, she doesn't. Unless you count John Rossmore, which she'd definitely like to. Boy, has she got the hots for him. The poor guy. Everyone can see how embarrassed he is by it, but he has to play along, you know, flirt with her and stuff, because it's what he does with everyone else, and she's the producer, so he can't afford to upset her, can he?'

'I thought he had a reputation for being difficult and egocentric,' Chrissie said, darting a look towards Ryan as Jilly made her squeal with laughter. 'You're making him sound as though he's just the opposite.'

Rosa shrugged. 'He is. At least, so far. But we've still got a way to go, you know, with the filming and everything ... We're going to Zanzibar, did I tell you that?'

Chrissie's eyes widened, then her mouth gave a slight tremble as she said, 'No, you didn't mention it. When are you going?'

'January.'

Chrissie leaned closer to Richard, who covered one of her hands with his own, and squeezed it. Rosa glanced at Jilly, who was still engrossed in the baby, so probably wasn't noticing all the weird body language taking place on the sofa. Pity, because Rosa wanted to get her take on it after they'd left.

'Did I tell you,' Chrissie was saying to Richard, 'that the

man with the grey hair's back? I saw him yesterday and today, walking past with his eye on your car. He loves it so much I think we should ask him if he wants to buy it.'

Richard smiled. 'I saw him earlier,' he said. 'He was telling me about his trip to North Wales.'

'You spoke to him?' Chrissie said, surprised.

'Not for long.'

Chrissie turned back to Rosa. 'There's a man we see outside sometimes,' she said, 'we think he might be a reporter.'

Richard's eyes were back on Rosa, and she felt the tingling heat of indignation burn right into her cheeks. 'You know, I'd almost forgotten that spread in one of the Sundays,' she declared stiffly. 'Makes you sick, all that stuff they print that's none of their damned business, especially when they got into those really sensitive parts of your past . . . Of course they made half of it up, we all know that, but those things Carla said about you . . . Well, all I can say is, if we didn't know she was a bitch before, we certainly do now.'

Richard's lazily raised eyebrow made her want to shout in his face. Just what was his problem, sitting there staring at her like that? But of course she didn't ask, possibly out of fear of him telling her.

Jilly was getting to her feet. 'Got to go to the loo,' she said, passing the baby to Richard.

As Ryan settled down with her daddy Rosa made a mental note to go to the bathroom too, if only to get a better look round, though she was already pretty certain that the big cream leather furniture and Oriental rugs and cushions in this room, and the futuristic design of the kitchen, was about as far as they'd gone towards making this dream house a home. 'She really is lovely,' she said, smiling at the baby, and hoping her words might do something to soften Richard's attitude towards her. 'How old is she now?'

'Almost eight months,' Chrissie answered, as Richard's arm drew her into a picture of perfect family bliss, with Mum and Dad gazing adoringly at their perfect creation.

Rosa twitched with impatience. If it was all so damned perfect, then why did Chrissie look like hell?

'Her bottom teeth are almost through,' Chrissie said to Richard.

Smiling, he said, 'Why don't you hold her?'

Chrissie took the baby awkwardly in her arms, then almost shoved her back as Ryan gave an ear-piercing screech.

Rosa's curiosity mounted, for she hadn't missed that split second of panic which suggested that despite their efforts to cover it, Chrissie was in as bad a state as the last time they'd seen her, she could even be worse.

'Would you like anything to eat?' Chrissie offered.

'Oh, no, thanks,' Rosa answered. 'Jilly and I are going on for dinner after. There's a new restaurant, just opened, on Kensington High Street. Everyone's going there, so we thought we'd try it.' She looked at Richard, and gave a quick, reflexive smile, which elicited no change in his own expression. 'Do you manage to get out much?' she asked, certain the answer had to be no.

'Richard does more than me,' Chrissie answered. 'His research takes him all over the place, though thankfully not out of London any more.'

'So how's the book going?' Rosa asked him.

'I'm still roughing out a first draft,' he answered. 'And it's proving more challenging than I expected, but there are a lot of foreign correspondents and film crews based in London who I can use to double-check dates and detail.'

Surprised, and encouraged by the lengthy reply, Rosa said, 'Have you limited yourself to a certain number of crises to write about, or are you approaching it as an autobiography, you know, from the cradle to the campfire where you sit down and look back over the whole of your life?'

He seemed amused by the question, which annoyed her, when she'd considered it to be a good one. 'Actually, I'm focusing on three crises in the Nineties,' he answered. 'The Gulf, Kosovo and East Timor.'

'Fascinating,' Rosa responded, knowing already that she wouldn't be buying, and by the look on his face he knew it too, and cared not a jot. Again she felt irritated, and couldn't work out for the life of her why women like Chrissie and Carla seemed to find him so compelling, when all she found him was arrogant, aloof and downright condescending. He wasn't even sexy if you asked her, though it seemed she was in the minority, because, if the gossip she'd been hearing

259

lately was true, he was not only supposed to be screwing some female producer over at the Beeb, but, according to a freelance cameraman she knew, he'd recently restarted an affair with the same air stewardess he'd been seeing while he was living with Carla. Fleetingly Rosa wondered if Carla knew about that now, or even if Chrissie did, since he must have been sleeping with Chrissie as well at the time, so it could be said that he'd been cheating on Chrissie too. However, if you were the air stewardess you might view it that he'd been cheating on you. Whatever, Rosa would lay money on every word of it being true, and she happened to know that Jilly thought so too.

As Jilly came back into the room, Rosa decided to let her take over for a while, and merely listened and watched as Jilly declared, 'I must say, you're not like most other couples with their first child, who just can't stop talking about them.'

Richard seemed amused. 'Believe me, we can talk about Ryan all day, if that's what you want.'

'Certainly Richard can,' Chrissie said teasingly. 'He's totally besotted, in case you hadn't noticed. And it's mutual, because Ryan's so mad about her dad that her mum hardly gets a look-in.'

Jilly continued to smile, so did Rosa, while Richard and Chrissie made silly clucking noises at Ryan, who produced adorable gurgling noises back, while waving her chubby little arms and legs.

At last, after a further half-hour of excruciating pauses and ludicrous politeness, Chrissie closed the front door behind Jilly and Rosa and went back into the sitting room to find Richard lying on the sofa with Ryan hoisted in the air above him. She watched them for a moment, then, going to sit in the chair Jilly had vacated, she said, 'Was I OK?'

Richard lowered Ryan on to his shoulder, then holding out an arm to Chrissie he waited until she was sitting on the floor beside him before he said, 'You were more than OK. They're a couple of old witches, at least Rosa is, and you handled it beautifully.'

Chrissie's blue eyes softened with pleasure. 'It was a bit of a shock finding them on the doorstep like that,' she confessed.

'I almost shut the door on them. In fact, if you hadn't been here, I probably would have.'

Richard said, 'Did you know Rosa was working for Carla?'

Chrissie shook her head. 'If I had, I would definitely have shut the door,' she responded. 'What about you? Did you know?'

'No. But I think we did her a favour, because she was obviously bursting to sound off to someone.'

Chrissie smiled, and waited for the sound of a passing motorbike to fade before slotting a finger into Ryan's fist and saying, 'I've got a confession to make. It wasn't Carla who always blocked Rosa's casting, it was me.'

His eyebrows went up. 'Sounds like a wise decision,' he remarked. 'So how come she thinks it was Carla?'

Chrissie grimaced. 'Because I told her it was. I know that's terrible,' she rushed on, 'but I've known her for years, we're supposed to be good friends, and Carla only met her when we started the programme. And believe me, I would have happily given her a part if I hadn't known what a menace she can be . . .'

His finger on her lips stopped her as, laughing, he said, 'It's OK, I get the merits of the decision. I'd probably have done the same myself. But there's something else that occurs to me here – do you think she could have been behind the newspaper story?'

Chrissie looked at him. 'What makes you think that?' she asked cautiously.

'Well, for one thing, her tone was much too defensive when she talked about it, as though she was trying to justify herself, and if she's got a grudge against Carla, which she obviously has if she thinks Carla's had it in for her all this time . . .'

Chrissie's colour was deepening. 'As a matter of fact I do think it was her,' she admitted. 'I did almost as soon as we saw it. Which means that it was my fault that Carla had all those horrible things said about her . . .'

He smiled and stroked her cheek with his fingers. 'She'll survive,' he said gently.

Her eyes dropped, then, turning her face into his hand, she kissed it, while still circling her fingers round Ryan's. 'Did you mind hearing all that about her?' she said. 'I mean, what

Rosa said about John Rossmore. Does it bother you that Carla seems to like him?'

He gave a laugh of surprise. 'Darling, it's been more than eighteen months since I left Carla to be with you, so I'd be more upset if Carla hadn't met someone else by now, than I am to find out that she might have.'

Chrissie's eyes dulled. 'So you do still care about her?' she said.

'You know I do, but that doesn't mean that I've ever regretted my decision to leave her and marry you. I know you find it hard to believe, but I love you, Chrissie. You're the only woman I've ever wanted to marry, and you're the only woman I will ever marry. It's true, I could wish that you hadn't found it all so hard to cope with, but it doesn't make me love you any the less. If anything it makes me love you more, because you need me and because I know deep down that you love me too.'

Her eyes were shining with emotion. 'I do,' she whispered. 'And Ryan. I love you both.' Then she laughed, for it seemed incredible that little more than a week ago she'd actually thought he was plotting to kill her.

'So how about that dinner you promised to cook tonight,' he said, 'while I go upstairs and bath Ryan?'

It wasn't a difficult meal to prepare, just some fresh pasta to put into a saucepan and a ready-made sauce from M&S to heat in the oven. She even lit some candles, and found some pretty mats and napkins to liven up the table. When everything was ready she was about to go upstairs to see what progress was being made there, when a terrible, debilitating sadness washed over her and tears began streaming down her cheeks.

'Oh God, it's awful, just so awful,' she sobbed, and, slumping into a chair, she buried her face in her arms and wept as though her heart would break.

'Darling, what on earth's the matter?' Richard cried, coming into the kitchen some ten minutes later. Lifting her up from the table, he cupped her face in his hands and searched her watery, red-rimmed eyes with his own. 'What is it?' he said, his voice gruff with concern.

It was a moment before she could catch her breath, and

even then the words were fragmented as she finally forced herself to say, 'I was ... just thinking ... about Eddie, Valerie's and Carla's dog.'

Laughing, he held her tighter, and said, 'And there was me thinking that hell was other people, not their dogs.'

After a moment she drew back, and looked uncertainly into his face. 'Was it . . .' She sobbed. 'Was it Jean-Paul Sartre who said that?' she asked tentatively. 'That hell is other people?'

Laughing and hugging her again, he said, 'Yes, my darling. Yes it was.'

Carla was humming tunefully to herself as she stepped out of the bath and reached for a towel. It seemed absurd to have been so nervous about coming back here to the cottage, for nothing was in the least bit scary about the place, it was the same old home she'd always known, and even the creepy sensation of being watched had obviously just been a figment of her overactive imagination, for she certainly didn't feel it now. Which was why she'd been careful to avoid Maudie all weekend, not wanting to get her started with her spooky stories again, especially now she had more important matters on her mind.

It was incredible, and exhilarating, how this strange allure she and Richard shared seemed to continue working its magic even when she'd stopped believing in its existence. Though in truth she never really stopped believing, it was just that sometimes she was so busy it slipped from focus.

However, now, with the recce crew in Zanzibar, she had more time on her hands, and the response she had received when she'd told him she wanted to see him was causing all kinds of chaos inside her, for he'd told her to name the time and the place. She hadn't answered yet, but knew she would sometime today.

In fact, she didn't go online again until she returned to London, when she checked the email on her laptop to find yet another message waiting from Richard. 'The space inside me for words is taken up with emotion,' he'd written, 'leaving me bereft of expression, and abundant with feeling. I need to share all this with you, but you're denying me, and I love you for it, because your resistance is sharpening my desire, and plunging me into oceans of longing that I could never hope to fathom without knowing you will be there in the end. Keep me in suspense, punish me as I deserve, but know that you are mine, as I am yours, and nothing, not even you, will be able to keep us apart for very much longer.'

She answered right away with an equally impassioned speech, designed to excite and torment him in ways that were cruelly erotic and almost angrily dismissive. Then she clicked over to her other email address to find a message from John. They'd been in regular touch since he'd left, though today's report didn't only convey details of some impressive early successes, but a closing comment that made her heart jump.

'. . . so, thanks to Jaffah, our local chap, the availability of historical locations is really opening up, and things are progressing so well at the moment that the only thing missing is you.'

Annoyingly, for the rest of the evening and most of the next day that remark kept returning to the front of her mind, until, in the end, it started to make her angry.

'And you don't know why?' Avril laughed, when she rang to vent her wrath, or maybe seek help, she wasn't entirely sure. 'Come on, you know exactly what's making you like this, you just don't want to face it, is all.'

Carla's lips were pale and tight. 'You always think you're so clever,' she snapped, 'but believe me, if I knew why I was feeling this way . . .'

'OK, stop!' Avril interrupted. 'You're in some kind of denial over there, and it's not only getting on your nerves, which is why you're in this state, it's starting to get on mine too. So let's haul a few facts out into the open, shall we? First, you fancy the pants off John Rossmore, but you're afraid to admit it. And why would that be? Because it feels disloyal to Richard. So let me tell you this, the hell with any loyalty to Richard, because that man's playing some kind of sick game with your head, and you know it.'

Carla was too furious to speak.

Leaping straight back in, Avril said, 'There's no reality here, Carla. No *physical* affirmation of his feelings, or his commitment, or even his intentions. And every time you bring it up he either manages to avoid the issue, or waft off into some weirdly esoteric fantasy . . .'

'I think we should end this call right now,' Carla said through her teeth. 'I always knew you didn't really understand, but I never expected you to throw it in my face like this, or use it to ridicule me.'

'For God's sake, Carla, if I was doing what you're doing, what would you say to me? You'd tell me to get my ass in gear and get on with my life. You wouldn't just sit there and let me carry on fooling myself that there's a future at the end of the yellow brick road. You'd have me back on the straight and narrow by now, which is what I'm trying to do with you – and not before time, because I should have got on your case months ago about this. It's all bullshit, Carla. Complete and utter bullshit, unless he does something to prove he really does intend to find a solution to the unholy mess he's created, which might not be a mess at all the way he's seeing it, because he's getting some kind of mind-fuck with you, at the same time as he gets the physical fuck with Chrissie, and what do you do but try to be as understanding and accommodating as you can to his poor, tortured soul, that's as capable of making mistakes as the rest of us, but apparently more deserving of forgiveness.'

'I can't believe you're sounding off like this,' Carla raged. 'In fact, it seems to me that you've got more of an issue with this relationship than I have.'

'Oh, stick around, honey, I've only just got started.'

'Well I don't want to hear it. We all know you've got little or no respect for men, so . . .'

'It's got sod-all to do with how I feel about men,' Avril butted in. 'It's how concerned I am about you. So now, let's calm this down, shall we, and take a look at it once the hot air has cleared.'

Carla was still too worked up to agree, but she didn't disagree either, merely sat tightly in her chair, trapped by a punishing need to hear more, even though she was hating every word.

'OK,' Avril said, 'let's start by asking a few questions, shall we? Have you ever asked yourself why he never calls you on the phone?'

'I know why, it would be too painful, too . . .'

'Why? He's asked to see you now, hasn't he? Isn't that going to be more painful than just hearing you?'

'I don't know what you're getting at.'

'Nor do I, but there's something odd in there, wouldn't you say? Something that's not quite adding up. And tell me this, has he ever mentioned anything about you becoming godmother to his daughter again, since that first time?'

Surprised by the question, Carla said, 'No.'

'Did he ever tell you whether he has the rest of the letter your mother wrote?'

'No.'

'But you did ask him?'

Carla's head was starting to throb. 'Yes.'

'What about him coming to the cottage? When Graham's wife saw him. Did he ever confirm whether or not it was him?'

'No.'

'You do see where I'm going with this, don't you? You never seriously challenge him. You get no answers, or explanations, so you make up excuses for him, and carry on in your peculiar state of delusion, which you call spiritual understanding. Now, what about actually seeing him?'

'What about it?'

'Well, you haven't answered him yet, so is this really a case of *you* playing fast and loose with *him*?'

Surprised Avril would think that, Carla gave the question some thought. 'I want to see him,' she said in the end. 'I don't know if it's wise, but yes, it's what I want.'

'OK. So do as he says, name the time and the place and go. But think about this before you do: what are you expecting to come from it?'

Carla's eyes closed as her heart plunged into free fall.

'He's a married man . . .' Avril began.

The words were out before Carla could stop them. 'There's such a thing as divorce.'

'But he's not getting divorced, is he?'

'You don't know that.'

'Has he said so? In any of his emails, has he ever said anything about divorce, or Chrissie, or his daughter? He

266

hardly ever mentions them, except to use them as an excuse for not seeing you. But they're there, and guess what, they ain't just going away. So, let's go back to him seeing you. What happens after you re-establish your relationship? *You'll* be his mistress then, instead of Chrissie. You won't come first, and you'll hate it. Unless, of course, he gets you to read Rousseau's *Émile,* as a way of persuading you that you can all live happily together under the same roof.'

'If you're going to be sarcastic . . .'

'You think it's sarcasm? Then let me tell you, from where I'm standing there seems no end to that man's power over you, which, by the way, is more bullshit, because he's only got power as long as you allow him to have power, but we'll get into that another time. For now, let's say, for argument's sake, that he decides to leave Chrissie for you. What then?'

'What do you mean?'

'Well, he's still going to be the man who cheated on you for God knows how long with your best friend; who told so many lies we'll probably never know even the half of them; who didn't have the guts to tell you himself it was over; who was too spineless to give you any answers when you desperately needed them; who's now, for all we know, considering dumping the mother of his child and maybe the child too . . .'

'All right, all right,' Carla said. 'I get the point.'

'Do you? Are you really in tune with how many issues you two have to resolve, and how unresolvable they actually are? Personally, I think you are, but you don't want to face them, which is why you're having such a hard time at the moment. You're trying to get your head round the idea of finally cutting loose, and accepting that he's no longer in your life. And shall I tell you something, if you don't do it, he will.'

Carla's heart turned over again. 'Why do you say that?' she asked.

'Because, in my opinion, in his own weird way, he's having as tough a time letting go as you are, but in your hearts, or your joined-up spirits, or whatever arcane means of bonding you have, you both know you don't really have any choice.'

Several seconds ticked by before Carla, with some irony, said, 'Well, I don't feel angry any more.'

267

Avril laughed. 'I'm almost afraid to ask how you do feel.'

'I might need some time to work that out.'

Avril's tone softened considerably then, as she said, 'Don't think I don't understand. It takes a long time coming to terms with the shock of finding out someone's betrayed you, especially the way he did it. Maybe worse is having to face the fact that all the dreams you've had just aren't going to come true. Shall I tell you something? More often than not it's the dreams we can't let go of, not the person. So maybe it's a good idea to see him, talk to him, and then you might very well come to realize that your dreams are already changing in ways that actually don't include him any more.'

Though Carla wasn't convinced, she didn't take issue, because, in her heart, this encouragement to see Richard was what she wanted. So all she said was, 'You never told me you'd been in love.'

Avril laughed. 'I haven't,' she said. 'But I've seen enough people go through what you're going through now to give me some understanding of the utter turmoil it puts you in, and how afraid you are of taking the new paths life is opening up for you. So,' she continued, 'are you ready to name the day?'

Carla looked around the lamplit room, at all the furniture and books that had once been theirs and now were hers. She thought of the empty office downstairs; of John and the crew in Zanzibar, and her here alone; of the last line of John's fax, and the Karen who called him more regularly than the others; of the weekend looming ahead that offered only the cold, empty cottage in Cannock Martin, and the occasional drink at the pub before going home, alone. Then there was Christmas and New Year on the horizon, the second that Richard would spend with Chrissie instead of her . . . There was so much to think about, so many pictures of togetherness for others, and hours of working to escape the loneliness for her.

So her answer to Avril was, 'I'll let you know when it's going to happen,' and after they ended their call, she opened her laptop and began composing an email. 'Though it hasn't always been easy deciphering your messages, and intuiting your meanings,' she wrote, 'I now understand how you've been using your knowledge of my psyche in subtly Machiavellian ways, sometimes resisting or frustrating me, often imploring or tempting me, but always guiding me gently and patiently towards the point where I am absolutely certain that I'm ready to take the next step in our journey. I'm at that point now, so I shall be at the Bluebird Café on Thursday at four.' And when she finally clicked on the box that sent the email she was amazed to discover just how right it felt.

At her end, Avril sat staring at the phone for some time after their call was over, wondering if she hadn't just made the most colossal error of judgement in what was needed to wrest Carla from her delusional state. But, for God's sake, something had to happen to start her emotional life moving forward again, and if getting some closure with Richard wasn't it, then she truly didn't know what was.

'You didn't mention you were going out today,' Chrissie said.

'Just over to the Groucho Club,' Richard answered, putting a scarf on over his raincoat. 'Ginger Buckley's back from Sierra Leone – he was with me in the Gulf, so he's got a starring role in that section of the book.'

'How long will you be gone?'

'A couple of hours, probably. If it looks like being any longer, I'll call.'

She gazed up into his eyes, and smiled with confidence, for she knew that her own were losing their dark shadows, even becoming blue again, and less tired. Her skin looked better too, and her hair was slowly regaining its curl as well as its shine. 'Would you like to invite him back for dinner?' she suggested. 'I can get Elinor to come to the supermarket with me. Or I might try going out alone.'

Laughing at the mischievous twinkle in her eyes, he pulled her into an embrace and said, 'If you're feeling up to it, then certainly I'll ask him. Just think it over for a while, then call me on the mobile to let me know what you decide.'

After he'd gone Chrissie remained standing in the hall, his kiss still warm on her lips, and the pleasure she felt at these few small steps of recovery glowing in her heart. This wasn't the first time he'd gone out without her feeling panicked about where he was going, or who he might be seeing, but each untroubled departure was proving a small triumph in itself. Since Rosa and Jilly had visited almost two weeks ago, there had been nothing but progress – so much so that Richard's mood over the weekend had been buoyant to the point of reckless, when he'd swept her off her feet in the middle of the park to swing her round and round in utter joy that she'd just completed her first session of therapy. Her second appointment was booked for tomorrow, and he was coming with her. After that they'd decide as each session came up whether or not it was necessary for him to attend too.

Wondering how she could ever have doubted his love, she took herself off to the kitchen to search out a recipe that would test her limited culinary skills to an extent that wouldn't embarrass them both. Then, after jotting down a list of ingredients she would need, she spent a moment trying to decide whether to go to Waitrose alone, or take Elinor and Ryan with her. First, though, she should call Richard to let him know that dinner, with a guest, was on.

'You're incredible,' he told her softly when she gave him the news.

'Will you bring some wine, or do you want me to get it?' she asked.

'There's still some Puligny in the cellar. Let's have that.'

'Good idea. But I've just had a thought. Do you know if Ginger's vegetarian?'

'He wasn't the last time I saw him, but I'll check when I get there and call you back.'

She sat down at the kitchen table to wait, and continued flicking through her recipe books, looking out for meatless dishes that sounded appetizing and cookable, just in case.

Half an hour later the phone rang. 'Darling, it's me. I'm with Ginger now, but I'm afraid he's not free tonight.'

Chrissie's spirits plunged. She'd really been looking forward to attempting this hurdle, and now it had been removed the race didn't seem worthwhile any more. 'Oh,' was all she said.

'But I am,' he told her, 'and I'm not vegetarian.'

It wasn't the same, and her disappointment was still crushing.

'Chrissie?'

She didn't answer.

'Chrissie, we can always invite someone else. It doesn't have to be Ginger.'

'I never meet any of your colleagues,' she said.

'We can invite him another night.' She heard a muffled voice at his end, then coming back on the line he said, 'Ginger says that if you're that keen to meet him he'll cancel his arrangements and come. And he's not a vegetarian.'

'Tell him I love him already,' she laughed, and, ringing off, she skipped up the stairs to help Elinor get Ryan ready to go out. She was feeling so exuberant, and proud of herself for wanting to entertain this much, that for one delirious moment she considered calling Carla to ask her to make up the four. What a shock that would be for Richard, but of course she'd never do it, it was just this madcap idea she had that one day they could all be friends again.

The hum and bleat of Christmas carols drifted out of the café and market, seeming somehow to warm the chill, late after-noon air, as Carla walked slowly through the arrangements of holly, mistletoe, elaborate wreaths and twinkling lights that were laid out on the Bluebird forecourt. The traffic on the King's Road roared past, while the delicious smell of roasting chestnuts evoked memories of when she and Richard had come here together, to shop in the exotic market that was a part of this old garage complex that had been converted into a nursery, food store, cafe and restaurant, all to serve the refined tastes of London's elite. Here they'd purchased foods from all over the world, which they'd experimented with at home, after drinking tea or something stronger at the café.

She'd chosen the venue because it was where he'd first asked her to move in with him. She knew he'd remember that, though he hadn't mentioned it in the email that had come back within hours of hers being sent, telling her how relieved and happy he was to know that she was finally ready to take this next step.

'I was going to ask if you're sure,' he'd written, 'but I know you are, and I'm so glad that you understand the worthier machinations of Machiavelli's mind-play. Do you understand how, in your own way, you do it to me too? The Bluebird Café

271

at four on Thursday. We have so much to discuss and I have more forgiveness to ask than one man could ever deserve. *Mais, on n'a rien pour rien.'* Nothing is had for nothing.

She didn't know who'd said that, nor was she entirely sure of its meaning in this context, though she suspected it was his way of saying that unless he asked her forgiveness he could never hope to attain it. Would she give it? Maybe she already had, though she knew very well that the wound still burning inside her, dimmed by nerves at present, was apt to flare into anger at any moment, and was likely to make this meeting even harder than she already feared it would be.

After she was shown to a corner table in the café, where a dozen or so Christmas shoppers had come in from the cold to sip hot chocolate and indulge themselves in cake, she ordered a cappuccino and stared out at the dismal, darkening afternoon. When he arrived, she would see him before he saw her. The mere thought of it twisted the knots in her stomach. This was how she had been since she'd got his email, unable to eat, or concentrate, or even sleep very much. She was glad John was away, he was too much of a distraction while she had this on her mind.

A waitress brought her coffee, asked if she wanted anything else, then went away.

Carla stirred the chocolate into the foam, and looked out to where a young couple in long black overcoats and light-coloured scarves were pondering over which Christmas tree to buy. This was where she and Richard had bought the exquisite blue pine for their first Christmas together. They'd decorated it entirely in silver. She felt suddenly strange as a horrible scenario came into her head, of him insisting on buying a tree today, for him and Chrissie and their baby, and asking her to help him choose it.

Looking around the brightly lit room she wondered what on earth she was doing here. Her nerves were so stretched now that her feelings were far closer to fear, as she began desperately to wish she hadn't come. Avril was right, there would be no going back after this, and she had no idea of the way forward. All she could see, as she sat here waiting, was more disruption at a time when it could do most damage, more heartache when she was finally starting to get over the last, and the total betrayal of her colleagues for even attempting this emotional minefield when they'd made their commitment to a programme that was hers. She pressed her fingers to her lips as the horrible nightmare of how she had suffered before swept through her with a frightening clarity, reminding her of just how devastated, and even deranged, she had been. She couldn't take that chance again. Not right now. It wasn't that she didn't want to see him, or even that she expected it to be that bad again, it was simply that the risk was still too great, when her responsibilities were so pressing. It was already four fifteen and the fear that he was going to stand her up was pulsing so hard through her head that she had to get out now, before the rejection became real and prevented her being able to tell herself later that there was a chance she'd let him down instead of the other way round.

By the time her taxi pulled up outside the *ménage* she'd drawn breath a hundred times to tell the driver to turn round and take her back. But she was here now, paying the fare, and bracing herself to face whoever was inside.

Mercifully no-one seemed to notice anything odd about her, and why would they when she looked exactly the same as when she'd left? Taking off her coat, greeting Eddie and turning on her computer was about as normal as her work day got. She went straight online, expecting to find an email explaining why he hadn't made it, but there were no new messages waiting. Quickly she typed in her own message, apologizing for not waiting – she had to do that in case he had turned up, and the waitress accurately described her – but she'd just rushed over there to tell him that something urgent had come up, which meant she had to go and join the crew on the recce. One of the best things about the email, no-one ever knew where you were!

His reply came the following morning, by which time she'd spent a near sleepless night trying to decide whether she was an appalling coward for running off like that, or one of the planet's most professional women for putting her pro-gramme first. She guessed it hardly mattered now it was done. However, when she read that he'd arrived at four twenty, after getting snarled up in traffic and calling the café to let her know he'd be late, only to find she hadn't waited, she not only felt calmer, she also, surprisingly, felt she had been right to leave.

Of course, she was annoyed with the waitress for not passing the message on, but this morning the relief she felt at having no catastrophe to deal with was so overwhelming, it made a mockery of her belief that she was ready to see him. So in answer to his request that she set another time and date as soon as she returned from the recce, she rather cruelly said.

'It seems destiny was not with us yesterday, though I still feel as secure in the mystery of its plan as I do in your love. Of course we shall meet, we both know that, it's what we want, so if need be we shall coerce the fates into making it happen. Nothing can stop me wishing you were with me now, and the stronger I wish it the more I feel it. I hope you're feeling it too, and will still be as eager to see me when I return as I know I will be to see you.'

Yes, that was definitely one of the better aspects of the email – that no-one ever knew exactly where you were.

Chapter 17

With the crew's return from Zanzibar everything shifted into a much higher gear, as preparations for the January departure had to be finalized before the Christmas break. Two more researchers were brought on board to help with the setting up of the rest of the series, while Carla concentrated on roughing out the scripts, furthering deals with various travel companies and apportioning the budgets accordingly. She was also becoming heavily involved in a search for the right web-site designers in order to take the company online, and was booked to attend an e-commerce conference in Geneva, with Avril, immediately after the New Year holiday. This meant that she and Avril would arrive in Zanzibar a couple of days after the crew, but Avril was insistent that Carla had to be at that conference, since the future of interactive TV was on the agenda, and Avril didn't want Carla to be running down the track, attempting to leap on board, after the train had left the station.

Being so excited about all the opportunities the Internet was opening up, and what it could mean, not only for *There and Beyond*, but for all the spin-off programmes and back-up businesses she had in mind, Carla had no problem agreeing to go. John was right into the new technology too, so much so that, as often as he could, he was coming with her to talk to the computer geniuses who were showing them such means and methods of marketing and communication that they'd never even dreamed of until now. In fact, it so fired up their enthusiasm that they both found it hard settling themselves back into the old-fashioned way when they returned to the office.

However, the stress and challenge of arranging every last detail of the schedule, and dealing with the infinite number of problems that went hand in hand with a foreign shoot, carried them so fast towards Christmas that before Carla knew it they were only five days away, and she hadn't even thought about shopping. Nor had she given much thought to her birthday, which had come galloping up at its own breakneck speed, with only Richard remembering, making her feel pleased, and sad, and slightly wistful, as she read his email and thought of the birthdays they had spent together in the past.

The fact that no-one in the office knew wasn't a problem, until the end of the day rolled around, and everyone started to leave. Then, faced with the prospect of spending the evening alone, she started to regret not speaking up, for she was certain someone would stay for a drink, or even suggest they go out somewhere, if they knew. But how could she tell them now, when she'd left it so late. She'd make them all feel dreadful for not having realized sooner – and besides, she didn't want anyone to know that she had nothing to do on her birthday. Which wasn't strictly true, anyway, because she was celebrating with Mark and Sonya at the weekend, then Avril was flying in on Monday, which was Christmas Eve, so there was no reason to feel entirely bereft.

However, as the door began opening and closing with increasing regularity, swallowing everyone into the dark winter's night, she could feel herself sinking deeper and deeper into such a childish glut of self-pity that she was finding it hard to keep smiling as she repeatedly called goodnight.

'You taking Eddie for a walk?' John asked, still looking at his computer screen, though starting to turn towards her.

Surprised, Carla said, 'Yes, in a minute. Why?'

'Thought I might come with you,' he answered. 'I don't have to be anywhere until eight, and a few things came up while I was over in Zanzibar that I want to run past you.'

'Sounds intriguing,' she said, her eyes playfully narrowing. Then, suddenly afraid it might have something to do with Richard and Chrissie's trip there, she looked quickly away.

When they left, a few minutes later, Hugo, Verna and

Felicia were the only ones remaining in the office, and Felicia was already putting on her coat. Guessing they'd all be gone by the time she got back Carla called goodnight, then, tucking her scarf warmly around her chin, she clipped Eddie onto his lead and followed John, in his thickly padded climber's coat and preposterous blue bobble hat, out into the cold.

'I've got to tell you,' she said, falling into step beside him, 'that only you could get away with wearing a hat like that. The rest of us would look utterly ridiculous.'

'And I don't?' he said in surprise.

'Actually, yes. So perhaps what I really mean is that only you would have the nerve.'

Grinning, and still managing to look devastatingly attractive, despite the absurd way he pulled the hat right down over his ears, he said, 'My mother knitted it. I could get her to rustle one up for you, then we could both look daft.'

Carla laughed, then paused as Eddie doused the foot of a lamppost, while John started running on the spot and puffing out clouds of white air.

'I've got a question,' Carla said, when they began walking again. 'I've been wondering when I'm going to meet the tantrum-throwing egomaniac we read about in the papers? I only ask because I've yet to catch a glimpse of him, and if he's going to make his debut in Zanzibar, I'd like to be prepared.'

When he didn't answer she glanced up at him. His eyes were shining with laughter, which didn't exactly surprise her, since she'd suspected for some time that the bad-boy image was all a hoax.

'He doesn't exist, does he?' she said.

His grin widened. 'What makes you say that?'

'Easy. Nice guys don't get the same kind of publicity bad guys get, and as far as I'm aware there's been nothing about you in the press since the first episode of *Beyond* was transmitted. Meaning, you haven't needed any publicity, so Lionel hasn't cooked any up.'

Though he was frowning now, there was no disguising the humour in his tone as he said, 'Are you doubting my skills as a gambler and womanizer? Because if you are . . .'

'Never let it be said,' she interrupted. 'I'm sure you're spectacularly accomplished in all areas of excess and carnality, but I still say Lionel is feeding the press the scandal in order to get you coverage when you need it.'

'You don't honestly think we could hoodwink the British press like that, do you?' he challenged.

'As a matter of fact, that's all that bothers me – how you manage to get away with it. Anywhere else in the world it might be different, but here the press is so cynical, and so hot on scams of any sort, that they must know they're being had. Unless, of course, they're in on it too, because scandal and excess sells more papers than . . .'

'Hey, I'm liking this,' he suddenly cried, 'because I've just realized it means you think I'm a nice guy. What a breakthrough!'

Rolling her eyes, she crossed Eddie over to the triangular island of Orange Square, and waited while he cocked his leg again, this time on a statue of Mozart. 'Don't get carried away,' she retorted. 'What I'm saying is, I think you're a con.'

'Did you hear that, Eddie?' he demanded. 'She definitely knows how to wound a bloke. I just hope she goes easier on you, little fellow.'

Eddie gazed up at him, eager to comprehend.

Smiling, Carla said, 'So, am I right?'

'When are you ever not?' he teased, dodging out of the way as someone suddenly swung out of a telephone box.

Carla's irony was audible as she said, 'Can't think of a single occasion, and I'm willing to stake big money that I'm right on this one.'

Stopping with her as she pressed a button on a pelican crossing, he said, 'Are you disappointed?'

Her eyebrows went up. 'That you're not a temperamental drunk with a babe on each arm, a gambler's debts threatening your kneecaps, and a penchant for major wobblies threatening my shoot? No, I don't think disappointed's the word.'

Laughing, he said, 'Should I press to know what is?'

'If you did, I'd probably say duped,' she responded.

'Ah,' he commented. 'Very cautious. Very Carla.'

She threw him a quick look and was about to ask him to expand, when she thought better of it, and crossed over to the pavement that ran alongside St Barnabas Church. 'OK, now

278

we've got your inimitable charm established as real,' she said a few moments later, 'and your dastardly alter ego as bogus, we can look forward to a happy shoot in Zanzibar, which brings us to the purpose of you being out here on this freezing walk.'

'But before we get into that, I want to tell you about a couple of venture capitalists you should meet, who could be willing to get you fully launched into the world of advanced technology.'

She was immediately interested.

'They're Swiss,' he told her. 'They approached me after we'd had a meeting with Dynamix last week. The chief exec. there must have told them about your interest, and now they're showing theirs.'

Carla inhaled deeply, as her excitement yielded for a moment to curiosity. 'So why did they approach you? No, don't tell me, you're the man, so they all presumed you were in charge.'

'I've put them right,' he assured her.

By the time they returned to the *ménage* they were so deeply engrossed in the discussion of yet another electronic spin-off that the subject of Zanzibar had still not been touched on.

'If your new ideas are going to involve any drastic changes,' she said, going up the front steps ahead of him, 'we'd better discuss them now. And if they call for an increase in budget . . .'

'They don't,' he assured her, waiting as she unclipped Eddie. 'Just some artful camera work on the part of non-professionals.'

'You mean equipping the researchers with DVDs to go and get shots the main unit won't have time to cover,' she said, pushing the door open. 'I think it's a great idea . . .'

'HAPPY BIRTHDAY!'

She stopped dead, so stunned she couldn't get her head to connect up with this totally unexpected turn of events. Confused, she turned to look at John.

'Surprise,' he said, his dark eyes simmering with humour.

She started to laugh. Then, turning back, she went on laughing, and gasping, as she saw that amongst all her

279

colleagues, who obviously hadn't gone home, were not only Sonya and Mark, but Avril too.

'Oh my God! When did you get here?' she cried, throwing her arms around her.

'This morning. Happy birthday.' Avril looked almost as thrilled as Carla, and very Californian, with her smooth golden tan and shining blonde hair.

Carla had tears in her eyes as she looked round at everyone's beaming faces. 'This is ... Oh God, it's... It's wonderful,' she declared, laughing at Frazer, Russell and Hugo who were still frantically pinning up streamers and birthday balloons.

'Champagne,' Sonya declared, pushing a full, fizzing glass into her hand.

'I can't take it in,' Carla gasped. 'I thought no-one knew. Oh God, whose idea was it?'

'Whose do you think?' Mark said, looking at Avril.

'Of course,' Carla laughed. 'Oh no, look at me crying. What an idiot. I don't know what to say.'

'Happy birthday,' Mark said, giving her a hug.

'OK!' Avril cried. 'Get that coat off, then let's get this party started!'

Right on cue Felicia hit a button on the sound system, filling the room with a deafening chorus of Happy Birthday, which they all sang along to, then Carla's breath was taken away again as they showered her with gifts, while the irresistible dance numbers of the moment began blasting out of the CD.

For a while, as she opened her presents, and drank champagne, she was too dazed to do much more than gasp and laugh, and throw things at Hugo and Kit who kept teasing her about all the hints she'd dropped that today was her birthday. In next to no time Felicia, Donna, Jackie and Sonya were dancing in the middle of the room, then John grabbed her hand and dragged her over to dance too, and very soon the place was alive with the beat and ringing with laughter.

It had been so long now since she'd partied that Carla had been half-afraid she'd forgotten how. But the way she entered into the madness of loud music and flashing lights, with all the careless flamboyance of a disco diva, showed that she wasn't even out of practice. It was so exhilarating and liberating, throwing herself around like this, music pulsing through her body, champagne fizzing through her veins, and everyone she knew and cared about dancing, laughing and drinking along with her. It didn't matter that she wasn't wearing a party dress, or make-up, or sparkling high-heeled shoes, no-one else was either, and her clumpy black boots, blue jeans and navy fisherman's sweater were just fine for cavorting around the desktops with one partner after another, after another, until she finally spun breathlessly into the kitchen where the food was laid out and more champagne awaited.

'This has got to be the best birthday I've ever had,' she told Donna, the make-up designer, whose fleshy cheeks were stuffed full of cheese vol-au-vent.

'Another glass for our illustrious exec.,' Frazer declared, passing over more bubbly.

'Where's my dancing partner?' John demanded, banging in through the door. 'Ah! What happened to you? You abandoned me in the middle of my favourite Ricky Martin.'

Laughing, Carla helped herself to some pâté, and said, 'Have you ever seen yourself dance?'

'Have you?' he retorted, making her laugh again.

'Ah! Food!' Avril cried, staggering in with Sonya. 'And more wine!'

'Mark's fallen in love with Phoebe,' Sonya declared. 'She's got to be at least three feet taller than him, but married to me, he's used to looking up to a woman.'

As everyone laughed, Carla said, 'Who's got the kids?'

'My mother. We're staying here tonight, by the way. John, please dance with me so I can make all my friends sick with jealousy and ruin their Christmases when I keep on and on about it for the next year and a half.'

As he tangoed her off Avril dived into the food, while Carla hiccuped and refilled her glass. 'Did I ever tell you I love you?' she said, wobbling slightly as she looked at Avril.

'I'm not sure how I feel about that,' Avril responded, 'not when we're supposed to be sharing a bed tonight.'

Carla spluttered with laughter, and, turning to Hugo and Frazer, said, 'If she tries to talk you into making it a foursome, as your executive producer, I forbid it. OK?'

'We don't take orders after six o'clock,' Hugo responded.

'You don't take them before,' Carla countered, sipping her drink, and turning to see who'd come into the kitchen now. It was Yale, followed by Rosa.

Carla's smile was dazzling, though her eyes weren't quite focused as she cried, 'Rosa! How are you?'

'Happy birthday,' Rosa said, smiling through her teeth.

'From me too,' Yale declared, sweeping Carla into a dramatic embrace. 'Sorry we're late. Got stuck in traffic. So, the big three-oh, eh?'

'And she doesn't look a day over forty,' Avril chipped in.

Carla flashed her a smile and turned back to Rosa and Yale. 'Have you got a drink?' she asked, grabbing a bottle and thrusting it at Yale. 'There're glasses over there, next to the sink.'

Rosa's expression was sour as she stood aside for Hugo and Frazer to go off and rejoin the dancing.

Carla winked at Avril, then said, 'Tell me, Rosa, I'm interested to know what I've done to upset you. I only ask because you've been so hostile towards me since you were cast, that I'd like to know why?'

Rosa's face was pinched as her small eyes darted between Carla and Avril. Though she was outnumbered, it was already evident that she intended to stand her ground. 'Why are you pretending not to know?' she responded bitterly.

Carla's smile started to fade. 'As a matter of fact, I don't know,' she responded.

Rosa scoffed her disbelief.

'Why don't you just answer the question?' Avril suggested.

'Hey, come on, the atmosphere's getting a bit tense around here,' Yale chipped in.

'And we can't have that, not on my birthday,' Carla declared, sipping her champagne. 'So that's why we're trying to clear it.' She looked at Rosa. 'Now, do you want to tell me what's bothering you, or do we have to go on playing guessing games?'

Rosa's face was becoming tighter all the time. 'You're making it sound as though I'm the one with the problem,' she snapped. 'But don't think I don't know how much it's galling you to have me on the cast.'

Carla's head tilted to one side. 'Why do you say that?' she demanded.

'You know why.' Her eyes were so harsh, and her manner so contentious, that Carla felt a moment of sobriety, as it dawned on her that she didn't actually want to pursue this. But it was too late to back down now, so, steeling herself, she said, 'Would I be right in assuming it has something to do with Chrissie and Richard?'

Rosa's eyebrows made a haughty arch. 'Amongst other things.'

Carla frowned and glanced at Avril to see if she'd understood, but Avril didn't seem to have either. 'Listen,' Carla said, starting to feel angry as she turned back, 'you were the one who cut me dead the day you walked in here, and it's you who's come very close to being offensive in your manner ever since. So yes, I'd say that you're the one with the problem round here, so either you tell me what it is, or leave your damned baggage at home, OK?' Her tone became so sharp towards the end that Rosa's face turned scarlet.

'Chrissie told me everything,' she seethed. 'So I know how you blocked my casting, and I know you wouldn't have let me in this time, if it weren't for John and Yale.'

Carla started to speak, but nothing came out.

'You could have given me a job a dozen times over,' Rosa hissed, 'but you never did. Do you have any idea how it feels, when your own so-called friends won't give you a part? And now you have you're expecting me to be grateful! Well, forget it. As far as I'm concerned I'm working for John on this production, and *you* can just go fuck yourself.' With that, she slammed her glass down on the table and stormed out of the room.

Stupefied, Carla turned to Avril, then Yale, who appeared equally as shocked.

Coming to first, he said, 'Listen, I'm really sorry. I don't know what went on before between you two, but she was well out of order with that. I'll talk to her. It won't happen again.'

'You're damned right it won't,' Carla fumed.

'No, please,' Yale said, holding up his hands for calm. 'She's obviously got the wrong end of the stick about something . . .'

'She certainly has,' Carla told him.

'So let me get her to apologize,' he said. 'If she won't, then OK, she's off the production. If she does, it's going to save you having to find someone else and prepare them for the role at this short notice.'

Realizing that to continue this would only spoil the evening, Carla said, 'I don't want to hear her apology tonight, but you can tell her from me, she'd better make it good in the morning.'

'Got you,' Yale said, and headed so fast out of the kitchen he slammed himself with the door as he yanked it open.

Carla and Avril giggled, then Carla said, 'So she thinks I was the one who vetoed her casting, when, did she but know it, it was her good friend Chrissie.'

'Are you going to tell her that?'

'I don't know. I might. We'll see what happens. But let's forget her now, or it'll only start me thinking about Richard, and I was having such a great time before she slithered in.'

'As you shall again,' Avril declared, and, linking arms, she marched them both back out to dance.

Not until after midnight did the first people start to leave, by which time Avril had exhausted her second wind and was well into her third, as she and Carla joined in an hilarious conversation with Phoebe and Sonya, neither of whom seemed to be listening to the other. One lamented the ties of motherhood, while the other wondered if it would be a bad career move to accept a modelling job in Milan. Frazer, who was swaying about in the confusion, managed some sympathy for both, while Mark fell asleep, and Hugo and Felicia pressed up against each other, supposedly smooching, to a dreamy ballad by the Back Street Boys. For the moment John was nowhere to be seen, but as Sonya hotly declared that no-one cared as much about their kids as she did, and Phoebe responded with a vehement demand that her credibility as an actress should remain intact, he came out of the kitchen and joined them.

No-one, except Carla, seemed to notice when he slipped an arm round her shoulders, and even she pretended not to, which was probably safest considering the way her body was responding. Besides, it was simply an idle gesture, and to start making something of it would be ridiculous. So she just carried on with the others, laughing and chatting, as they mimicked Sonya and Phoebe with non sequiturs of their own, while tossing back what was left of the champagne.

She wasn't sure at what point she became aware of John looking at her, all she knew was the strangeness of feeling her attention being drawn from the crowd. Nothing physical had happened, his embrace hadn't tightened, nor had her body moved, yet, when she tried to carry on with the madness, she found his magnetism too strong to resist, and the heat in her body too intense to control. In the end, unable to do anything else, she turned her head, and as their eyes met the burn of desire surged through her so powerfully that her lips opened to catch her breath.

'Happy birthday,' he said. His voice was almost drowned by a sudden whoop of laughter, but she heard him.

She continued to look at him, and did nothing as his mouth came softly to hers in a kiss that felt so intimate her breath simply stopped. Lifting his head again he gazed into her eyes, and smiled when she gave a small gasp for air, which made her smile too.

'Thank you,' she whispered.

His eyes were still on hers. 'Time to go,' he said. 'See you in the morning,' and without a word to anyone else, he left.

It was Christmas morning and bedlam reigned. Carla and Avril had decorated the cottage like a grotto, with presents hidden everywhere for the children, who swooped on them with rowdy delight when they arrived with Mark and Sonya, bringing a mountain of other new toys with them. In no time at all they were hooting, squawking, jangling and boom-boxing around the place, trampling festive paper, bows and ribbons all over the floor, while Sonya and Mark attempted to make breakfast, and Carla and Avril writhed, wriggled and jived in time to Courtenay's drums. Eddie was having a whale of a time too, with his new chewy bones, and a set of four dog boots that Avril had brought him from the States. Watching him high-stepping around the garden in these peculiar contraptions had been the funniest spectacle of the day so far. Now, Santa's singalong was blaring out of the TV, not quite drowning out Steps on Kitty's new CD player, while along the road the church bells were going at full pelt while they all rushed to get ready.

'Come on, we're going to be late!' Sonya shouted over the din.

'I don't want to go to church,' Kitty shouted back.

'Get your coat on!'

'Can I take Buzz Lightyear?' Courtenay asked, looking up at his dad with big blue eyes.

'Has anyone checked the turkey?' Carla called, coming down the stairs.

'I just did,' Avril called back from the kitchen.

'Dad! You just trod on Barbie's head!' Kitty wailed. 'Oh, *Dad*!'

'I'm sorry,' Mark responded.

'Fancy treading on Barbie's head,' Carla snorted as she passed.

Mark shot her a look. 'Come on,' he said to Kitty, holding up her coat. 'Arms in.'

'Bloody hell!' she grumbled. 'I don't want to go to church.'

Carla's and Sonya's eyes met as they both suppressed a smile, before Sonya launched into the necessary reprimand.

'Can we go to the pub?' Courtenay wanted to know.

'On the way back.'

'I want to take my drums,' he cried, jumping up and down. Then, 'Auntie Avril, I can see your knicks.'

'Oh, you told her,' Carla groaned, and laughed as Avril tugged the hem of her skirt out of her panties.

Five minutes later they stumbled out of the house, still dragging on coats and scarves, and headed off to church. After putting their hearts and souls into the carols, and shivering through the sermon and prayers, they surged back out into the crisp, sunny morning and made for the pub. Everyone from the village was arriving, with the exception of Fleur and Perry, who'd gone off to Sedona, in Arizona, for a fortnight's commune with all things spiritual and spatial.

'They took us out in their transit before they left,' Gayle told Carla and Avril, shouting to make herself heard above the jostling crowd in the pub.

'Not UFO spotting?' Carla cried, laughing.

'You can mock, but I'm telling you, I never had any idea so many people were into it. There must've been a hundred or more, all in their earthbound spacecrafts watching out for ET and his mates. And you should see all the flippin' technology they've got, computers, scanners, radios, transmitters, satellite dishes . . . Must have cost them a fortune.'

Avril was laughing too. 'Where did you go?' she asked.

'Stonehenge. Where else?'

'So, did you see anything?' Carla wanted to know.

'Did we heck. But it was dead spooky, I can tell you. You really got the impression something could happen with all that bleeping and pinging and crackling going on. Isn't that right, Joe?' she said to her husband, who was squeezing through the crowd with a couple of drinks. 'I was just telling them about our night out with Fleur and Perry.'

Joe was about to answer when Maudie poked him hard in the back. 'You got a nerve putting your face in a Christian church, you devil-worshipper, you!' she snarled.

Carla and Avril grinned.

Joe turned to Maudie, his eyes rolling in their sockets, his lips trembling as he let forth a sudden stream of gibberish. 'Okee anocki abo bluba,' he chanted.

Maudie shrank back, and rapidly made the sign of the cross, as he raised his arms and loomed after her like a monster.

'Get back here,' Gayle laughed, grabbing his collar. 'You're such a wind-up with all that. She really believes it, you know.'

'No, she doesn't,' he replied. 'She loves it. Gives her something else to have a go about.' He took a sip of beer and, turning to Avril, said, 'So, how's Hollywood?'

'Dull compared to Cannock Martin,' she responded. 'At last!' she cried, as Mark broke through the congestion with drinks for her and Carla.

'They're from Graham,' Mark informed them. 'He's over by the bar, apparently buying for everyone.'

'He does that every Christmas,' Carla reminded him.

'Hey! Carla!' Sylvia shouted from behind a beer pump. 'Phone for you!'

'For me?' She looked at Avril, mystified. 'No-one knows I'm here.'

'Well obviously someone does,' Avril responded.

Curious, Carla handed Avril her drink, then shoved her way through to the bar.

'Take it round the back,' Sylvia said. 'Can't hear yourself think out here.'

Slipping through to the storeroom, Carla unhooked the receiver on the wall, and put it to her ear. 'Hello?' she said, pressing a finger to her other ear.

All she could hear was the noise of the bar, until Sylvia put the extension down, cutting off at least some of it.

'Hello?' she said again.

'Carla?'

'Who is this?' Carla said. 'Can you speak up, I can hardly hear you.'

The voice was faint, and definitely female, but it was impossible to distinguish the words fully as she said, '. . . speak to . . . The house . . . You've got . . .'

'I'm sorry,' Carla shouted. 'I can't hear you. You'll have to speak louder.' She waited, but there was no response. 'Hello?' she shouted. 'Are you still there?' But it didn't seem anyone was, so in the end she hung up and returned to the bar.

'Bizarre,' she remarked to Avril and Sonya, who'd left Mark in charge of the kids on the swings outside. 'No idea who it was, I couldn't make out what she was saying.'

'But it was a woman?' Sonya said.

'Yes, it was definitely a woman.' Her nerves were on edge as she thought of the intruder Maudie had seen and wondered if there was a connection.

Avril was watching her closely, remembering the intruder too, but she let it go when Carla suddenly smiled brightly and said, 'Well, if it's important she'll call back.'

'Whoever she is,' Sonya added, staggering as someone pushed past her. Carla grabbed her and said, 'Did you hear from Greg, by the way?'

'No. Did you?'

'Who?' Avril wanted to know.

'My other brother,' Carla reminded her. 'I spoke to him just before I left London,' she told Sonya. 'He's not coming down over Christmas.'

'Well, there's a surprise! Wifey won't let him, I suppose?'

'I think that's about it,' Carla responded. 'Apparently they're going to her parents, as usual. Anyone would think he didn't have a family the way she carries on.'

'She's such a bitch,' Sonya commented.

'I know. But not everyone can be as perfect a sister-in-law as you.'

Sonya nodded gravely. 'True,' she responded.

Laughing, Avril said, 'Come on, who's for another G & T before we get slung out of here?'

'I'll get them,' Carla insisted, swiping the glasses.

Pushing a path back to the counter, she squeezed herself in next to Graham and shouted, 'Merry Christmas!'

'Merry Christmas,' he shouted back, his face lighting up.

'The pen was fantastic,' she told him, referring to the gold Cartier he'd given her. 'I'll really treasure it.'

'And I loved the socks,' he grinned, 'especially the ones that play "Rudolph the Red-Nosed Reindeer", and shed opal cufflinks when you put them on.'

Laughing, she admired the cufflinks as he flashed his wrists to show her, then raised his trouser bottoms to reveal his jazzy socks.

'What are you doing tomorrow?' she wanted to know. 'Would you like to come for lunch? Leftover turkey, chips and pickled onions?'

His eyes crinkled with laughter. 'How can I resist?' he said. 'And as Betty's gone to her sister's, I shall be happy to have the company.'

Carla was aghast. 'She's left you on your own at Christmas!' she cried. 'Then you must come today. We can always make room for one more.'

'No, no,' he protested. 'Tomorrow's fine.'

'No. I'm putting my foot down. You're coming back with us today. We can't have you on your own at Christmas. It's simply not allowed.'

He was smiling at her fondly. 'OK, if you insist, but you must let me bring something.'

'Like what? We've already got enough food to feed half of Somerset.'

'Ah, but I have some very fine bottles of wine in my cellar. Perhaps I can contribute a few of them.'

Carla rolled her eyes. 'I don't think you'll get any objection to that,' she told him. 'Oh God, Teddy! What happened to you?' she cried, as Teddy Best appeared with a black patch over one eye.

'I was Santa, over at the school,' he grumbled, 'and one of the little buggers nearly poked my eyeball out with some radio-controlled gadget.'

'Well, you look very rakish,' she told him. 'Now, what are you having to drink?'

Not until the pub was ready to close did everyone start spilling out on to the street and making their way home. By then Mark had already taken the kids back to the cottage, so it was left to Carla and Avril to help a carol-singing Sonya weave her way across the road, while Graham popped home to get the promised wine.

At last, just after four o'clock, the seven of them were squashed around the table in Carla's kitchen, plates piled high with turkey, roast potatoes, roast parsnips, cabbage, peas, carrots, sprouts, big dollops of cranberry sauce, and a delicious chestnut-flavoured gravy made by Avril. Even Eddie had a helping, though his was served in his usual bowl, over in its usual spot by the back door, where Carla had put a special little Christmas tree just for him.

'OK, who's saying grace?' Carla wanted to know, as Sonya finished dishing up for the children.

'Grace!' Kitty shouted.

'Very funny. You do it, Mark.'

Mark started, got interrupted by Eddie, barking, then by his son feeling sick, then by his wife telling him to hurry up. So he gabbled the last couple of lines and hoisted up his glass. 'Toast!' he declared. 'Merry Christmas to one and all. And to Graham for supplying this tasty vintage. And to the rest of us for drinking it. And to . . .'

'Shut up and drink,' Sonya told him, busily clinking glasses with everyone else.

'Nectar,' Mark declared, after rolling the first sip around his palate.

'Can I have some?' Courtenay asked.

'No,' Mark answered. 'Drink your Coke.' Then, turning back to Graham, 'So, you were telling me about your new book. You reckon it's about finished?'

Graham chuckled. 'Oh, still a couple of months away yet,' he answered. 'But for me, that's almost finished.'

'How long have you been working on this one?' Avril wanted to know.

'A couple of years.'

'What's it about?' Sonya asked, taking a mouthful of food.

'Oh, it's the usual detective-thriller stuff.'

'He's so modest,' Carla said. 'All his books are best-sellers, and no-one, but no-one, writes like he does. That's what makes his work so unique and compelling – I'm quoting now from . . .' she looked at Graham, 'the *Guardian*? Or was it the *Independent*?'

'I don't know,' he smiled, tearing his eyes from the photograph of Carla's mother that was on the dresser beside him. 'One of them. It doesn't really matter, as long as people go out and buy.'

'So how come you didn't go up north with Betty?' Sonya asked.

'Oh, she's happier up there without me hanging around. Goodness knows, we see enough of each other, and it's not much fun living with someone who's shut up in his study all day, and never talks about anything real at the end of it.'

'What do you mean, real?' Mark said.

'We tend to talk about my work a lot. She's got a first-class mind for detail, and I try most things out on her before I get to work on them. Then we go over them after they're written . . . Gets a bit tedious, I imagine, especially when she doesn't have many friends to break the monotony with. Now, that's enough about me, let's put someone else in the spotlight. How about you, young man?' he said to Courtenay. 'What did you have for Christmas?'

'I've got some drums,' Courtenay told him.

'And I got a pushchair, and a cot and three dolls and a CD player,' Kitty piped up.

'You had a lot more than that,' Mark grumbled.

Sonya was helping herself to more cranberry. 'So what's John Rossmore doing for Christmas?' she asked Carla.

With a mouthful of food, Carla shrugged and looked at

Avril, glad that no-one could know how the mention of John's name had just caused her insides to flutter.

'He's in France,' Avril answered.

'France, eh?' Sonya said, sounding impressed. 'What, he's got a house there, or something?'

'I think so. Or someone in his family has. They're all going, apparently. His mother and father, his sisters and their husbands, brother and girlfriend.'

Carla wondered if the girlfriend belonged to the brother, or John, but didn't ask.

'Where in France?' Graham enquired.

'South. Théoule-sur-Mer,' Avril told him, looking at Carla and attempting not to grin.

Noticing, Sonya looked at Carla too.

'What?' Carla said.

Sonya's eyes moved from one to the other. 'OK, what's going on?' she demanded. 'What haven't I been told?'

'Nothing,' Carla said. 'I don't know why she's looking at me like that.'

Sonya turned to Avril. So did Mark and Graham.

Avril's eyes were dancing, 'She didn't tell you about the birthday kiss?' she said to Sonya.

Carla immediately reddened. 'What about it?' she cried. 'It was no different to anyone else's. Anyway, Sonya was there.'

'Was I?' Sonya said, bemused.

Avril grinned. 'You were. So was I. And from where I was standing, it was a lot different to everyone else's.'

'How did I manage to miss it?' Sonya demanded. 'Did you see?' she asked Mark. 'What am I talking about, you were asleep. So what happened?' she said to Avril.

Carla jumped in first. 'Nothing happened,' she said firmly. 'He just gave me a quick peck, like everyone else, and said happy birthday.'

'And the atmosphere was so charged up,' Avril added, 'you'd have electrocuted anyone who touched you. And I mean both of you.'

'She's exaggerating, as usual,' Carla retorted, glancing over at Graham. Then seeing the way he was beaming at her too, she cried, 'Honestly, I don't know what's got into everyone. So John Rossmore gave me a quick kiss for my birthday. I

292

expect he's down there in France now, giving lots of other people quick kisses for Christmas, and they'll all mean just the same.'

'Oh come on,' Avril said. 'You know he's nuts about you.'

Carla's heart took a dive, as the colour flooded back to her cheeks. 'I know no such thing,' she said sharply, 'and nor do you.' Then, *Why are you doing this?* He's a colleague – and a friend, I suppose. But much more of a colleague, and we have to work together, so let's just drop this shall we?'

'OK. OK,' Avril responded. 'Keep your hair on. But there's nothing wrong with finding the man attractive, you know? After all, the rest of us do, and we're not trying to hide it.'

'I'm not hiding anything!'

Everyone looked at her.

Carla took a breath, then surprised even herself as she started to laugh. 'OK,' she said, picking up her wine, 'he's an attractive man, and the kiss was . . . nice. But let's not get carried away, all right?'

'Oooh, Auntie Carla had a kiss,' Courtenay was singing.

'Does that mean she's got a new boyfriend?' Kitty demanded of her mother.

'No, it doesn't,' Carla said forcefully.

'It might,' Sonya corrected.

'All right. I give up,' Carla said. 'You all think what you want, and I'll know the truth. Now, can we please change the subject?'

'More wine?' Graham offered, holding up the bottle.

No-one refused, and as the conversation finally moved on to who'd had what in their stockings that morning, Carla, though glad the teasing was over, found herself enjoying the moment when Avril had claimed John was nuts about her – not because it was particularly what she wanted, simply because of how good it made her feel to hear it.

Since the night of her birthday they'd seen each other only twice, and though nothing had been said, she'd known instinctively that he was remembering the kiss too. Whether it had had quite as powerful an effect on him, as on her, she had no idea, though she guessed not. His sex life was undoubtedly a lot more active than hers, so it was highly unlikely that a simple kiss had thrown him into the same fever of lust as it had thrown her. And the fact that the next time she saw him would be in Zanzibar wasn't helping much either, for the very idea of being in such exotic and romantic climes, feeling the way she was now, was just too unsettling for words. As was the chance of somehow finding out that she was sleeping in a bed Chrissie and Richard had shared. The mere thought of that was enough to send her into a state of near-panic. There were just too many emotions attaching themselves to this trip, and most of them seemed to be running out of control, so she could only try her level best not to think about any of it until she had to.

'Have you told Richard yet that you're going?' Avril asked, when Carla finally confessed some of her fears. It was Boxing Day morning now, and they were both still snuggled up in their dressing gowns, hot tea cupped in their hands as they watched the sitting-room fire smoke and flicker into life.

Carla shook her head. 'He thinks I was there before, remember? On the recce. He didn't say anything about it then, thank God, because the last thing I want is him telling me all the places to visit or things to do, or anything about when he was there. Can you imagine?' She shuddered, then, sighing, let her head fall back. 'Ow,' she groaned, as her hangover throbbed. 'I think we should go for a long walk with Eddie,' she suggested. 'If nothing else it might blow away some of these cobwebs.'

'Good idea. You go, and then you can tell me what it was like.'

They sat quietly for a moment, then Avril said, 'Is he still asking you to see him?'

'All the time.'

'So how's he dealing with your reticence?'

'The way Richard deals with most things, patiently, non-judgementally.'

'Did he say what he and Chrissie were doing for Christmas?'

'Spending it at home, just the three of them.' Carla's eyes closed as her heart caught on the image. Then, forcing a smile, she said, 'I wonder what sort of time John's having in France?'

Avril grinned. 'I'm more interested to know what sort of time he's going to have in Zanzibar,' she teased.

294

Despite herself Carla laughed, and Avril ducked as a cushion came flying her way. 'That'll be Sonya,' Carla said, glancing at the clock as the phone started to ring.

'You get it, the bath should be full by now,' Avril said. 'Then I might join you on that walk.'

Going into the study for the portable phone, Carla was in the process of picking it up when she noticed Betty driving past in her car. Surprised she was back so soon, then thinking no more of it, she said into the receiver, 'Good morning, Sonya.'

There was a pause, then the voice at the other end said, 'Not Sonya.'

Carla's heart jolted. 'John?' she said, already knowing it wasn't.

'Try again.'

She was in such a commotion now that she could neither speak nor think. It couldn't be Richard, it just couldn't, yet she knew it was. 'Richard?' she whispered.

'How are you?'

Her heart was thudding, her mind racing. This was the first time she'd heard him in over eighteen months, yet the warmth of his voice, the intimacy of his tone, made it feel like yesterday.

'Are you still there?'

'Yes, I'm here.'

'I can't stay,' he said, 'I just wanted to hear your voice.'

Her hand went to her mouth as a strange sound erupted from her throat. 'I wish you hadn't done this,' she said.

There was a moment's hesitation before he said, 'I'm sorry. I didn't mean to upset you.'

'You haven't. I mean, you have, but . . . Oh God, don't you realize how much harder this makes it?'

'I do now. Are you all right?'

'I don't know.'

'It's been so long.'

Her heart felt so tense it might tear itself apart. 'Richard, please, don't do this again,' she said, hardly knowing what she was saying.

He didn't answer.

'It's not that I don't want to hear you,' she continued, 'it's just . . .'

'It's all right. I understand. I just want you to know that I'm sorry, and . . .'

'No, don't,' she gasped.

'I have to go,' he said.

There were a few moments of silence, then the line went dead.

She remained where she was standing, still so caught up in the shock of it that her body could only shake, while her heart increased its pounding. 'I don't believe it,' she mumbled. 'I can't believe that just happened.' Then, without really thinking, she snatched up the receiver and dialled 1471, but the message told her that the caller had withheld their number.

Though it didn't surprise her, it angered her, and, slamming the phone down, she ran up the stairs and burst into the bathroom.

'Jesus Christ!' Avril cried.

'No, me. You'll never guess who that was on the phone.'

Avril's tone was dry. 'Evidently not Sonya.'

Carla shook her head. 'Richard.'

Avril's eyes and mouth opened, then, groaning, she sank beneath the bubbles.

Carla waited for her to surface.

'So what did he say?' Avril asked.

Carla repeated what she could remember. 'It was all such a shock,' she said, 'I mean, I can still hardly believe it was him. If I hadn't heard him with my own ears . . .'

'Shit,' Avril said, for lack of anything else, though it was clear she was a lot less delighted with this surprise than Carla was. 'Where was he calling from, do you know?'

'I presume home, but he'd blocked the dial-back.'

Avril's lip curled.

'I know, it pissed me off too. But actually, I don't want his number. I don't want the temptation.'

Avril picked up a sponge and began smoothing it over her arms. 'I wonder why he chose now,' she said. 'What makes today different from any other, that he should have picked up the phone now?'

Carla was shaking her head.

'I mean, why has he never done it before? God knows

there's been enough opportunity, and you can't tell me Chrissie's with him every minute of the day.' Her eyes started to narrow. What was coming into her mind wasn't making much sense, but she was going to try it out anyway. 'Tell me,' she said, 'do you think there's any chance that call you got yesterday, at the pub, could have been from Chrissie?'

Carla's eyes widened with amazement. 'What on earth makes you say that?' she asked.

'I don't know,' Avril answered truthfully. 'But could it?'

Carla shook her head. 'No, I don't think so. It was hard to hear, but I know Chrissie's voice so well, and . . . No, it wasn't her, I'm certain of it.'

Avril shrugged.

'I'm intrigued to know what made you think it might be,' Carla pressed.

'To be honest, so am I. I suppose it's just one of those hunches you get sometimes . . .' She looked at Carla again. 'What if she's found out about you and Richard? That might make her call, mightn't it?'

'I suppose so. But I'm sure it wasn't her.' A few seconds ticked by, then she said, 'You're not thinking it's her who the children and Maudie saw, are you?'

Avril looked perplexed. 'I don't know what I'm thinking,' she answered. 'I suppose it doesn't seem very likely, does it, unless she's lost her marbles.'

'But even if she has, the kids know her. So does everyone in the village. Someone would have recognized her.'

'Mmm,' Avril responded, ponderously. 'I guess you're right. Anyway, what are you going to do now, about this call?'

Carla shuddered with nerves, then laughed. 'Nothing,' she said, 'except thank God we're going to Geneva right after the New Year, before we go to Zanzibar, because I feel very much in need of distancing myself, even if only for a couple of days, from everything to do with . . .' She stopped, as Avril's eyes started twinkling. 'What?' she said.

'Nothing. I was just waiting for you to admit that this distance has to be taken from John, as well as from Richard.'

Carla's expression was full of irony. 'Well, I don't need to, now you've just said it for me, do I?' she retorted, and, flashing a grin, she turned and walked out of the door.

'Everything all right?' Graham said, coming into the kitchen where Betty was kneading dough on the big pine table.

Nodding, she said, 'Barry's coming for dinner. He likes freshly baked bread.'

Graham watched the pull and twist of her hands for a moment, then, helping himself to a mince pie from the pile on a plate, he sat down to eat it. 'Why didn't you stay longer?' he asked her.

Her pale, tawny eyes came briefly to his. 'I suppose I didn't like to think of you here, on your own.'

He carried on chewing the savoury tart, apparently absorbed in thought, until she said, 'Did you have a nice time at Carla's yesterday?'

'Very nice,' he answered. 'Though no-one cooks quite as well as you, my dear.'

Betty smiled. 'How is she?' she asked.

Graham's eyebrows went up. 'Apparently she's got a new boyfriend.'

'Oh?' Betty responded.

'Well, perhaps that's rather overstating it,' he confessed. 'What I should say is, it seems there's an attraction developing between her and John Rossmore.'

'He's a handsome man,' Betty commented. 'Wild though, if you believe the papers.'

Graham's lower lip jutted forward as he considered that.

Betty said, 'It should please you to think she's getting over Richard at last.'

Sighing, he said, 'I thought she was, but apparently he called her on the phone, which seems to have unsettled her rather.'

Betty's surprise showed. 'What did he say?' she asked.

'Not much, other than he wanted to hear her voice.'

Slapping the dough down on the table, Betty began to shape it.

Finishing the tart, Graham brushed the crumbs off his fingers, and got up to go and gaze out at the grey, bulbous sky that was descending over the apple orchards beyond their garden.

'Do you think there's any chance of them getting back together?' Betty asked after a while.

With his back still turned he shook his head. 'I don't know,' he answered.

'But not if you can help it?'

Turning round in surprise, he said, 'What on earth could I do to stop it?'

Betty merely looked at him. Then, carrying her loaf over to the oven, she opened the door and popped it in.

'I just wish I could believe being back with Richard would make her happy,' Graham said. 'But after everything that's happened . . .' He sighed and shook his head.

Betty came over to pat his shoulder. 'I know you care for her, but she's not your daughter,' she reminded him. 'And even if she were, she's a grown woman . . .'

Graham's eyes went down.

Betty watched him, then, seeming to read him, said, 'You're afraid he's found the letter Valerie wrote, aren't you? That's what you're thinking. He might have called to tell Carla . . .'

'If he'd found it, he'd contact me first,' Graham assured her.

Betty's eyebrows rose. 'Well, I suppose we'd better hope you're right,' she responded.

There was a barely discernible tightness to Graham's voice as he said, 'I don't want to remind you, that were it not for you that letter wouldn't even exist.'

They stood looking at each other, tension starting to crackle in the air, until a kind of weariness seemed to crumple him, and, returning to the table, he dropped into a chair.

They didn't speak about Carla again until later that night, when Barry Fellowes was dining with them, and Betty told him about the call Carla had had from Richard.

Fellowes's wide jaw and sharp grey eyes turned immediately to Graham. 'Well, that's incredibly bad timing,' he commented. 'Do you think she told you everything he said?'

Graham nodded.

'If she didn't, we can always . . .'

'No,' Graham interrupted. 'She told me everything. Let's leave it at that.'

299

Fellowes looked at Betty. 'I hope you haven't . . .'

'Let's leave it!' Graham barked.

Fellowes seemed startled by his tone, but said no more.

'So where did Chrissie and Richard spend Christmas?' Betty asked, after a while.

'At home, apparently,' Fellowes answered. 'Though I'm told they went out for dinner, the two of them, on Boxing night. Last night? Yes. I'm losing track of the days.'

'After Richard had called Carla,' Graham said almost to himself.

'It would seem so.'

A long, pregnant silence ensued, broken only by the clatter of their cutlery, and the wind blowing outside. A car went past, then the sound of a dog barking carried from somewhere distant. Fellowes finished his wine and looked pointedly at the bottle, but Graham didn't seem to notice. Then, quite suddenly, Betty got to her feet.

'I'm tired of this,' she declared. 'I tell you, I'm tired of it.'

Graham and Fellowes looked at her agitated face, though neither man appeared surprised when she stormed from the room.

The candles flickered in the draught as the door closed behind her, and a small cloud of smoke billowed out of the hearth. Graham looked across the table at Fellowes, then, refilling their glasses, he said, 'She'll calm down in a moment. Probably just gone to get the pud.'

Chapter 18

Zanzibar. As if the name weren't evocative enough, the island itself, with its proud and shameful history, oozed such mystery and charm that the sun-dazzled reality of present-day life seemed to merge with centuries past and cultures forgotten as though the vast, disorienting swell of sound, smell, colour and heat were as imagined as true. Narrow cobbled lanes zigzagged erratically through the heart of the town, a confounding maze of grand Islamic style and Indian splendour, with lacy balconies and bulbous domes winking in the sunlight, though succumbing now to their years of neglect. Oblivious to all but their purpose, men in crisp white kanzos and intricately embroidered kaffiyehs – the Islamic prayer caps – rode motorbikes with dangerous abandon, swerving through the hustle and bustle, skidding and shouting urgently for a path to open. The bitter, musky scents of spices, and the stench of drains hung in the humid air, while the haunting wail of Arabian music harmonized with the throb of African drums and the persistent blare and buzz of car horns and bicycle bells. Hawkers whose wares made a sea of riotous colour, and whose baubles glittered like a child's eyes, beckoned in languages as diverse as Swahili, Italian, Afrikaans and English. Clusters of seepingly ripe fruit passed from one hennaed female hand to another, and the flamboyant swathing of smiling women who toted baskets on their heads and jangled bracelets on their wrists made a striking contrast to those in the flowing black robes and secretive veils of their faith.

To Carla, as she and Avril observed it all from the back of a car, it seemed that everything the senses touched was part of a potion brewed for intrigue and seduction. Even the tragedies of history seemed to have yielded up their misery to combine with the heady, hypnotic amalgam of now. As easy as it was to imagine pirates and slaves, it was as easy to envisage sultans and princesses, harems and palaces, hovels and dungeons. Ghosts of red- and blue-coated soldiers tramped the dusty streets with European ladies in crinolines and bonnets. Echoes of Eastern traders jumped around the dirty, decaying walls, along with the agonized wailing of captured men, women and children, chains clanking at their wrists and ankles, despair and terror preying on their hearts.

'Unbelievable,' she muttered, trying to absorb the sheer potency of it all as their air-conditioned Land Cruiser pressed a precarious route through the teeming masses of pedestrians, cyclists and open-air buses that Jaffah, the unit's Mr Fix-it, had just told her were called *dala-dalas*. Jaffah's enthusiasm for the shoot, and power to galvanize the indolent as well as to circumvent officialdom, were proving the unit's most valuable assets, according to John's latest report. Despite his dignified appearance in an old Etonian tie and starched white shirt, Carla knew already that he hadn't escaped the crew's irreverence, for he'd told her himself, with the sunniest of smiles, that if she liked she too could call him Orange.

Beside her Avril stifled a yawn. 'All this sun, after London and Geneva,' she said, 'I feel as though I'm about to break out in bloom.' Her eyes were roaming the billowing blue expanse of the sea where humble fishing boats and rusting container ships jostled about on the waves.

'See, over here,' Jaffah told them excitedly, 'is House of Wonders.' He was indicating a splendid old building that was a curious combination of the colonial and Islamic styles with its sturdy white pillars, filigree balconies and impressive clock tower that soared from the red-tiled roof tops – no doubt a perfect lookout point for days gone by, when ships had sailed in from both east and west to trade in ivory and jewels, spices and teas, silks, muslins, gold and ambergris – and, of course, slaves. 'Was palace of Sultan Barghash,' Jaffah explained. 'Is called House of Wonders because it first in Zanzibar to have electricity lights, and first in all of East

Africa to have lift.' He beamed with such pride that he might have installed this wizardry himself. 'Was office of British government from 1911 until 1964,' he continued, 'when we have coup in Zanzibar and boot out British and sultan. After it office of Party of Revolution.'

'And now?' Carla asked, already knowing from the research, but not wanting to steal his moment.

'Is magnificent, magnificent museum,' he told her with rapture. 'Or will be when is finished.' As they were already five years past the completion date, it was anyone's guess exactly when that might be, though Carla couldn't help being impressed by such heartfelt pride in something that didn't yet exist. 'And next door is old palace of Sultan Said,' Jaffah gabbled on, as they moved slowly past the high white crenellated walls, now heavily smudged in soot and grime. 'Is very beautiful, no? See the Arabic ramparts, and Indian-style arches. Inside is old Sultan's furniture, and original lavatory, and many portraits of family. We film there, tomorrow. It close to public, and tomorrow Jaffah, that's me, make it so unit can film. Oh, and Masud, here, he your driver all time you in Zanzibar. Masud from very noble tribe in Kenya. He second son of powerful Masai chief. He have education in France and soon he become very important doctor here in Zanzibar.'

Avril slanted a look at Carla whose eyebrows went up, for Masud's limpidly intelligent eyes and hard physique lent a very potent edge to an almost breathtaking beauty.

'Does he speak English?' Avril asked.

'Little,' Jaffah apologized. 'But you want something, you tell Jaffah, I fix.'

Avril turned away as with a smile Carla said, 'Maybe we should start making for the hotel now?'

'Oh, yes, yes,' Jaffah answered quickly. 'They film today in beach. You go beach first, or hotel?'

'Hotel,' Carla answered, then turned to Avril, whose head had turned in her direction. 'What?' she said.

'You look fine, if you want to go and see him right away,' Avril told her.

Though Carla let her head fall back against the seat, there was no ignoring the response Avril's words had set off, and she was already anxious enough about the aphrodisiacal. powers of exotic locations. 'OK, let's stop this now,' she said. 'This is an expensive shoot, and there's definitely not going to be time for all that. Nor, after the kind of days we've got scheduled, is anyone going to have the energy, or inclination, to do anything but eat then fall into a comatose sleep.'

'Sounds fun,' Avril commented. Then to Jaffah, 'Are we going to be able to power up our mobile phones?'

'Oh yes. All fixed,' he assured her. Then excitedly declared, 'Over here, is most famous tree in all of Zanzibar. Is called Big Fig Tree.' Which indeed it was, for it rose a good forty feet from the ground, and extended vast, leafy branches over a group of dhow-builders who were working in the blistering sun. 'This tree plant by Sultan Khalifa in year 1911,' he told them. 'In Swahili we say *Mtini* – the place of the Tree.'

Their guided tour continued as they made a slow, circuitous journey to the hotel, passing the old dhow harbour, several ox-drawn carts, a garishly painted blue and white mosque and many side-stall cafés with English football results chalked up on boards outside. Most impressive of all, however, were the huge, hand-carved doors that were to be seen everywhere, both Indian and Arabic in style and made from teak. The fearsome brass studs, Jaffah explained, were to stop the elephants breaking the doors down. Too tired to take out her writing pad, Carla made a mental note of this colourful detail, a must for the script.

Finally they rejoined the main road and began heading back towards the airport, where the Fisherman's Resort Hotel was situated at the end of a bumpy track in a secluded bay, just south of the town. A dusty-looking guard in a red fez and white tunic let up the barrier for them to sweep into a rectangular courtyard which was enclosed by long low white buildings with high coconut-thatched roofs and dark wood pillars. The moment they stepped out of the car the hot, steamy air embraced them again, though a breeze was wafting its way in from the sea, across a vast, shimmering blue pool surrounded by palms, through the open-air bar with its coco-thatched roof and bamboo chairs, across the decorative ponds and fountains in the reception and out to where they were standing under the thatch-canopied entrance.

'Heaven,' Avril declared, as Masud and Jaffah began hauling luggage from the car. 'How long are we here for?'

'Three days, then we go north to Mapenzi Beach,' Carla answered, tearing her eyes from the heady romance of the setting and turning to drag her laptop off the back seat. 'After that, we're over on the east coast for three days at the Sultan's Palace.' Though she'd vowed not to torment herself with images of Chrissie and Richard being here, they'd come flooding in of their own accord and for a horrible moment the deception and pain seemed to well up anew.

'Are you OK?' Avril asked, accurately reading the situation.

Carla nodded. 'He knows I'm here now,' she said. 'I emailed him a few days ago.'

'And?'

'I haven't heard from him since.' She forced a smile, then started into the hotel as though to escape the unwelcome reflections. The truth was, she'd only heard from him once since he'd called her on Boxing Day, when he'd told her that hearing her voice had changed many things for him. Quite what he'd meant by that she wasn't sure, and the extract he'd added, in French, from a work she didn't know, had rambled inconclusively about a man's confusion between dream and reality, so hadn't been much help. Though she guessed the author was Descartes, as yet she hadn't had the time to find out, and wondered if it was her failure to interpret it that was causing his silence. It didn't seem likely, but maybe the reassurance of knowing how similar their minds were was something he needed much more than she'd realized.

After checking in, and receiving a warm welcome from the manager and staff, they were led out past the pool, along a path that dissected the carefully tended lawns with the sea rushing up on to a rocky shore to the right, and rows of two-storey guest cottages to the left. Theirs was at the far end, with a wooden staircase on the side, taking Carla up to a spacious veranda with two cushioned chairs and glorious views of the ocean, then on into the cool, air-conditioned darkness of her room.

Before disappearing inside she leaned over the gnarled wood of the railing and called down to Avril. 'Remember,

305

this place is predominantly Muslim,' she said, 'so keep it covered up while we're out in public.'

After tipping the porter she turned into the room and gazed at the large, Iroko wood bed with its exquisite Zanzibari carvings and copious folds of muslin draped from a hanging frame above. The rest of the furniture was in the same dark wood, the walls were washed in white, and the floor was coolly tiled in terracotta and stone. Finding herself imagining Richard and Chrissie lying together on the beautifully canopied bed, she quickly opened her suitcase and started to unpack.

Less than an hour later, after showering and washing her hair, she wrapped a brightly coloured sarong around her waist, turning it into an ankle-length skirt, pulled on a plain short white T-shirt, and slipped her feet into a pair of flip-flops to go and turf out Avril.

'Perfect,' she declared, when Avril came out in pale blue pedal-pushers with matching loose shirt, and modest sleeveless top. Then, grimacing at the pile of messages Avril was holding, she waved her own, and carried on reading them as they headed out to find Masud. It didn't take long to drive to the location beach, though it was a noisy journey as both Carla and Avril shouted into their mobile phones, returning calls from London and LA, while holding on to the front seats to stop themselves bouncing around too violently.

Finally they arrived at the beach where the bulk of the unit was clustered at the water's edge. Remembering to turn off their phones, they climbed from the car, but didn't get far before the second assistant signalled for them to stay where they were, as the camera was rolling. Silently they watched the take, though weren't able to make out much of what was happening through the bodies surrounding the action. A minute or two later Hugo yelled cut, and as the grips started pushing the camera back along the tracks the unit began to break apart.

'What's happening?' Carla asked, as Verna came to meet them.

'We're doing the scene where the slave trader's wife and pirate captain fix a price for the slave girl,' Verna answered.

'There're a couple more set-ups, then apparently we're doing the romance shots.'

'Romance shots?' Avril said curiously.

'Of the dashingly handsome Sultan riding manfully along the beach on his trusty white stallion,' Carla said drolly, while looking up to see where the sun was. Satisfied that the shots were likely to coincide with the sunset, she looked around for John.

'Isn't that Rosa?' Avril said, nodding to where a straw-hatted woman in a tight lace bodice and voluminous skirts was talking to Gary Houseman, the pirate captain.

'Mmm,' Carla responded, thinking what a good job Jackie had done with the costume, and how insufferably hot Rosa must be in it.

'So I take it she apologized after that scene in the kitchen,' Avril said.

Carla nodded. 'Grudgingly, it has to be said,' she answered.

'Did you tell her it was Chrissie who'd blocked her casting?'

Carla's eyebrows went up. 'As a matter of fact, I did.' She hadn't felt too proud afterwards, but it was done now, and hardly worth losing sleep over.

'How'd she take that?'

'Don't know. Didn't ask, and haven't seen her since. However, she did send me a New Year's card, which I presume was some kind of peace offering.'

'She's a snake,' Avril commented, looking at Rosa with distaste, while taking the cold drink an assistant was handing her. She sipped it, then almost choked as she caught sight of John striding across the beach towards them. 'Jesus Christ,' she murmured.

Following her eyes Carla started to laugh, though she could only feel thankful for the sunglasses covering her eyes, since the image he created, in his long white flowing robes, intricately wound turban and high leather boots, had to be every woman's wildest dream. And from the irony of his expression he not only knew it, but was loving it.

'I don't know if a man's ever made my knees go weak before,' Avril told him, as he embraced her, the way everyone on the unit embraced, with a kiss on either cheek. 'And at the risk of a ribald response, aren't you hot in that?'

'Surprisingly no,' he responded.

'He's an outrage,' Jackie, the costume designer, declared, joining them. 'I can't get him out of this stuff now. I swear he wears it to bed.'

'Well, there's one way to find out,' he teased her.

Jackie's hands flew to her cheeks. 'Oh my God, did you hear that?' she gasped. 'Do you think he meant it?'

As the bantering continued, John's eyes kept going to Carla, and she knew that his decision not to greet her with the standard kiss was deliberate. Though disappointed, it excited her too, for she knew that the chemistry between them was becoming too powerful for them to engage in the careless physical contact they had with others.

'How was your flight?' he finally asked her.

Once again she was glad he couldn't see her eyes, for the way he was looking at her felt so intimate that she almost lost her smile. 'Fine,' she answered. Then, indicating his costume, 'Devastating.' He swept her a bow, and with a droll lift of an eyebrow, she said, 'I imagine there's quite a queue to be swept on to horseback when you gallop the beach at sunset.'

'Phoebe's started a lottery,' he answered, his smile doing things to her that she knew would prey on her mind later.

'Then I'll have to get myself a ticket,' she responded.

His eyes seemed to narrow as they moved over her face, bringing a faint colour to her cheeks and causing Avril to give a polite little cough.

'I think you're wanted,' she told him, nodding towards the unit. 'Something to do with a film shoot.'

Laughing, he tore his eyes from Carla, saying, 'I'll catch up with you later. I want to hear all about Geneva,' and he strode back across the sand to where the actors were waiting to rehearse the next shot.

'Do you know what I think?' Avril said, linking Carla's arm and walking her on down the beach into the cooling swirl of the waves. 'I think it's going to do you a power of good being here. Or it will if you, Miss-Got-To-Remain-Professional-At-All-Times, are sensible enough to take my advice.'

'Which is?'

Avril inhaled deeply, and as they both took a moment to gaze out at the glorious panorama of nothing but blue, sun-dappled sea and a perfectly cloudless sky, she said, 'My advice to you, Carla, is: detach and float.'

In the end it was Angelica Reed, the travel writer acting as guest presenter, who was swept up on to horseback and carried off into the sunset for the final shot of the day. The image was so perfectly romantic, with John's robes trailing in the wind, the thundering horse's hooves kicking up sand, and the fiery wash of the sun as Angelica was seized up into the saddle, that everyone agreed there was no point in going for another take. So after a close-up on John's face and a cutaway of the galloping hooves, a wrap was called. By then Carla had been briefed by the researchers on who was going where with the hand-held DVDs to get the footage that the main unit wouldn't have time to cover. She was also impressed by the amount of information they'd already collected regarding hotel and transport deals, all of which were necessary for the statements to camera, and she could see that she would have more than enough to do to catch up on the two days she'd missed.

Leaving the unit to pack up she and Avril rode back to the hotel in Masud's car, both shouting into their phones again, and all but oblivious to the stunning scenery they were shouting about, as Avril attempted to give an interview to a weekly magazine in London and Carla talked to a researcher who was at Nungwi, on the northern tip of the island, trying to find out what kind of material he was getting so she could prepare a covering script. When they finally arrived back they made straight for the bar, where they slumped down in a couple of capacious bamboo chairs under wildly whirring fans and loudly lamented the fact that they couldn't have ice in their drinks.

It wasn't long before the fleet of Land Cruisers carrying the unit began pulling up outside, depositing a hot, tired and dusty crew who were in dire need of refreshment before going off to shower. Presuming John had gone straight to his room, Carla asked Frazer if there was any chance of seeing the past three days' rushes, only to be told that John had already given instructions for them to be sent to her room so she could view them at her leisure.

Not wanting to get into whether he intended to come and view them with her, she decided to leave it till morning, as she was jet-lagged and hungry now, and probably wouldn't stay awake long after dinner.

'Hi, mind if I join you?'

Carla looked up to where Rosa, now wearing a loose cotton dress and sloppy sandals, was hovering with a tall glass of beer and a sunburned face. 'Feel free,' she said, avoiding Avril's stare as she airily waved Rosa to the chair Kit Kingsley had just vacated.

'Well, everything seems to be going to plan,' Rosa commented, helping herself to a handful of freshly roasted peanuts. 'Have you seen any rushes yet?'

Carla shook her head, then covered her mouth as she yawned. 'The best part, so far,' she said, 'is that we're on schedule. If it stays that way, we get Sunday off.'

'I hope so,' Rosa said. 'It'll be the only time we have for ourselves, except we'll be a long way from town.'

'Don't worry about that,' Carla assured her. 'I'll get Frazer, or Jaffah, to arrange some buses to bring back those who want to come. For anyone else there'll be plenty of snorkelling and swimming and diving up at Mapenzi Beach. Or so I'm told.'

Avril was staring hard at Rosa, not bothering to conceal her dislike, as the conversation fell into a brief and vaguely uneasy silence. In the end Rosa turned to Avril and treated her to such a scathing look that Avril almost laughed.

'So how was your Christmas?' Rosa asked Carla.

'Great. How was yours?' Carla answered, lifting her face to the fan.

'Oh, you know,' Rosa shrugged. 'New Year was better. What did you do?'

'We were in Somerset,' Carla replied.

'Oh.' Then, when no-one asked her, Rosa said, 'I went to a party at Chrissie and Richard's. There were only a dozen of us, and it was a bit, you know, but it was OK.'

Though Carla's expression didn't change, she was suddenly very tense inside and her heartbeat had noticeably altered.

Avril said smoothly, 'So you're still friendly with Chrissie, despite knowing she refused to cast you?'

Rosa's nostrils flared. 'I don't know if friendly's the word,' she responded haughtily. 'It's hard to be anything with someone who's in the kind of state she's in.'

Carla desperately didn't want to have this conversation, but for the moment seemed unable to steer herself out of it as Rosa continued with, 'She's so screwed up, I mean like *seriously* so. I really thought she was going to lose it altogether, not so long ago. Everyone did.' She shrugged. 'I have to admit she seems a bit better lately, but it makes you wonder how Richard puts up with it.'

Avril's and Carla's eyes met.

'I can't make the man out at all,' Rosa blundered on. 'I mean, on the one hand he's all over her, won't let her out of his sight, you know like he really, genuinely cares about her, and on the other, he's having affairs with at least three other women.'

Carla's heart stopped, as the blood drained from her face.

Avril said, 'How do you know that?'

'Jilly knows someone who knows one of them,' Rosa answered. 'She's an associate producer, or some kind of editor I think, at the Beeb. Then there's some waitress or other at the Groucho Club, and apparently he's still seeing that air stewardess he's been with for years. What *is* the man like, I ask you? But, hell, you know him better than most,' she said to Carla. 'I'll bet you're glad you're shot of him now. I know I would be.'

Carla's voice wasn't quite steady as she said, 'Rosa, just take your gossip somewhere else, OK?' Though she smiled there was no mistaking the chill in her tone.

Rosa's eyes widened with shock. 'Gosh, I'm sorry,' she cried. 'I didn't mean to upset you. Oh God, I thought you were over him by now. I mean, with the way things are between you and John . . .'

Carla's anger flared. 'What the hell are you talking about?' she demanded. 'There's nothing between me and John, and if you're spreading it about the unit that there is . . . Jesus Christ, I see what Chrissie meant now by how disruptive you are. You're a menace, Rosa. Now just go.'

Rosa was on her feet. 'Carla, I'm really sorry,' she said earnestly. 'I didn't mean any offence . . .'

'On your way,' Avril interrupted.

Rosa had barely left before Hugo's gangly frame flopped into the empty chair, and as he began talking about the shoot Frazer joined them too, then Kit returned with Phoebe and Yale, and before long John arrived, having swapped his Arab attire for khaki shorts and a white Ralph Lauren polo shirt, his hair still wet from the shower.

'OK, who's having what?' he demanded. 'Fraze, you can get them, and put them on your room. I don't want the producer on my case over a giant bar bill, she terrifies me witless as it is.'

As he looked at her, Carla felt the knots starting to loosen inside her, and a renewed warmth returning to her smile. 'Not quite so dashing,' she told him, meaning his clothes.

'But still utterly ravishing,' Phoebe finished.

His eyes remained on Carla's, as though she, not Phoebe, had spoken.

To break the moment Carla said, 'What are you going to drink?'

Pulling up a chair to sit between Kit and Yale, he said, 'I'll have one of those Kilimanjaro beers.'

After taking everyone else's order, Frazer transferred it all to a barman, then came back to join in the increasingly raucous exchange that was going on now that John was there. As the director, his presence seemed to sharpen everyone's wits and created such an eagerness to impress that the entire proceedings were heading fast towards the outrageous. Though she joined in from time to time, Carla was content to admire the way he handled himself, and the crew, with such guilelessness and humour. He was such an easy man to like, and seemed so unaffected by his looks and fame, that no-one ever had a problem relaxing with him – if anything, they all appeared so remarkably stress-free that they might have been on holiday, rather than in the grip of a punishing schedule.

As she watched him, listening and laughing, she began wondering about the man behind the charisma, since no-one's life escaped the vagaries of fate, and as untroubled, even blessed, as he appeared, she didn't imagine that

312

heartache and pain were unknown to him, for the simple reason they were strangers to no-one. But whatever his particular difficulties had been, or even were, he certainly didn't wear them on his sleeve, nor did he exhibit any signs of the bitterness or cynicism that so often settled over the scars of emotional wounds. He was simply there, in the thick of whatever was going on around him, with that wonderful gift of making everyone feel special, or incisive, or accomplished, or just plain entertaining. And she knew how heady a feeling it was to make him laugh, for she'd done it plenty of times herself, though probably not as often as he'd done it to her. It suddenly struck her how rarely Richard had made her laugh. They'd done so many other things together, but the kind of laughter and light-heartedness she experienced with John hadn't been a part of what she'd known with Richard. He was much more serious and cerebral, deeply into the pathos of life's recondite meanings, and the mind's unfathomable depths of knowledge and understanding. All of which made him extremely stimulating, and in many ways amusing, but he was never fun, the way John was fun, nor did he ever exhibit the same kind of interest in others, unless they were French and dead.

Realizing her criticism was a way of punishing him for what Rosa had said, she let the thoughts go and returned her mind entirely to John, who she knew was aware of her scrutiny. He winked at her, and as she smiled she felt an almost overwhelming affection for the way he flirted and fooled with her, and invariably stopped her taking herself so seriously. How much easier life seemed when he was around, she reflected, and what a gift it was to make someone feel that way. Even when they went into dinner, and began discussing the conference she and Avril had just come from, he made it all seem so exciting and achievable that her eagerness to get started on their new interactive project was only surpassed by her need, at that moment, to sleep.

Finally leaving him to go and join the others, she and Avril meandered back through the lamplit gardens to their rooms, too jet-lagged to hang on any longer. Though they talked, idly, neither of them mentioned Rosa, or what had been said earlier. It was as if, by unspoken agreement, they would treat

313

it as the unfounded gossip it probably was, though Avril knew she was much more inclined to believe it than not. However, she wouldn't mention that to Carla, for there was no point spoiling what was promising to be an extremely enjoyable shoot.

The following morning the crew left at six to make an early start filming the town. Though a few were starting to fall victim to the African diet already, their absence from the unit wasn't going to prove disastrous, though what they'd do if John or one of the main cast went down certainly would prove a problem. Already the temperature was soaring into the nineties as the Land Cruisers rolled out of the hotel's courtyard, heading for a complicated day, with a lot of crucial sequences to get through, and no doubt plenty of interested crowds to keep quiet and out of shot. Jaffah had hired some local men to help with the security, and apparently a few government officials were promising to show up too, to make sure things didn't get out of hand.

Carla didn't join the unit until lunch time, staying behind with Avril to watch rushes and discuss what they should do with Gus Ringborne, the freelance reporter, due to fly in later. Avril's London team had booked him to cover the shoot, while Jaffah had organized a photographer locally, who was already out there taking stills of the action.

Finally ready to leave, Carla picked up her hat, heavy bag and sunglasses, and trotted downstairs to where Avril was preparing to go and meet Gus at the airport. They'd already agreed that Masud would take her, while one of the unit cars was on its way to get Carla.

Reaching the bottom of the steps and hearing Avril still banging about inside her room, Carla paused to gaze out at the ocean that was shimmering white beneath a hot, milky sky, and inhaled deeply of the wonderful fragrances that wafted through the tropical gardens. An unexpected flutter of happiness stole through her, and the soothing warmth and light seemed to stir anew the feelings of anticipation and excitement she'd awoken with earlier. Avril was right, it really was doing her good to be here, for not only did the low grey skies and wintry darkness of England seem a whole world away, so too did the confusion of her relationship with Richard. It surprised her that Rosa's rumour-mongering last night hadn't had more of an effect, but once past the initial shock and anger she'd found herself unwilling even to think of him, which was why she hadn't checked that particular email address since arriving, nor would she for a while. She'd decided that this trip wasn't about him, nor his time here with Chrissie, it was only about her, and the programme, and, she had to admit it, the thrill of being around John.

Hearing the clop of Avril's mules she turned to ask what time she expected to be back, but got stuck on a gasp of laughter.

'What?' Avril asked.

'You're going like that?' Carla cried.

Avril looked down at the yellow T-shirt and cotton wraparound skirt she was wearing. 'What's the matter?' she demanded. But her eyes were sparkling with mischief, for the wide slash across the front of her T-shirt more than amply revealed the tops of her breasts. 'The plane's not due in for hours,' she said, slipping a sheer cotton shirt on over the T-shirt and fastening a few buttons, 'so I've agreed to go and get some shots of the bay John was talking about last night, and hopefully the dolphins too.'

With an undisguised wryness Carla made no further comment, simply followed her through the gardens and out to the front of the hotel where they found Masud looking more arresting than ever, in a long white tunic which was buttoned up to the neck, white cotton trousers and expensive leather sandals. He was chatting with the driver who'd come for Carla, but the moment he saw Avril his astute brown eyes were entirely on her.

'Incidentally, what kind of camera are you using?' Carla enquired, taking out her mobile as it started to ring. 'Stills or video?'

'Both,' Avril responded.

Grinning, Carla answered the call, while Avril attempted to tell Masud that she had to pop into the production office to pick up the cameras.

'Oh, hi John, how are you?' Carla said on hearing his voice. 'How's it all going?'

'Slowly. The heat's hard to deal with. When can we expect you?'

'I'm on my way now.' Handing her bag to the driver, she slipped into the back seat, and gave Avril a wave as the car began moving off down the drive. 'Where exactly are you?' she asked John.

'The old slave market. We finished outside Tippu-Tip's house about an hour ago. They're setting up the whipping post at the moment. It's pretty grim, and I think we should cut it.'

Carla thought about it, and quickly came to the conclusion he was right, for the inhuman practice of tying a man to a post and whipping him half to death – or even right to death – in order to test his strength, was indeed too horrific a part of the island's history to be re-enacted for the purposes of *There and Beyond*. 'OK, drop it,' she said. 'I'll take a look at the script and have it reworked by the time I get there.'

There was a pause before he said, 'Did you manage to see the rushes?'

'It's what I've been doing most of the morning. We'll talk when I get there.'

His smile was audible. 'That sounds ominous,' he responded.

She smiled too. 'I'm sure you know what I think,' she said.

'Reading your mind is a skill I haven't yet acquired,' he replied.

'Then maybe I should feel thankful for that,' she answered, and after hearing him laugh she rang off.

It took a little less than an hour for Masud to drive Avril to the south coast fishing village of Kizimkazi. They were met on the beach by an agile young boatman, who cheerily handed her into his vessel and sped her out into the bay where at least a dozen bottle-nosed dolphins were putting on quite a show for a small boatload of tourists who were already there. Using both cameras Avril easily and expertly captured the kind of shots even a wildlife programme would applaud, and was so entranced by the dolphins' performance that she stayed watching much longer than she needed, for the massive, graceful creatures with their silvery smooth flesh and happy smiles were hard to tear herself away from. Eventually, however, she signalled to the boatman to take her back to shore, where Masud was waiting to drive her on to the coastal spot John had circled on the map. Apparently it was a deserted bay with the kind of pristine beach and clear blue ocean views he needed for a special-effects sequence.

As they drove away, heading out of the village and along a badly pitted and rocky coast road, Avril casually shrugged off her over-shirt, and threw it onto the back seat. After a while she turned to look at Masud's imposingly regal profile, and gave him a quick smile as he glanced her way. For a long, anticipatory moment she allowed her eyes to linger on the hand he had resting on the gearstick, then feeling a deep, slow burn spreading all the way through her, she stretched out her limbs, before turning to gaze out of the window.

A while later the Cruiser turned off the road, and began a more cautious drive along a much narrower track that led finally to the bay. It was indeed breathtaking, and, seizing both cameras, Avril climbed out of the car to begin a series of wide shots to capture the backward curl of the spray as it was flung from the coral rocks. Then, repositioning herself, and refocusing the lens, she recorded close-ups of the foaming surf rolling on to the sand. There were no stills required for this location, so the film she loaded into the Nikon, after returning the DVD to the car, was her own, to take shots of whatever she wished. When the camera was ready she raised her eyes to Masud, who was still in the driver's seat, watching her every move.

Smiling, she turned away, and, with her back to the car, began taking random shots of the spectacular sun-drenched beach with its small clusters of orange and pink rock and impossibly fine sand. After a while she glanced back over her shoulder, then held the camera out to Masud, asking him to take some pictures of her. Obediently he stepped down from the car, and, taking the camera, remained standing on the grassy bank as she descended the gently sloping beach towards the waves.

The first shots he took were of her standing in the surf, hair and skirt blowing in the breeze, wicked abandon shining in her eyes. Then, after beckoning for him to come closer, she began striking a series of sultry and outrageous poses, until finally she tugged down the hem of her T-shirt so that her breasts were fully revealed through the gash. His only response was to carry on clicking, as though he did this every day of his life, and even drop to one knee as she removed her skirt to expose her nakedness beneath, then sat down in the waves, legs slightly apart, to allow the flowing water to soothe her burning flesh.

When the film was used up she walked towards him, carrying her T-shirt and skirt, and keeping her eyes on his as he lowered the camera to watch her come. Though there was no question he was as aroused as she was, he merely gestured politely for her to return to the car and followed on behind. When she got there he began speaking in what she presumed was Swahili, and turning round she saw that he had a hand outstretched, asking for her clothes. Dutifully she handed them over, and watched as he folded them carefully, then laid them on the back seat, before opening the passenger door for her to climb in.

After turning the car round he headed back to the road, and didn't speak again for several miles, only looking at her from time to time, seeming to admire her body, though making no attempt to touch it. They passed few other vehicles, though saw plenty of men toiling the land, who might or might not have noticed her bare breasts as Masud slowed the vehicle to plunge carefully into potholes and bring them smoothly out the other side. For Avril, the whole experience was so unspeakably erotic that when finally he stopped, a mile or so from the airport, and handed her her clothes, the last thing she wanted was to put them on.

Laughter rang around the old marketplace where the grassy centre island with its succulent red dwarf palms and leafy rain trees provided the only cover from a blistering afternoon sun. The unit base was behind the church, shielded by parasols and stocked with ice-cold drinks. These were regularly ferried out to the actors, who were suffering nobly in the heat now that the sun had appeared over the crenellated ramparts of the slave-market building that had earlier provided some shade. Yale Winfield, as Tippu-Tip the infamous trader, had just, in the middle of an extremely tense stand-off with a customs official, threatened to 'lip out' the man's 'river' instead of rip out his liver, which was what had prompted the laughter, and Hugo's ensuing 'Cut!'

'Sorry John,' Yale bellowed across the square, 'but these feeth don't quite tit!'

Laughing, John signalled Hugo to reset from the top, and walked over to join Yale and Phoebe, who, as the prized slave girl, was heavily adorned with bracelets, necklaces and earrings, which were just a part of the package to make her more attractive to buyers.

Running a cool damp towel around her neck, Carla watched as they reset for the third take of this particular shot, in which Phoebe's ears, eyes and teeth were crudely inspected by a potential buyer, while the customs official harangued her trader for unpaid taxes. This was a very dark note in the island's history that rang so long and discordant that it simply couldn't be ignored, but John was right, it wasn't necessary to dwell on it.

'What do you think?' John murmured as he came to join her in the shade of a passenger palm, so called because it was a tree everyone paused under to take shelter.

'I'm not sure,' she answered, as an assistant handed him a bottle of chilled water.

'Me neither.' He drank deeply, then, wiping his mouth with the back of his hand, he said, 'Let's just get it in the can, then decide when we edit how much to use.'

Carla took the bottle he was offering, and drank too, then looked up as she realized he was watching her. Raising a humorous eyebrow, she walked off in answer to Frazer's yelled demand to know where she was, and wondered what it was about the heat that made such commonplaces as the sharing of water feel as intimate as an embrace, and unspoken attractions seem to find their own voice.

By the end of the day, which, even despite the cuts, went two hours beyond schedule, everyone was tired and more than ready to return to the relaxing, uncomplicated ambience of the Fisherman's Resort. Carla and John rode in the same car, sharing it with Phoebe and Kit Kingsley, talking over the exceptional material they'd managed to capture, and how it

319

was going to cut together. When they got back Carla waited as John talked to the sound-recordist about the local Taarab music he wanted taped, then before he could disappear to his room she stopped him and said, 'We haven't discussed the rushes yet.'

His eyes remained on hers.

'What I saw this morning is making me wonder how it's all going to look when you put it together. You've got some unusual ideas.'

He continued to look at her in the moonlight, and her heartbeat quickened as the expression in his eyes seemed to intensify the moment, and maybe, had it not been for the arrival of another crew car, bathing them in light, one of them might have taken that fateful step across the invisible barrier they'd drawn that forbade all physical contact for fear of where it might lead.

She was the first to turn away, her senses blurring and her breath shallow as she attempted to remind herself that this was only the first of six programmes, so for them to become involved now could prove not only complicated, but potentially disastrous.

'So did you meet Gus all right?' she asked Avril later, as they strolled over to the dining room.

'Yep. He's here,' Avril answered. 'Went straight to bed, so we might not see him till morning.'

Carla allowed a couple of seconds to pass, then in a nonchalant tone asked, 'And did you manage to get much footage this morning?'

Avril feigned surprise. 'Of course,' she answered. 'The dolphin display's going to blow your mind, and I think John's going to be very happy with the deserted tropical beach.'

They walked on, watching the moon shimmer a path along the sea, and listening to the harsh buzz of cicadas rising up from the gardens. 'You know what I admire most about you,' Carla suddenly said, 'is how honest you are with yourself.'

Avril accepted the compliment with a laugh. 'I'll let you into a secret,' she said, 'being honest with yourself is easy once you stop being afraid of the truth.'

Carla winced. 'Is that what you think?' she said. 'That I'm afraid of the truth?'

320

'Yes,' Avril responded, 'but you're not on your own, because most people would rather hide behind self-deception and delusion than face up to reality.'

Carla didn't know what to say to that, so she remained silent, watching the fireflies drifting in and out of the bushes, their tiny lights seeming as elusive as her thoughts. Then with an abrupt recall of where the conversation had begun she cried, 'Just a minute, how did we manage to go from your morning excursion to a deeply depressing dig at my psyche?'

Avril grinned. 'Funny how one led to the other, isn't it?' she quipped.

Carla's eyes narrowed, then, following her into the bar, she was about to order a drink when she was waylaid by Jaffah who was asking for a quiet word.

Once out of earshot Jaffah said meekly, 'Is OK for me to ask question?'

Carla smiled encouragingly. 'Of course.'

Jaffah smiled too, then with a nervous glance down at his hands, he said, 'I want to ask why is lady who come here first time not come again? She very lovely lady. My family like her very much.'

Knowing exactly who he meant Carla felt the warmth drain from her smile, but there was no way of avoiding the question, so in as neutral a voice as she could muster she said, 'I'm afraid she doesn't work with us any more.'

'Oh,' he said, clearly disappointed. 'I hope you gonna say she coming soon.'

Carla shook her head.

'What happen to her?' he asked. 'Why she not work with you now?'

'She . . . She got married and had a baby,' Carla answered, the words only just making it past the dryness in her throat. 'She married the man who was here with her. I expect you met him.' Her heart sank at such stupidity, for he was now going to tell her everything she didn't need to hear, like what a wonderful man Jaffah thought Richard was, and so lucky to have such a beautiful woman as Chrissie. And how it was in this very hotel that Chrissie had first told Richard she was pregnant, then they had shared their good news with Jaffah. In fact, Carla could almost see the tenderness in Richard's

321

eyes as he folded Chrissie in his arms and asked her to be his wife. How she wished that no longer had the power to hurt, but it did, and now she was probably going to find out that the proposal had happened in this very bar . . .

'I sorry, I no understand,' Jaffah said, frowning. 'There no man here with her. I only man with her.'

Carla looked at him, her self-torment coming to such a sudden stop that it was a moment before she registered what he had said. But obviously he hadn't understood.

'Why you say man with her?' he pressed. 'I see her every day. All time she alone.'

Carla was still staring at him. Maybe she was the one who didn't understand, though his words couldn't have been simpler, nor his certainty more convincing. 'Alone?' she echoed.

He nodded.

No, he'd obviously got it wrong, because she knew Richard had been here, so maybe they were talking about different people. 'You do mean Chrissie?' she said. 'Tall, blonde hair . . .'

'Yes, yes, Chrissie,' he confirmed.

Carla was beginning to feel light-headed. 'And she was here alone?' she said. 'You didn't see the man who was travelling with her?'

'No-one travel with her,' he said. 'I meet her from plane, and I with her all the time.'

Carla's eyes remained on his, as she tried to remember exactly how she'd found out that Richard was in Zanzibar when he was supposed to be in Kosovo . . . It must have been Chrissie who'd told her, on that terrible morning when her mother had died and Chrissie had come to tell her she was pregnant . . . She couldn't actually remember Chrissie's words now, but she was sure she'd mentioned Zanzibar. Or had she? It was all such a blur, and the shock had been so immense that maybe she only thought she remembered . . . Maybe Chrissie hadn't mentioned it at all and she had just assumed . . . She looked at Jaffah, whose confusion couldn't appear more genuine, and as she began to realize that there was a very good chance he was telling the truth she felt the stirrings of relief lightening her heart, as though in some way she was being set free. Of course, even if he was telling the truth, it didn't change anything – the betrayal and duplicity had still happened, so had the wedding, so had the baby – but if Richard really hadn't been to Zanzibar . . .

'Will you excuse me,' she said, and, after signalling to Avril that she wouldn't be long, she ran back to her room and quickly set up her computer.

Minutes later she was reading a message from Richard that was making her heart thud with confusion. 'Zanzibar is a truly beautiful island,' he'd written, 'and much more worthy of your programme than it ever was of my visit with Chrissie. We thought it would allow us some freedom in our affair, a brief respite from having to shroud ourselves in secrecy, but how wrong we were, because neither of us forgot you for a moment, and now I wish with all my heart that I could be there with you.'

She stopped reading and gazed blankly at the wall. What on earth was going on? Jaffah had seemed so sure, yet this message couldn't be more clear. He'd been here, with Chrissie, but for some reason Jaffah hadn't seen him.

'It doesn't make any sense,' she said to Avril when she returned to the bar. 'Why would he have hidden from Jaffah?'

Avril rolled her eyes. 'Why would Richard do anything?'

'Richard who?' Kit demanded, coming to join them.

Carla looked up and smiled. 'No-one,' she answered, and, sliding effortlessly into her producer's role, she said, 'I'm glad to see you, because I want to talk about these extra lights.'

Leaving them to it, Avril wandered over to join John and Phoebe who were on their way in to dinner. This news about Richard was making her more suspicious and uneasy than ever, for nothing about the man, or the way he'd behaved these past few months, was making any sense at all, and the fact that Carla seemed unwilling to do anything about it was frustrating in the extreme. After all, it wasn't as if Carla had no doubts of her own, but getting her to act on them, or even voice them, was proving damned near impossible. Well, Carla could keep her head buried in the sand for as long as she liked, but there was no way in the world Avril was going to join her. She wanted to know what that man was about, and the minute they got back to London she was going to start finding out.

Chapter 19

After five full days of shooting in the main town and surrounding spice plantations the unit travelled across the island and north to Mapenzi Beach, where a strong and constant breeze blew in from the ocean, making the forty-degree temperature slightly easier to handle than the oppressive humidity of the dense and malodorous town. For those whose digestive systems were still in trouble, life definitely became more bearable, as this part of the shoot was concentrating on the sprawling white hotel with its typical coconut-thatched roofs and the exquisite silvery stretch of beach beyond. Since there were other guests staying, some members of the unit were having to double up, so it wasn't long before the inevitable jokes about their partner's sleeping or hygiene habits started to abound. And as for the blossoming affairs, well, Carla didn't ask, though she was in no doubt of their existence – she just hoped they didn't end up causing any problems.

The quaint little ocean-front bungalow she was sharing with Avril was simply furnished: two single beds with mustard-coloured covers and white muslin drapes, a large minga-wood chest of drawers with dull brass handles, a set of narrow, leaded-glass French windows that opened onto the beach, and a cooling clay-tiled floor with a couple of green and purple rush mats next to the beds. It was where they were now, taking refuge from the sun, much like the rest of the unit who'd been more than happy to take advantage of the unscheduled siesta, before shooting again this evening.

While Avril dozed Carla stared at the joyously contorting figures of the colourful 'batik' painting that was facing her bed, and thought about going online to check if there was any more mail from Richard. The idea had no appeal, however, for the pleasure of lying there, beneath the fan, feeling her body responding to thoughts she should really be avoiding, was simply too blissful to give up.

Smiling sleepily to herself she turned onto her side and wondered if John ever thought about her the same way, and if he did, was it possible that their thoughts, in some other dimension, were morphing into reality? An interesting idea, but too artificial to rival the very physical pleasure she was experiencing now. Better still would be if he were to come quietly into the room, lie down beside her and start to undress her. A small sigh shuddered from her, as her mind moved on through the exquisite feel of his hands on her skin, his tongue in her mouth, his legs between hers . . .

Sighing as someone knocked on the door, she swung her feet to the floor and went to see who it was, half-annoyed and half-relieved to have been torn from such a crucial moment. 'Gus?' she said, surprised to see the reporter. 'You're not still interviewing, in this heat?'

'No,' he answered, dabbing his face with a towel. 'I've just been for a swim, and I thought, while no-one else is around . . .' He looked anxiously past her to where Avril was still sleeping. 'Is there somewhere we can talk?'

Carla's eyebrows went up. 'Is everything all right?' she said.

'I'm not sure. Nothing to panic about, but there are certain things you should know . . .'

Curious, and not a little concerned, Carla said, 'I'll meet you in the bar. Say, five minutes?'

After he'd gone, she went into the bathroom for a quick freshen-up, pulled a T-shirt on over her shorts and crop top, then, letting herself quietly out of the room, she wandered along the beach to the steps that zigzagged up to the hotel. There was hardly anyone around, though she soon spotted Gus, on the half-moon terrace that overlooked the glistening blue pool with its surrounding loungers and parasols.

'You've got me worried,' she told him, sitting down and signalling the waiter to bring her a passion-fruit punch as she stretched her legs out into the sun.

'Sorry,' he said, stubbing out a cigarette and immediately taking another from its packet.

She watched him light it, noticing the awkwardness of his movements, though this was typical of Gus, whom she'd known for several years, so there was no need to read anything into it – right now though, she was finding it hard not to. 'Come on, don't keep me in suspense,' she chided.

'No. No,' he said, waving away a cloud of smoke. 'It's just . . . Well, I've managed to talk to a few of the cast and what I'm getting's going to make a pretty good piece. The local photographer's been getting some good still shots too. Obviously John's the one everyone wants to read about, so nothing's going to pull together until he can spare me some time, then I'll need to talk to Avril about where she wants me to sell it . . .'

'Gus, come to the point,' Carla said softly.

He nodded, took another puff and said, 'We're friends, Carla. I like you, and I don't want to write anything bad about this shoot, which is why I'm telling you what I've been hearing. If it were anyone else, I'd be filing an exclusive.'

Carla's smile was fading. 'So what have you been hearing?' she prompted.

'Things about Avril. You too, and about how some of the crew are taking drugs . . .'

'What!' Carla cried. 'Gus, this is serious. If you even so much as hint that drugs are being taken on this unit, my programme's finished. We'll never get permission to film anywhere else, our sponsors will pull out . . .'

'It's OK,' he assured her. 'I'm not going to do it. And to be honest, I don't think it's happening, and even if it is, it's probably the locals, which you can't do anything about. I just want you to be aware that someone's spreading these rumours, and though I might not intend going to print with them, there's a good chance she'll find someone who will.'

'She?'

His eyes fixed on hers.

Carla stared back, then her eyes closed, as, sighing, she said, 'Rosa Gingell.'

He nodded.

326

'That damned woman!' she muttered. 'So what's she been saying about me and Avril?'

His eyes went down as he flicked ash from his cigarette. 'It's mainly about Avril,' he said. Then with an embarrassed laugh, 'I don't want to spell it out, but she's putting a pretty sordid spin on whatever Avril's got going with that driver. For the right publication it might make sensational copy, especially with the pot-smoking allegations, and the bribery of local officials . . .'

'Bribery?' Carla cried.

'That's what she intimated you're up to. And I mean you personally. She's making it sound as though you're paying them to turn a blind eye to the drugs.'

Carla's eyes closed. 'We pay facility fees, just like any other unit,' she told him through her teeth. 'You know that.'

'Of course. I just want you to know the way she's telling the story.'

Carla turned to look down at the pool, watching the clear blue water glisten and ripple, as she considered the best way to handle this. To fire Rosa and send her back would be favourite, were it not the kind of knee-jerk reaction guaranteed to bring the worst results. Besides she had further scenes to shoot, so they couldn't get rid of her now. But something had to be done, so maybe she should discuss the problem with John – and Avril – before coming to a decision on what action to take.

'Gus, I really appreciate you telling me this,' she said, looking up as Jaffah wandered into the bar. 'I know you'll keep it to yourself, but if you hear anything else . . .'

'You'll be the first to know,' he assured her.

'Is OK for me to sit with you?' Jaffah said, respectfully holding back.

'Of course,' Carla assured him. 'In fact you're just the person I want to see. Will you have a drink?'

He glanced over at the barman. 'Same,' he said, indicating the glasses of passion-fruit juice already on the table.

'Don't take it personally,' Gus told him, getting up, 'but I'm in need of a shower. See you later,' he added to Carla.

After he'd gone Carla waited only until Jaffah had his drink before asking him bluntly if he knew anything about the local crew members taking drugs. To her relief he couldn't have looked more shocked, as his hand froze in mid-air and he stared at her in horror. Then, setting his glass back on the table, he spoke very earnestly as he said, 'I don't think is true, but Jaffah will make certain, and if is true, I call my cousin in the police and he arrest them.' He was shaking his head gravely. 'Is very bad thing, drugs. Is problem all over . . .'

'Yes, but hopefully not on this shoot,' Carla interrupted, more sharply than she'd intended, and he looked so chastened that she immediately said, 'It's OK, I know you'll take care of it.'

'Oh yes, yes,' he assured her. 'I take care of it now.'

'No,' she laughed as he started to get up, 'finish your drink. Everyone's asleep anyway. And besides, I think now is a very good time to tell you how indebted we all are to you for the way you've helped us with this shoot. In fact, we couldn't have done it without you, and if we do manage to get Sunday off, it'll be largely down to you and your outstanding organizational skills.'

His cheeks flushed with pleasure. 'Ah, yes, Sunday,' he said. 'I arrange for all equipment to go to Sultan's Palace Hotel, early in morning. Then all the people can take bus into Stone Town for the sightseeing and shopping, or stay here and make diving. Later Land Cruisers take everyone to Sultan's Palace when shopping and sports is finished.'

'Perfect,' Carla smiled, wondering how to broach the subject of Chrissie again.

Brimming over, he said, 'Mr John, he ask me to rent him car on Sunday. So car coming early, same time as bus.'

Carla's insides fluttered as she wondered where John was intending to go. 'Good. Very good,' she said.

Jaffah raised his glass, and after saluting her, drained it in one go.

At the sound of a splash Carla looked down at the pool, and watched the diver glide along the bottom, then slowly surface, to begin lapping with a grace and style it was hard not to envy. She'd barely had time for any swimming herself, and secretly she'd been hoping that on Sunday she and John might go somewhere together . . . But she had to stop thinking that way, it was the route to disaster, and besides, the hire-car obviously meant he had other plans, which was good, because if they were alone, and so scantily dressed, it would be just about impossible to suppress the physical yearning of her body, and as powerfully as she wanted it . . .

'Mr John!' Jaffah cried, suddenly leaping to his feet.

Carla started, then turned to look over her shoulder, and, seeing John coming towards them, felt a wave of pure pleasure coast over her heart. 'I thought you'd be sleeping,' she said.

'Funny, that's what I thought you were doing,' he responded, sitting down next to her. Then to Jaffah, 'Any luck with the car?'

'Oh yes. I tell Miss Carla. It come Sunday, early, when bus come.'

John nodded. 'Good man. So did you manage a siesta?' he asked Carla.

'Of sorts,' she answered, meeting his eyes and remembering those few minutes she'd spent lying on the bed. 'Actually, there's something I need to talk to you about,' she told him.

'You please excuse me,' Jaffah said, with several little bows. 'You talk in private.'

'It's OK,' Carla assured him, as more crew began strolling up from their beach-front bungalows. 'Stay and finish your drink.' Then to John, 'Let's go over to my room.'

His eyebrows waggled, making her smile – and only wish that it could be that easy.

As they strolled along past the pool, and down the steps to the peppery-white beach, he began talking about the drama sequence they were shooting the next day. 'I'm not worried about our guys,' he said, 'most of them will have done this kind of thing before. It's the extras we might have a problem with, so I'm going to try to shoot it in a way that calls for no more than three, and just have them wading ashore.'

She nodded thoughtfully. 'That should work,' she said. 'In fact, we really only need to see Gary, don't we?'

'And Phoebe,' he reminded her.

'Of course.' Then she added, 'Do you think I've been over-optimistic telling everyone they can have Sunday off? I mean, if we run over tomorrow . . .'

'If we do, we'll just have to cancel the day off,' he said. 'But we won't.'

She looked at him. 'You seem rather definite about that.'

'I'm trying to be,' he responded.

They walked the next few paces in silence, winding through the palms and mangroves that were growing up all over the beach, and feeling the soft warm sand seep in between their toes. She was wondering about the hire-car, and if it would seem too inquisitive to ask what he had planned for the day. Probably not, though in the end all she said was, 'Well, I hope we don't have to cancel. Everyone needs a break, and it's going to be a bit tough coming to a place like this and not having any time off.'

After glancing at her briefly, he said, 'So what are you planning to do with Sunday, if it does stay free?'

'I haven't really thought about it,' she answered. 'Maybe work. Sunbathe. I'm not sure.'

It was a moment before she realized he'd stopped, and, turning round to see why, she felt her heart leap when she found him looking at her with the same intense dark eyes that haunted every one of her dreams.

'Spend the day with me,' he said. 'Just the two of us.'

Immediately her insides turned weak and as her heart started to pound she said, 'You mean . . .?'

'Yes,' he said quietly, 'that's exactly what I mean.'

Desire seared through her, and, knowing she was incapable of any other answer, she nodded, then turned to walk on.

Though she questioned her decision a thousand times over the next twenty-four hours, the dread she harboured that the shoot might run over was so beyond a producer's normal concern that really, there was never any doubt Sunday morning would find her right where she was, in a state of high anticipation, as she showered and dressed for the day ahead. Though she'd been awake half the night, concerned by the way her self-protection was rolling back like a tide, leaving her vulnerable and exposed, she kept reminding herself that John wasn't Richard, in fact was nothing like him, and the last thing she wanted was to give in to the fear of ever trusting again.

'Am I mad? Am I completely insane?' she demanded of Avril, as she plugged her mobile phone into her computer's modem. 'I mean fantasizing about it, and longing for it is one thing, but actually going through with it, when there's so much at stake . . . Shall I wear that hat, by the way, or does it look a bit OTT? God, this thing takes ages to connect. Do you have any sunblock, I've used all mine?'

'Here,' Avril said, tossing a tube of Clarins on to Carla's bed. 'What time are you leaving?'

Carla glanced at her watch and felt her stomach turn over. 'In fifteen minutes.'

'Do you know where you're going yet?'

'I know the Jozani Forest Reserve is our first stop,' Carla answered. 'After that . . .' Her breath gave out, and, laughing, she said, 'So what are your plans today? Has Masud managed to find a few square inches you haven't yet explored?'

Avril grinned. 'Actually,' she said, 'I'm going diving with Kit and a few of the others.'

Carla looked up in surprise, but Avril was already disappearing into the bathroom. 'So the romance is over?' Carla called out, picking up a brush and pulling it through her hair.

'No,' Avril answered, 'though I wouldn't call it a romance.'

'Really? Then what would you call it?'

There was a moment as Avril thought, then she said, 'An understanding. Yes, that's what I'd call it. Masud understands me in a way most men fail to, and the remarkable part of that is that we don't even speak each other's language.'

Carla was intrigued, though probed no further, as she watched her computer making the on-line connection.

'By the way, I talked to Gus about Rosa,' Avril called out.

'Good!' Carla shouted back. 'Is he willing to do what you're suggesting?'

'Yep. He's a good guy.' She popped her head round the door. 'Do you need any condoms?'

Carla's insides dissolved. 'Stop that,' she laughed.

'I'm sure John'll have some,' Avril said, already back in the bathroom. 'Any mineral water left? I need some to clean my teeth.'

'On the nightstand.'

There was only one message, from Richard.

'I don't know why you're doing that, when you're about to go off with John for the day,' Avril remarked as she came back into the room. 'Or are you looking for an excuse not to go?'

Carla's eyes were on the screen. 'I'm going,' she said firmly.

Avril picked up the water, and was about to return to the bathroom when Carla murmured, 'That's so strange. He's still saying he was here.'

'Did you talk to Jaffah again?' Avril asked.

'Not yet.'

Tucking her towel in tighter, Avril went to read over Carla's shoulder. '". . . wish with all my heart that I could be there with you, watching your face as you drink in the island's beauty, and feeling your heart beat with the pleasure of discovery. Maybe you are now in places that I have already visited, when in my foolishness I thought I loved another woman more than I loved you. So much has changed for us, and the love I feel . . ."' She stopped as Carla suddenly closed down the screen.

'I don't know what's going on,' she declared, 'whether he was ever here or not, but I've got no intention of spending a single moment of today trying to work it out.'

'Good for you,' Avril cheered. 'You just go have yourself a wonderful time with a wonderful man, because God knows you deserve it.'

Carla's eyes softened, and, getting up from the chair, she turned her back on the computer and thought of John, whose reality as a man was so much more appealing right now than Richard's poetic, but disembodied attempts to keep their love alive. 'I'm *so* looking forward to this,' she confessed.

Avril smiled, then took a step back to cast a critical eye over the sleeveless silk georgette dress Carla was wearing, which fluttered to the ankles, but split right up to the thigh, the soft pale green fabric of the bodice and shoestring shoulder straps showing that there was no bra underneath. 'He's a lucky man,' Avril told her. 'But I don't think he needs me to tell him that.'

An hour later Carla was beside John in the car, gazing out at the passing countryside, where local women, shrouded in brightly coloured robes, drew urns of water from wells, while others ground maize on primitive stone wheels, and still others transported fraying baskets of fruit, or charcoal, on their heads. The small villages of mud-and-stick huts were mostly tucked into the shelter of trees, where cows with flesh like worn rags stood silently enduring the heat, and children scuffed footballs about in the dust. Overhead the sky blazed an impossible blue, while plantations of mangos, papayas, coconuts and bananas soon gave way to those of cloves, cumin, ginger, coriander and saffron.

Since the road was hard to travel with so many boulders and potholes, they rarely spoke, though occasionally their eyes met, and knowing they were thinking the same thoughts seemed to intensify the already charged air between them.

'Did you tell Avril about today?' he asked, when finally they began travelling a smoother road.

She turned to look at him. 'Do you mind?'

His eyes lingered a moment on hers before he turned back to the road. 'Why would I mind?' he said, pulling out round an ox-drawn cart.

Her eyebrows drew together. 'I'm not sure how to answer that,' she responded.

'I don't mind,' he told her. Then, looking at her again, 'I'm glad you came.'

Her chest felt tight, and a spasm of desire cut through her with such force that she started to wonder how she was going to get through the next few hours without begging him to take her right there on the roadside, or in the car, or against a tree, or . . . Reaching into her bag for the guidebook, she quickly flicked through to the relevant pages and began reading aloud. '"The Zanzibar red colobus monkey is one of Africa's rarest primates, and is to be found in the Jozani Forest . . ."'

'Are you nervous?' he interrupted.

'Yes. Are you?'

'No.'

She turned to find him laughing; then, laughing too, she tossed the book over her shoulder and, lifting her feet onto the dashboard, returned to gazing out of the window, where the trees were becoming denser now, and the ramshackle mud-and-stick dwellings ever more humble. Yes, she was nervous, and excited, and very glad she'd come, despite the occasional thoughts of Richard that made her feel strange about being with another man. Fortunately, they were easily ignored, though she wasn't naive enough to believe that the damage of past experience wasn't going to try playing some kind of part in the day. However, she wasn't going to encourage it, so maybe it would help pacify her concerns about trust and honesty, and any other issues that might be lurking, to try taking her mind off it for a while. The guidebook hadn't worked, so maybe the programme would.

'OK,' she said, 'I know we weren't going to talk shop today, but I'm breaking the rules. Has anyone been out to the forest yet to get some footage? Maybe we should have brought a camera.'

'Verna did it before you arrived,' he answered. 'You haven't seen the rushes?'

'I've only had time to see the ones you've shot. Did she get any monkeys?'

'About a dozen. Apparently they're not hard to find, or not for the guides.'

'What about a dhow under sail, and footage around the reef?'

'Avril and Kit are doing it, possibly as we speak.' He glanced over at her. 'Did anyone give you a copy of the schedule?'

Chuckling, she said, 'I just want to make sure it's all happening. So how about giving me a rough rundown of how you're intending to put all the modern sequences together?'

As they continued to talk she felt at least some of the tension leaving her body, and before long they were both so absorbed in the programme's structure that they were still discussing it when they turned into the Jozani Forest Reserve, and bumped along the track to the ranger's station.

The instant they stepped out into the thick, humid air the noise of the forest assailed them, twittering, chattering, squawking, buzzing, a symphony of tropical sounds that was both haunting and shrill. Carla looked around at the rickety palm-thatch hut and various wooden boards that made up the station, where sketches and photographs of the forests' inhabitants were pinned up alongside grubby T-shirts and oversized shorts that were presumably for sale. While John went to negotiate with a guide she picked up a few brochures and postcards that would help with writing the commentary, then, after taking them to the car, she strolled over to where he was just closing a deal.

'This is Akili,' he said, introducing the gangly, solemn-faced youth who was to be their guide.

'Akili mean wisdom,' the boy gravely informed them.

Carla held out a hand to shake. *'Jina langu ni* Carla,' she said. *'Ninatoka* England.'

John's eyes were dancing. *'Jina langu ni* John,' he added, but didn't attempt to shake hands, since Akili was shouting something at one of his colleagues.

'You follow,' he said, apparently unimpressed with their Berlitz Swahili.

Carla glanced at John, whose ironic smile matched her own, then she started after the boy who was already moving off along a narrow, shady trail that twisted through the rubbery foliage of giant banana palms that overhung the path like fat green tongues. Though Akili wiped away the cloying nets of spiders' webs, Carla was glad of her hat, since many of the silvery strands were left dangling and seemed all too keen to make her acquaintance. However, the trail soon widened, and they were better able to see the way trees and vines writhed and tangled in a choking struggle to reach the sun, while tiny blue butterflies flitted amongst the shrubs like confetti. With Akili's expert guidance they soon began identifying the high-pitched screech of hornbills, and the rich fluted tones of a red-capped robin, even the click and trill of a dark-backed weaver. The boy certainly knew his birds, Carla reflected, as she listened to him mimicking their calls, and apparently getting along rather well with a little greenbul. Since a host of other creatures could be heard bleating and hissing and scuttling about in the underbrush, she tried not to think of snakes and trod carefully into Akili's footprints as he finished making a date, or whatever he was doing, and moved on.

Finally, about three-quarters of a mile in, they came upon a cool, sunny glade, where an old tamarind tree had entwined its limbs with those of a wild fig, to provide a blissful shelter from the midday sun. Akili was at the foot of the fig gazing up into the shadowy umbrella of leaves. 'See, there,' he said glumly.

Removing her hat, Carla stepped round behind him, frowning as she tried to find what he was pointing at.

'There,' he said, pointing harder. 'You see him. He see you.'

'I see him,' John said softly.

Then Carla did too, and broke into a smile, for the monkey's leathery black face and startling shock of spiky white hair were exactly like those she had seen in the guidebook, so she knew it was a red colobus – though quite what he might be making of the strange faces staring up at him was anyone's guess. 'Do you think he considers us to be another species of animal?' she whispered.

'No, he knows we're humans,' John answered glibly.

She turned to look at him. 'What I meant was, do you think he feels threatened by us?'

John looked at Akili, who shook his head. 'He know we not hurt him,' he said. 'He used to people. Maybe family in almond tree, over there.'

As he lumbered off Carla returned her gaze to the monkey above and was about to whisper again when John moved closer and her breath was lost in a sudden swell of desire. Her eyes remained where they were, able to make out the long red tail now, and lugubrious blink of his eyelids, though all she could hear was the thump of her heart. When she finally felt able, she said softly, 'You can't look at him without wondering if we were like that once, can you?'

'I was never that ugly,' John assured her.

Choking back a laugh, she said, 'I think he's cute.'

They continued to look up, though were so intensely aware of their closeness that it startled them both when the monkey suddenly swung itself up to a higher branch. 'I wonder how evolution fits in with reincarnation and past lives,' Carla said, in a voice that wasn't quite steady.

He didn't answer, and she was almost afraid to look round.

'Do you believe we've lived before?' she said. 'In another place, another time?'

'I think it's possible,' he answered.

336

'What about soulmates? Do you think that's possible?'

'Do you?'

'I don't know. I used to.' She turned to look at him, and found his mouth so close she could almost feel his breath. Seconds ticked by, filled with the hiss and scream of the forest, as he took in every curve and hollow of her face, every plane and shadow. Then he was looking only at her lips, watching them part in readiness for his own . . .

'Family over here,' Akili said, making an untimely return.

Carla's breath expelled in a laugh, as John rolled his eyes, and laughed too.

Obediently they went to look at the family, most of whom were sleeping, though the babies were curious and playful, and might, at any other time, have been even more enchanting than they seemed right now.

'What I think,' John said, later, as they wandered along the raised boardwalk of a mangrove swamp where sunlight streamed through a ceiling of fleshy green leaves to fall in small, quavery splashes on the water, 'is that we connect with a lot of different soulmates throughout all of our lives. Sometimes they're friends, sometimes lovers, members of our families, people we work with . . . They can be anyone.'

'So you don't think there's just one special connection?' she said, glancing back over her shoulder.

He shook his head. 'I can think of plenty of connections I've made in my life that I'd term special, so it would seem, well, dismissive, or just plain inaccurate, to say there was only one. But I know what you're driving at, and sure, sometimes it can feel as though just one person, the one you love so much you can't imagine existing without them, is connected to you in a way that goes much deeper than the simplicity of conventional understanding.'

'You don't sound convinced,' she prompted, when he didn't continue.

He stopped to copy the way Akili was dropping mangrove shoots into the swamp, trying to get them upright so they'd plant in the mud. 'No matter how much you love someone, or how much they love you,' he said, as she came to stand beside him, 'they'll never be your sole reason for being on this earth, and without them life doesn't come to a stop.'

337

Carla watched as one of his shoots balanced. 'Sometimes it feels like it might,' she said.

'Sure, because coming to the end of a journey with a soulmate can be one of life's most painful experiences. So, isn't it more helpful to believe that there are others out there who can mean every bit as much, if not more, than the person who has chosen, or is maybe destined, to leave the path you've been sharing?'

Sensing he was speaking as much to himself as he was to her, she glanced over at him, and wondered whom he had loved that much. Whoever she was, it was hard not to feel jealous, for she was obviously in his thoughts now and her presence was altering his mood. Then he looked at her, and the roguish light that came into his eyes relaxed her and made her laugh.

Their tour of the forest and swamp went on for another hour, by which time they were more than ready to tip Akili and return to the air-conditioned coolness of the car, where they set upon the packed lunch they'd got from Mapenzi, attempting to eat it, and drink beer, as they bumped, rocked and rattled along the dirt road towards the Sultan's Palace Hotel on the south-east coast of the island. The plan for the afternoon was to go snorkelling, an activity Carla adored, and since the unit had exclusive use of the hotel's fifteen suites and long white stretch of beach for the next three days, the prospect of having it all to themselves for a few hours, before the rest of the crew arrived, was more than appealing.

Though Carla had heard a lot about the hotel during the build-up to shoot, and had even seen photographs, her first sight of it, when finally they rounded the curve in a drive where shiny green succulents bristled amongst brilliantly blooming flowers, almost took her breath away, for the sheer splendour of the combined Islamic and Indian styles was like nothing else they had encountered on the whole of the island.

'It's beautiful,' she murmured, gazing at the gently curving coral and limestone walls with their onion-domed archways, and stained-glass windows of purple, yellow, red and green. The roof tops were edged in glossy white crenellations, where the starburst tops of coconut palms swayed in the breeze, and the cloudless sky provided a dazzling backdrop of blue.

338

Already she was in no doubt that as far as hotels went this was the jewel in Zanzibar's crown, and, stepping out of the car, she took a moment to enjoy the welcome of a wayward sea breeze that brought the heady perfume of frangipani flowers along with it.

Having been here before, John watched her with humorous eyes as she turned slowly around, taking everything in, from the flame red blooms of the flamboyant trees, to the young gardeners who were clearing the grass with palm brooms, to the shimmering allure of the ocean that stretched out endlessly beyond the hotel. Then she looked at him, and felt her heart expand, for he'd obviously known how special it was here, and by deliberately underplaying it had turned it into the most wonderful surprise. She wished she could think of the words to thank him, though he must know how she was feeling, and as she looked at him she could think only of their first kiss and just how magical it was going to be.

At the sound of footsteps, they turned to see a petite, elegant woman coming out of the entry courtyard to greet them, two porters in long white tunics and red waistcoats close behind her.

'Paola,' John said, taking her outstretched hand and shaking it warmly. 'This is Carla Craig, the programme's producer.'

'It is a pleasure to meet you,' Paola said, in Italian-accented English. 'I have heard about you, from John and the others, and I am very happy that you are going to make some of your programme here. We are only one year old, so I think you will help us a great deal. Now, please, come inside. We shall find you something to drink, and maybe a little pasta . . .'

'It's OK, we've already eaten,' John said, as they followed her into the circular courtyard, where a giant coco palm soared from an island of gazania, right up through the open roof.

'Then perhaps a little Italian coffee,' Paola said, with mischievous eyes.

Both Carla and John smiled, for she'd clearly guessed that the powdery brew they'd so far been offered meant that neither of them had actually drunk any coffee since their arrival.

'Oh my,' Carla breathed, coming to a stop at the threshold of the foyer.

Paola smiled with pleasure as Carla looked around the gleaming white rotunda, with its brass birdcage lamps, exquisite Indian sofas, vibrant African paintings, and huge French windows whose pointed bulbous domes and colourful stained glass were so redolent of the *Arabian Nights* it was easy to imagine Scheherazade herself, spread out on the sumptuous scattered cushions, spinning her endless tales for King Shahriyar. Then Paola led them up a central staircase of minga wood to another circular room, where huge calico sails were draped around the vaulted ceiling making it feel like a tent, and red-and-white-robed tables were already set for dinner.

'And now I leave you to get the coffee,' Paola said, waving them towards an open veranda.

As she disappeared Carla wandered onto the veranda, where more cushions were thrown casually against the walls, and the view down to the ocean could be freely glimpsed through the garden's tropical extravagance of trees and shrubs. A tremor of excitement coasted across her heart, for the whole place exuded such an air of romance that it was impossible not to be affected, and she could only feel sorry that the crew were arriving so soon.

'Have you decided how to shoot it yet?' she asked John, as he joined her.

With an ironic lilt, he said, 'From every angle.'

Smiling, she was tempted to lean into him, as he too gazed out at the ocean.

'It's a good place to make memories,' he said.

'Only very special ones,' she whispered, turning to look at him.

His eyes were suffused with more than laughter as he said, 'Oh, I think they'll be that,' and, hearing Paola's footsteps, they moved apart to watch her set the tray down on a low wooden table.

They drank the delicious dark coffee from tiny porcelain cups, while lounging comfortably on the cushions and informing Paola of their plans for the next few days. Finally, when the pot was empty, she took them back downstairs and out to a thatch-canopied walkway that led to the suites, all of which were in their own private gardens, and named after a tree. Since the crew was doubling up again, Carla was sharing the Papaya suite with Avril, while John and Kit Kingsley were further along in the Eucalyptus.

After they'd agreed to meet in twenty minutes, John walked on with a porter and Carla followed Paola into an Eden of hibiscus and bougainvillea to a set of heavy teak doors that opened into a sweeping crescent-shaped room with long cushioned banquettes, polished rosewood floors, and two double beds swathed in copious folds of muslin and lace. As Paola threw open both sets of French windows to let the sunlight stream in, Carla wandered through the arch that was between the two beds to find herself in an oval dressing room, where her suitcase was already laid out, and a vase of fresh flowers spilled over a central table. Beyond the dressing room was a crescent-shaped bathroom, and the secret niche for the bath and double shower made her think of an opium den.

After Paola had gone she lowered the straps of her dress, and let it slide to the floor. Then, removing her panties, she went to stand under the shower. The water was cooling, and soothing, and when finally she stepped out she wandered into the bedroom, dabbing herself gently with a towel, and feeling the anticipation of what was to come fluttering through her like currents of air. On the private veranda she gazed down at the view and seeing the tide ebbing back to the horizon gave her a moment's unease, for it reminded her of her thoughts in the night, when she'd felt as though her defences were rolling back like a tide, leaving her vulnerable to growing emotions. However, this tide had drawn back to reveal a vast blue lagoon where white-topped waves were spilling over the coral reef that she and John were about to explore, so perhaps there was no bad omen there at all.

Turning back into the dressing-room she dropped the towel and began coating her skin with a protective lotion. Then, taking out the silver and black bikini she'd never yet had the courage to wear, she stepped into the bottom, drew it up over her thighs and hooked the elastic high onto her hip bones, making her suntanned legs appear even longer than they were.

The bikini top had no straps, only strategically placed bones and a back loop fastener. Cupping it around her breasts, she linked it together behind, arranged the supporting bones, then turned to the mirror. Her heart gave a leap of shock and excitement to see just how sexy it made her look, though the way her large breasts were pushed up and together, and were so daringly revealed, made them seem so likely to burst free that she bent double, shook herself about, then stood up again to make sure they wouldn't. To her relief she was still decent, though only just, so pulling a T-shirt dress on for the walk down to the beach, she picked up a towel and her snorkelling mask, closed the French windows and left the room.

She found him sitting at the beach bar, which was in a palm-thatch gazebo, wearing khaki shorts and an open blue shirt and drinking a beer. She saw him before he saw her, and to her surprise she was overcome by such a sudden rush of emotion that she almost couldn't go on. She wanted him so much, yet dreaming about it and longing for it was so much safer than actually going through with it. Then, as abruptly as it had come, the doubt disappeared, and she was still walking towards him.

'OK?' he asked, as she joined him.

She nodded, glad for the moment that she'd worn the dress. 'I'll have a beer too,' she said to the barman.

When her drink came they got up and walked along the deserted beach, past the coconut-wood loungers and parasols, to an overhanging rock where the shade was deep and the sand cool.

'We can walk out to the reef,' he said, using his beer to point to the walkway that led to the edge of the lagoon. 'Have you got fins?'

She shook her head. 'Only plastic shoes,' she said, showing him her feet.

Finishing his beer, he put the bottle down with his towel and mask, then stripped off his shirt and shorts. His navy trunks were brief and tight, showing the hard masculinity of his body, and a bulge that betrayed his state of semi-arousal. Raising her eyes to his face she smiled as he winked, then, taking the hem of her dress, she pulled it over her head and let it drop to the sand.

The sun was hot on her skin and her breasts rose and fell with her laboured breath, as his eyes caused such desire to burn through her it was as though he was already holding her. But though she ached for him to, she knew he wouldn't, despite his increasing arousal. Nor, when his eyes came back to hers, did he speak, but she saw a tightness round his mouth that told her just how hard he was finding it to hold back now.

They swam and snorkelled for almost an hour, pointing out all the many wonders of the reef where black-and-orange-striped clownfish, long yellow trumpet fish, wavery, blue-spotted stingrays, sea urchins, jellyfish and a whole plethora of other marine life glided and darted about the crystal clear waters in a kaleidoscope of colour. They moved quietly, pulling gently at each other's arms to indicate new and more spectacular sights, careful not to touch the reef itself, while stretching out their fingers for the fish to nibble.

When finally they waded back to shore they towelled themselves dry, then Carla sat down in the sun, leaning back on her hands, to stare out at the gentle roll of the lagoon. He sat next to her, his elbows resting on his knees, as he too gazed out at the view. Time drifted on with only the rustle of palm fronds in the breeze and occasional screech of a bird breaking the silence. Beads of water dripped from her hair and rolled between her breasts, while dustings of crystal white sand clung to the taut, dark skin of his legs with their covering of curling black hair, and sinewy curves of muscle.

Then he turned to look at her.

For a moment only their eyes conveyed the desire that engulfed them, until his mouth came slowly to hers, touching it in a soft, lingering kiss that seemed to gather up her heart and send so many sensations through her body that she could no longer breathe. It was a long, sensuous and tender embrace, his lips moulding hers, covering them, sucking them, then gently biting them. When finally he lifted his head, he watched her, waiting for her eyes to flutter open, then he kissed her again.

As he stood up he didn't even attempt to hide the enormity of his arousal, simply took her hand and pulled her to her feet. He put on his shirt and shorts and gathered up their masks and towels as she slipped into her dress. They walked back along the beach and up through the gardens to her suite, where he closed and locked the door while she opened the French windows.

Going to stand behind her, he took her shoulders between his hands and kissed her neck. Her head fell back against him, and turning her round he kissed her with a potency that made her go weak. The sound of a blues piano began to drift in on the breeze, as, taking the hem of her dress, he pulled it up over her head. Reaching behind her to unfasten her bikini top, he peeled it from her breasts. They were heavy and swollen, and her nipples were so enlarged and tender that just the feel of the breeze was like an erotic caress. Then he was drawing down her bikini bottom, holding it as she stepped free, then removing her shoes. When he stood up again she felt brazen in her nudity, and so aroused that she could hardly bear it.

He undressed himself quickly, casting aside his shirt, shorts and trunks, and stood apart from her, allowing her to see just how great his desire was for her. She looked at him, big and hard, straining up to his navel, and felt her heart turn over to think of it going inside her. Closing the space between them, he found her lips with his own, filled her mouth with his tongue and with his erection against her belly, began moving her gently in time to the music. After a while he slipped his penis between her legs, using it to rub her most intimate part as they continued to dance. Then he ran his hands over her breasts, cupping them, squeezing them, tugging her nipples and rolling them, before stooping to suck them deep into his mouth. Such a brutal onslaught of sensation was making it hard for her to stand, as her fingers twisted his hair and her breath escaped in tormented groans of pleasure.

The bed was behind her, the muslin drapes fluttering in the gusts of an overhead fan. Lying her down, he parted her legs and knelt on the floor between them.

'Oh yes,' she murmured, as he began stroking her gently, while watching the effect on her face. Then his tongue was there, and his lips, starting her on the exquisite journey to a place she hadn't been in so long she was almost afraid to go. But he was persistent, and strong, and the pleasure was so intense, and the sensations so great that all too soon she could feel herself soaring . . .

'John, please, please,' she gasped, reaching for him.

But he only increased the pressure, holding her wide, and forcing her on until finally the sheer power of the explosions that began ricocheting through her caused her to cry out over and over, as though she were in pain, which she was, an overwhelming ecstasy of it that seemed to have no end.

Her body was still shaking and her eyes were closed as, lying down beside her, he drew her into his arms and waited for her to relax. There were tears on her cheeks, and her heart continued to pound, but when a small gasp shuddered from her and she turned to look at him he could see she was regaining control.

'Shall I tell you something?' he whispered. 'Almost from the first time I saw you I've wanted to make you come like that.'

Laughter sprang to her eyes. 'What a very worthy ambition,' she commented. Then she was serious again as she saw the way he was watching her lips, and knowing he was going to kiss her she pressed her body in harder to his, and as his tongue entered her mouth she felt the thick, solid stem of his erection between them, and reached down for it.

'Mmm,' he groaned, as she squeezed it. Then he was kissing her again with a mounting urgency and passion, until she slipped from his arms and, pushing him onto his back, began kissing her way down over his body.

He lay very still, eyes closed, muscles tensed, as she sucked gently on his balls and stroked him with her tongue. Then she was taking him deep into her mouth, and he was so hard, and she was so good, that within minutes he was dangerously close to losing it, and grabbing her quickly, he rolled her on to her back and lay between her thighs.

It had been so long that she knew it was going to hurt, but she didn't care, she wanted him so badly she could endure anything except not having him. And when at last he began lowering his hips, watching her as she watched him, the sensation of him filling her started to move her beyond anything she'd known before.

'Are you OK?' he murmured.

'Yes. Oh yes,' she breathed.

He drew back a little, then pushed in again.

345

She was so tight that they could both feel the unsurpassable pleasure of him opening her up, slowly, deeply, until finally he was all the way in, then pulling back, he began the exquisite penetration all over again.

'This is blowing my mind,' he told her, rocking gently in and out of her. 'Can you take it any harder?'

'Oh God, yes,' she gasped, then cried out as he suddenly slammed all the way in, before slowly easing back, only to slam in hard again.

'Keep doing that,' she panted. 'Oh God, just keep doing that.'

'Can you come this way?' he asked, driving even faster and harder.

'I don't know. I . . .' He changed rhythm, and as he hit the place that would do it, she cried, 'Yes. Oh God, oh God, yes!'

He rode her brutally, manipulating that place and feeling her match his pace, until suddenly she thrust herself at him so hard that his own climax began erupting violently into the very heart of hers. They clung to each other, shaking and shuddering in the powerful tremors of release, kissing and gasping for breath, jerking their hips, and knowing every moment of each other's blissful abandon.

A long time later they were stretched out, side by side on the bed, basking in the cooling air from the fan as it drifted over their bodies. The piano had stopped long ago, and the sun had moved round. The crew would arrive soon, if they weren't already there. Someone would come looking for them, but neither of them made any attempt to get up.

Staring out at the milky white sky Carla knew that this was the moment she'd been dreading, when the mystery of how it might be was over, and she had to admit that her emotions had become entangled with the yearnings of her body. So where did they go from here? She turned to look at him. His eyes were closed, and the shadow on his jaw was darkening. Her heart contracted, but as she started to look away his eyes opened and, reaching up, he turned her face back to his.

'Let's eat dinner here. In the room,' he said.

She nodded, and felt only relief as her eyes fluttered closed and his fingers began trailing over her breasts.

'They're even more beautiful than I imagined,' he told her.

She smiled and watched him stroke and kiss them, his skin seeming so dark against the paleness of hers. She was becoming aroused all over again and knew that he was too. She turned to look at him, then moaned softly as his tongue moved into her mouth.

'Tell me it doesn't get any better,' he said, gruffly, 'because I don't think I can handle it if it does.'

Smiling, and rolling on to her side, she said, 'You know, we could be in danger of allowing this to mean more than we intended.'

He stopped for a moment, then, pulling her in tightly against him, he said, 'Well, I don't know what you intended, but I'm in no danger of shying away from what this means to me.'

Chapter 20

Early the following morning Carla left John in the shower and went in search of Avril, whom she'd spoken to on the phone the night before, to ask her if she'd mind finding somewhere else to sleep. Typically of Avril, she hadn't minded a bit, and had obviously been expecting it, but Carla still felt she owed her an apology.

She found her on one of the main verandas having breakfast alone, her shiny blonde hair being tousled by an ocean breeze, and her mobile phone pinning a couple of faxes to the table next to her tea.

'Hi,' Carla said, hugging her from behind, and dropping a kiss on the top of her head. 'Where is everyone?'

'A few of the guys have just gone off to start setting up on the beach,' Avril answered, 'and Phoebe's due to join me any minute.' Her eyes were already sparkling as she waited for Carla to sit down. 'So, where's the man?' she said.

Carla's heart swelled, as, unable to control her smile, she said, 'Still dressing. And listen, I'm really sorry about last night, I should have sorted something out before you got here . . .'

'Stop,' Avril interrupted. 'It's all taken care of, and the best of it is, yours truly has ended up with the Flamboyant suite all to herself. It's next door to yours, by the way, and I should warn you, if I climb up onto the second branch of my eucalyptus tree, then strain my neck around an oleander bush, and manage to keep my balance long enough for the breeze to toss aside a hibiscus, I can see the hammock in your garden. Just in case.'

Carla was laughing. 'Well, I'm glad it's worked out,' she

said, as a waiter brought her a glass of fresh pineapple juice and prepared to take her order.

'Have the lemon grass tea,' Avril recommended. 'Paola grows the lemon grass herself, and it's pretty damned good.'

Going with it, Carla added toast and fresh fruit to the order, then, inhaling deeply the jasmine scent that wafted around them, she let her breath go in a sigh of utter contentment.

'So, I take it you two had a good time yesterday,' Avril remarked, pouring more tea into her cup.

Carla's eyes glowed. 'An understatement,' she responded. 'But it's not going to get in the way of the shoot. We talked about it last night, and though it's pointless trying to hide anything from the crew . . . What are they saying, by the way? I feel so embarrassed for them to know . . .'

'Why? They've all been expecting it, and half of them probably thought it was already happening. So what was it like? I imagine he's sensational.'

Able to feel the tenderness inside her, and the strain of reawakened muscles, Carla smiled and said, 'Avril, I'm not sure that even your vivid imagination can get to just how sensational, but don't ask me to elaborate on that, because I'm already having a problem getting my mind to stay fixed on the day ahead, and talking about it's just going to make matters worse. So tell me, who are the faxes from? Is there anything I need to know about?'

Avril shook her head. 'Not really. Just that I'm staying on in London for another week when we get back. Apparently one of my clients is going to be there from LA, so I should be around to take care of him and his wife.'

'Well, that's good news,' Carla replied, after finishing her juice. 'The world always feels more complete when you're in it.'

Avril's eyebrows went up. 'Well, I'm so touched,' she said, mocking her own sincerity. 'Even if you do make me sound like an extraterrestrial.'

Though Carla laughed, she was already looking over the day's schedule, calculating how much there was to fit in and how likely it was to be achieved. 'Only two drama sequences today,' she commented. 'I thought there were more. Any idea where costume and make-up are setting themselves up?'

'No, but the production office is in Frazer and Hugo's suite, which, I believe, is the Frangipani.'

'You're right,' John confirmed, surprising them both as he came out on to the veranda.

Immediately Carla's heart turned over, and as she looked up at him, the urge to embrace him was so strong that she had to turn away.

'Good morning, Avril,' he said, kissing her on either cheek.

'Good morning,' Avril responded. 'I won't ask if you slept well.'

Laughing, he put a hand on the back of Carla's neck and ran his fingers into her hair.

Carla turned weak, as desire pulled through her like a magnet. Then he was saying to Avril, 'You won't mind if I do this, will you?' and lifting Carla's chin he covered her mouth lingeringly with his.

Seconds later, as he sat down, Carla said, 'You've got to swear to me you won't do that when any of the crew are around.'

'I swear,' he responded. 'Now, do you have a copy of today's script?'

'Not with me, but the two drama scenes aren't scheduled until late afternoon.'

'What about Angelica's statement to camera? I think that's up first.'

'It is, and I haven't actually written it yet, so I'm going to leave you now to go and get started.'

As she stood up the waiter arrived with her fresh fruit and toast, which she really didn't want, so telling him to give it to John, she said good morning to Phoebe and Yale who were just arriving, and went off to find Verna. Though her body ached for him to return to the suite with her, she knew he wouldn't, and was glad, for there was a lot to get through in the next few days that was going to need their full attention. Her decision to stay away from the set as much as she could had to be adhered to, for neither of them needed the distraction.

The morning sped by as she and Verna, working on the veranda of Frazer and Hugo's production office-cum-suite, scripted Angelica's first piece to camera, gave it to Hugo's assistant to run down to the beach, then began collating information from the various hotels they'd stayed at on the island, as well as others they hadn't. It was a complicated, as well as frustrating job, though it was helped by Carla having some idea of the way John was intending to put it all together. What was hampering her, though, was the way her thoughts kept drifting back to the night before, or down to the beach where the unit was shooting. She guessed she was on his mind too, though thinking that way was only making it harder to focus her attention on matters at hand.

'This is ridiculous,' Verna suddenly declared, making Carla jump.

Carla looked up, and was about to apologize, when she realized Verna was looking at her notes.

'I can't read my own flipping writing,' Verna complained. 'Do you remember the name of the Aga Khan's hotel in Stone Town? Was it Sedima? No, that doesn't sound right.'

'Serena,' Carla told her, her thoughts returning to where they'd been before her concentration dropped out. 'The eco-project on Chumbe Island is interesting,' she said. 'Do we have anything on it?'

'They sent us their own video,' Verna answered. 'I've got it here, in my bag. Haven't seen it yet though.'

'Well, we're never going to make any sense of anything unless we can see it,' Carla stated. 'Frazer!' she shouted over her shoulder. 'Has anyone got the TV and video working yet?'

'He's probably with the unit,' Verna said, when there was no reply from inside. 'I'll go and find out what's happening. Can you take a look at these hotel rates I've written down here? They start with beach bungalows, and go all the way up through the scale to here and the Serena. In other words from thirty to three hundred dollars a night, which we need to convert into sterling, then decide which ones we want to feature. We've got footage of them all.'

After she'd gone Carla pulled the notes towards her, and was about to get started on the currency conversions when Frazer's phone rang. It was Jackie from costume wanting to know what time the actors were called this afternoon. The information was on the magnetic board that Frazer never

351

travelled without, so Carla relayed it, then returned to the veranda to carry on where she'd left off. Minutes later she was distracted again, this time by the sound of voices coming from the footpath below the veranda. Recognizing one of them to be Verna's she didn't take much notice, until Verna said, ' . . . we're really close to where she is, she'll hear you.'

'Well, I'm just saying,' Rosa responded tartly, 'I think it's outrageous the way she's carrying on, going off for the day like that, and now not even trying to hide the fact they're sharing a suite. I'd like to hear what she had to say if anyone else did it . . .'

'She'd turn a blind eye,' Verna informed her. 'I know, because I've seen it happen on previous shoots.'

'Well, that's as maybe,' Rosa huffily responded, 'but I can tell you this, it's not going to develop into anything, because I happen to know that John Rossmore's not . . .'

'Stop!' Verna interrupted. 'I really don't want to know. OK?'

'I'm just saying, if she knew . . .'

'*Don't!*' Verna snapped. 'It's none of my business, and frankly it's none of yours either.'

Silence followed. Carla stared at her paperwork, fury vying with unease, as Rosa's words echoed in the warm air. Then her mobile phone rang, making her start. For a moment she only looked at it, until, pulling herself together, she picked it up.

'At last,' John said. 'Where were you?'

Instantly warming to the sound of his voice, she said, 'Actually I was eavesdropping. Not intentionally, but I was treated to Rosa's opinion of us sharing a suite.'

He sounded amused as he said, 'Do I need to know it?'

'You can probably guess,' she answered. 'How's it going down there?'

'We've just wrapped for lunch, which is why I'm calling. I know you didn't eat breakfast and must be starving, but I'm driving myself crazy thinking about you here . . .'

'You're not the only one,' she said. 'I'll meet you in the suite as soon as you can get there.'

Five minutes later, as they fell into each other's arms, anything Rosa might or might not know was forgotten, as

352

were the rules they'd made the night before that forbade all personal contact during the day, for all that mattered then was the precious hour they now had to spend together.

'I want you so badly,' he said, pressing kisses to her lips, 'that I don't know whether you staying away from the set is making it better or worse. Does it matter if they know what we're doing?'

'I don't know,' she murmured, her head falling back as his lips moved down over her neck, 'and right now I don't care.'

Behind them the phone rang, but neither of them attempted to pick it up as they undressed and collapsed onto the bed, unable to consider anything now beyond the burning needs of their bodies. ·

Though their passion was quick to climax, the tenderness lingered, holding them together in a tangle of limbs, and intricate fusing of emotions. Through the open French windows they could hear the sough of the ocean mingling with the rustling of palm fronds, and smell the perfumed flowers that clustered around the veranda.

'Happy?' he whispered, stroking her hair.

She smiled. 'You need to ask?'

Her head was resting on his chest, and as she turned to look at him he kissed her softly on the mouth. 'If only we could just stay here,' he said.

'Do you mean for ever, or just the afternoon?' she teased, though the seriousness of his tone had unsettled her slightly, for it made her think of Rosa's gossip.

'If either was an option,' he said, entwining her fingers with his own, 'I'd take the first. But since neither is, I'll just have to make the most of you while I can.'

Her heart gave a twist of unease. 'Does that mean we stop seeing each other when we get back?' she said, struggling to keep her smile.

He frowned in surprise. 'Is that how it sounded? Because it's not what I meant.'

'Good,' she said, relaxing and lifting a hand to his face.

Turning his mouth into her palm he kissed it, then, wrapping her in his arms, he said, 'Do you feel we're in danger of going too fast with this?'

'Probably,' she answered.

353

'Does it bother you?'

'I'm not sure. Yes, I suppose it does in a way. What about you?'

He sighed, and squeezed her. 'Lying here with you now, nothing bothers me,' he said.

Over the next couple of days, though Carla was occasionally tempted to confront Rosa and ask her what she'd been about to tell Verna, she resisted, not only because she didn't want to give Rosa the satisfaction of knowing she was concerned, but because she so detested the idea of going behind John's back. If she asked anyone, it should be him, and the reason she didn't was because she wanted to believe in him, and trust him, and not let her insecurities drive her to making a fool of herself. On the other hand, she'd made a terrible mistake with trust in the past, so she should at least discuss it with Avril.

'Well, there's bound to be a lot more to him than either of us know,' Avril admitted, when Carla told her what she'd overheard, 'there is to everyone, but we both know John's no Richard. In fact, they could hardly be more different. And as for Rosa, take it from me, anything she knows about John she's learned from the press. Which would be why she said it wouldn't go anywhere, because that's his reputation. But you know very well that he isn't the man we all read about.'

Yes, Carla did know that, and it helped no end to get Avril's view on it all when Avril's instincts weren't bearing the miserable failure of a Richard. Besides, there was mercifully little time to dwell on it, when by now the shoot had fallen three hours behind schedule. With a deadline of Friday, and today being Thursday, Carla was much more concerned with how they were going to get everything in before they left than she was with Rosa's gossip.

That night the production team worked until well after ten, totally restructuring the following day to try and fit in the three outstanding hours, as well as everything else that had been planned for Friday. As scenes and shots were axed, then reinstated, then put on standby, then axed again, Carla was frantically rewriting the script, trying to keep track of the cards, script pages and schedules that were being moved from noticeboard to desk, to floor, to bin, and back to the noticeboard. Her head was reeling as time and time again she pointed out discrepancies, bad continuity or gaping holes that made just about every suggestion unworkable. Finally, deciding she could no longer allow so much input, she ordered everyone except John and Frazer out of the room, and an hour later she'd managed to put together a script and schedule that at least had a fighting chance of working.

The following morning she woke at five with such chronic pains in her stomach that by the time John got up for the dawn call she knew she wasn't going to be able to move very far for a while. Of course, this was Africa, and since half the unit had already suffered it was unreasonable to expect that it wouldn't afflict her, but she could have wished it had happened to her earlier, when the schedule wasn't so fraught – and when she wasn't sharing a room with John. However, with such a hectic day ahead, he didn't hang around any longer than it took to shower, kiss her, and tell her he was in control, before leaving her to collapse back into bed the very second the door closed behind him.

At lunch time, after a morning spent on the phone and computer dealing with her own affairs, Avril picked up her bag and sunglasses and was about to go and check on Carla when Frazer told her that the unit had broken half an hour ago, and if she wanted to eat she should go right away.

'It's only a forty-five-minute lunch today,' he said, 'so I don't know how much food's going to be left. It's fish or pasta. I can recommend the fish. And don't worry, I've already checked with Carla, she was very definite about not wanting anything.'

Avril laughed. 'So she's still laid up, is she? How's it all going down on the beach?'

'OK,' Frazer answered. 'We're moving like lightning, so there's a chance we'll make it, but I wouldn't put a great deal on it. By the way, the photographer dropped in his contacts this morning, if you want to take a look at them.'

'I most certainly do,' she responded. 'I'll stop by later,' and, slipping on her sunglasses, she sauntered on along the path, then down to the beach. Its beauty was slightly marred by the stray limbs of equipment strewn about the sand, and casually dumped holdalls, shoes and drinks that clearly belonged to

355

those who were catching a few rays, or splashing about in the waves.

'Hey, Avril,' Phoebe called out.

Shielding her eyes, Avril peered through the brilliant sunshine and found Phoebe strolling towards her, still made up as a slave girl, though with a red and blue crêpe sundress covering the rags of her costume.

'Can we count on you to boost our numbers tonight?' Phoebe said, joining her. 'We're having a little party in the bar to celebrate the end of shoot, even though some of the guys are going to be out doing night shots.'

'Sure, I'll be there,' Avril answered, walking on towards the dining gazebo. 'So who's out with the camera?'

'I think only John, Kit, an electrician and a driver. How's Carla? Any chance she might join us?'

'Since it's the last night I doubt she'll miss it, no matter how bad she's feeling,' Avril responded, her mouth starting to water as she caught wind of the food. 'Do you see Gus anywhere?' she added, looking around the gazebo. 'I'm supposed to be meeting . . . Ah, there he is. God, who could miss that sunburned face? The man could stop traffic. Ah well, see you later,' and off she went to join him.

'So, how are you?' she asked, sitting down in the chair he was holding out for her. 'Apart from the face, I mean.'

'It looks worse than it is,' he responded. 'And the rest of me is in your debt, as ever.'

'Oh?'

'Well, it's thanks to you I'm here,' he reminded her, returning to his own chair and sweeping a hand out towards the horizon. 'It certainly beats being in London at this time of year.'

'I wouldn't argue with that,' she said, as a waiter filled her glass from a carafe of chilled white wine. Then to Gus, 'So did you manage to get an interview with John yet?'

'Half an interview,' he answered. 'We're doing the rest on the plane tomorrow. Have you decided where you want me to go with the article, when it's done?'

'Mm,' she nodded, picking up the menu to find out how the pasta and fish were being served. 'I've drawn up a list. We need it in print by the end of the month, because that's when the first series starts repeating.' Having made her decision, she put the menu down and took a crusty roll from the basket. 'Now, do we have Rosa sorted out?' she asked, breaking the roll open.

'We do,' he confirmed. 'It's all written up. I can let you have a copy as soon as we get back to England, unless there's a way of printing it out here.'

'There is, in the production office,' she said. 'I'd like to see it before we leave. Have you told her anything?'

'No. I thought you wanted to do that.'

'Oh, I do,' she responded with relish. 'She's going to regret the day the word drugs ever passed her lips.' After eating a morsel of bread, she dusted the crumbs from her fingers, saying, 'So, that's done, and again, thanks for coming to us before going to print.' She smiled brightly. 'Now, I expect you're dying to expose the new love affair.'

Chuckling, he said, 'You're not going to be able to keep this one under wraps, Avril.'

'Of course not,' she agreed. 'But it would be good to see it told with some delicacy and truth, rather than the usual bullshit and scandal.'

'So you don't want me mentioning anything about him going off to her room in his sultan's gear like he did just now, or making lewd suggestions about her belonging to his harem?'

Raising an eyebrow, she said, 'I'd rather you didn't say anything at all, because we both know that not many relationships fare well in the spotlight. But being a realist I'm prepared to accept that in this case it's unavoidable. So, in the hope of lessening the damage, I'm going to ask them to give you an exclusive, provided you give us copy approval.'

'I've never worked for you without giving you approval,' he grumbled. 'You're a control freak, and you know it. But how do you know someone like Rosa hasn't already contacted one of their chums back in London to give them the story?'

'I don't. But believe me, if anything had hit the papers already, or was even about to, I'd know. And Rosa's less of a problem than you think, or she will be once I've had a chat with her.'

His eyes sparkled with delight. 'You're not a woman to be crossed, Avril Hayden,' he told her.

'And don't you forget it,' she responded, picking up her wine.

He was laughing. 'OK, getting back to the lovers . . . No, maybe we'd better change the subject, because here they are and they could be heading this way.'

Turning to see Carla and John strolling along the beach with Kit Kingsley, Avril waited to catch Carla's eye and waved her over. 'How're you feeling?' she asked.

'Better,' Carla answered, picking up Avril's water and drinking it.

'Have you eaten?'

'No. But I might join you for coffee. I just need a quick word with John before they start setting up in the foyer.'

She caught up with him already on his way to the set with Kit and Hugo, and, falling into step with them, she listened to their discussion of the numerous costume and lighting changes that had to be got through by the end of the day.

'Do you think we're going to make it?' she asked him.

'We might,' he answered.

She turned to Frazer, who'd just joined them. 'Did you calculate the cost of shooting again in the morning?' she asked.

'Yes. It'll put us way over.'

'I thought so,' she murmured. 'But we have to get these night shots, and if we don't finish the foyer scenes this afternoon . . .'

'We should start looking at more cuts,' John told her.

'I know,' she responded. 'But let me go over the figures first. I'll be in the production office if you need me.'

A few minutes later, having seen first hand the prohibitive cost of an overrun, she sent a message to John informing him that the penultimate scene should be cut altogether, and if he could, he should reduce the number of set-ups for the rest of the day. She was on her way to inform costume and make-up of the imminent changes, when Yale stopped her to ask if the rumours were true that they were shooting tomorrow and might not get back to England until Monday.

'It's going to give me a big problem if it is true,' he said. 'I'm due to fly to Vancouver on Sunday to start a movie.'

'We'll finish today,' Carla assured him, guessing Rosa was being her usual helpful self in spreading the rumour. Then, spotting Frazer hurtling off to the set, she collared him and got him to go to make-up and wardrobe, while she went to drag Jaffah out of the shade of a tree he was sitting under with the drivers. 'Did you check about the drugs?' she asked, taking him aside so they couldn't be overheard.

'Oh yes, yes,' he assured her. 'No drugs. Nothing. But like I tell Mr Gus, the reporter, Sudi and Jumaane, they roll own cigarettes. Maybe someone make the mistake . . .'

'It's possible,' Carla said. 'Just as long as there's nothing illegal going on.'

'No. Nothing illegal. You have Jaffah's word.'

She smiled. 'OK. If I have your word, then I won't worry any more.'

Obviously pleased by the compliment he said, 'No need worry. Jaffah in control. No-one take drugs.'

'Good.' She hesitated a moment, then, deciding it probably wouldn't take long, she said, 'I want to ask you about Chrissie again. Are you absolutely certain she was here alone when she came?'

'She definitely alone,' he responded earnestly. 'I meet her from plane. I stay with her all time, and I take her back to plane. She even eat dinner with me and my wife some nights. We take good care of her. We like her very much.'

Carla was completely baffled, for Richard had specifically said that he and Chrissie had thought this trip would give them some freedom, so if he'd been here, how could Jaffah not have seen him? 'I'm asking,' she said, 'because someone I know, a man, says he was here with her.'

Jaffah was obviously confused. 'I not see how possible,' he said, starting to sound upset. 'She give me money at end of trip, I pay hotel bills, so I know no-one in rooms either, just her.'

'It's OK,' Carla said, keeping him calm. 'It's probably just a misunderstanding.'

Seeming a little happier with that, he took himself back to the others, while Carla, still disturbed by the mystery, started towards the front of the hotel, where the electricians were rigging for the next shot. She stopped to speak to them, wanting to know if the extra gels had been used. Satisfied that they had, she skirted round the side of the hotel to where the admin offices were hidden amongst the tasselled green foliage of casuarina trees. Either Richard or Jaffah was lying, they had to be, though why either of them would was totally beyond her, unless, of course, Richard had paid Jaffah to keep his trip here a secret, and had forgotten to let Jaffah off the hook. It didn't seem very likely, but it was the best she could come up with, unless Paola could shed some more light on matters.

'No, there was no-one here with Chrissie,' Paola said, frowning curiously, when Carla asked her. 'Only Jaffah, but of course he didn't stay at the hotel.'

So it had to be Richard who was lying. But why? His being here, or not, hardly made a difference all this time later, and besides, wouldn't it be more reasonable to lie about *not* being here, rather than the way it was now? Maybe she should read the rest of his email, see if it explained the puzzle, though it would have to wait. Right now she had more pressing issues to deal with, like making sure they finished today, and the wretched nausea that continued coming over her in waves.

A few minutes later she walked into the hotel's main foyer to find it crowded and totally transformed into the inner chambers of a harem. Two eunuchs stood where before there had been lamps; chaises longues replaced the Indian sofas; elaborate draperies covered the bare walls; and several fountains sparkled where ferns had formerly been displayed. The women – or Sarari as they were correctly called – were extras who'd been cast locally, and dressed in the exquisite brocaded silks and muslin that Jackie had brought with her, and had very cleverly stitched and pinned to make look like the genuine article. Since they were the Sultan's wives, Carla was already preparing to tease John later about just how very young and lovely some of them were.

Right now, she merely listened as he talked everyone through what was needed.

'. . . so this is the summer residence,' he was saying. 'We've done the establishing wide shot of how the foyer looks today, so when the electricians are done we'll start positioning you, and walking you through your moves. There's no dialogue in this sequence, it's simply the closing shot of the drama sketch, which I'll lay over the establisher in the edit, then fade out all of us in our costumes, as though bringing the palace into modern times. So it's going to be crucial that you all hit your spots. Did you call Angelica?' he said, glancing over his shoulder to Hugo. 'We'll need her in about an hour.'

'Done,' Hugo confirmed.

'OK. So give the guys, how long, Kit?'

'Just a couple more minutes,' Kit answered, from halfway up a ladder.

Knowing that meant at least five, John said, 'Where's Phoebe?'

'In her suite,' Hugo answered.

'Then get her over here. We need her for the rehearsal.' As he finished speaking he was starting to smile, for he'd just spotted Carla standing off to one side, in front of the billiard-room niche.

'Are you OK?' he said, going over to her.

'More or less,' she answered. 'Have you reduced the number of set-ups?'

'Yep. I don't think there's so much danger of an overrun now. But it'll be tight.'

'We have to be on that flight tomorrow,' she told him, 'because there's simply not enough time to renegotiate the deal with the airline, even if we could.'

'I hear you,' he responded. Then, after glancing around to make sure everything was going to plan, he eased her slightly back into the niche and said, 'Are you sure you're feeling OK? You look pretty pale to me.'

Her eyes sparkled with mischief. 'Maybe you should carry me off to your harem,' she suggested. 'That would make me feel better.'

Laughing, he said, 'How about if I kiss you? Would that help?'

'No-one's stopping you,' she teased, tilting her head to one side.

'Except a producer with a schedule to meet.'

Standing on tiptoe she whispered in his ear, then laughed as he groaned. 'How does that make you feel?' she said.

'What do you think?'

She spoke softly again, then watched his eyes close as he started to laugh, and ignored whoever was calling his name.

'I hope you're going to live up to that,' he told her.

'What time are you leaving for the night shoot?'

'Eight, I think, and we're due to wrap here at six thirty, and you, tyrannical producer that you are, have just made sure that I hit that six-thirty deadline, cos no way am I out of here tonight without making you go through with that promise,' and, throwing up his hands, he shouted, 'All right, I'm coming!'

'No, it's OK,' Frazer said, appearing round the corner. 'I've got your mobile here. It's Karen. She needs to speak to you urgently.'

Carla's eyes moved back to John's face, and her heart turned over when she saw how alarmed he suddenly looked. Grabbing the phone he began striding away. 'Karen? Is everything OK?' she heard him say.

She looked at Frazer, for a moment too bewildered even to think, then Frazer said he was going back to the production office, which was where she should go now. Her legs felt slightly leaden, and she seemed disoriented, as she asked herself why this woman was calling him here, and what had made him look like that when he'd heard her name?

'Do you know Karen?' a voice said behind her.

Carla spun round to find Rosa right there.

'Karen? His wife?' Rosa said.

Carla's head started to reel, as everything around her seemed to slip out of focus.

Rosa was smiling. 'She's an absolute saint,' she said warmly. 'But I suppose she needs to be considering the kind of life she leads. I went to drama school with her, back in the Seventies. She had an amazing talent. Everyone said so. But she never pursued her career, not after she met John. I went to their wedding, oh God, when was it? Must have been about twelve years ago now. They were so close . . . Well, they still are. He's so protective of her. I was over there just before we came out here . . .'

'Aren't you needed on the set?' Carla suddenly broke in.

Rosa glanced over her shoulder. 'Oh! I think I am,' she

responded, and with a jaunty little shrug she slid off into the chaos.

Going straight down to the beach Carla walked over to the gazebo where Avril was still sitting with Gus and said, 'Can you excuse us please, Gus? I need to talk to Avril alone.'

'Of course,' he said, jumping up. 'I'll take my coffee with me . . .'

He was barely out of the gazebo before Carla snapped, 'I take it you haven't dealt with Rosa yet?'

'I was waiting until she'd finished shooting,' Avril answered. 'What's going on? Sit down, will you? You look terrible.'

'Did you know John was married?' Carla blurted, hardly able to believe she was saying it.

'What?' Avril cried. 'Don't be ridiculous. He's not married!'

'So who's Karen?'

'Karen who?'

'I don't know. She calls him all the time . . . Here. At the office . . .' Her voice faltered, but forcing herself on, she said, 'She's on the phone now, and from the way he took the call it was plainly obvious that she's someone who matters.'

'That doesn't make her his wife,' Avril pointed out. 'But OK, obviously someone's told you she is. Who?'

Carla's eyes closed as she took another breath. 'Who do you think? Rosa,' she answered, wishing that the name alone would render it impossible.

Clearly thinking it did, Avril said, 'For God's sake, you're not listening to anything she says, are you?'

'How can I not, when I was there, Avril, I saw him when he took that call, and Rosa says she was at the wedding . . . Are you sure he's never mentioned her to you?'

'Of course not, if he had I'd've told you. Now, exactly what did Rosa say?'

Carla took a breath, then, pressing a hand to her mouth, said, 'Oh no, I'm going to be sick.'

'Come on, let's get you back to your room,' Avril said, starting to rise.

'No! No, it's OK. It's gone now. Where were we? Oh God,' she groaned, remembering. 'Rosa claims she went to drama school with this Karen, and that she was at the wedding, twelve years ago, I think she said. She even said something about visiting them just before coming here . . .'

'This has got to be bullshit,' Avril declared. 'I mean, if she was some kind of friend of his he'd have said so, for God's sake. And why would Yale have to twist his arm to give her the part if . . .'

'OK,' Carla interrupted, 'I really do have to get back to my room now.'

Seeing how green she was, Avril immediately leapt up and followed her back through the gardens to her suite. Once there, Carla headed straight for the bathroom, while Avril opened the French windows and walked out on to the veranda.

Carla emerged a few minutes later, dabbing her face with a cold wet towel, though still looking deathly pale. 'Sorry,' she said. 'Of all days to be feeling like this . . .' Then, seeing the bed, crumpled from where they'd been lying on it during the lunch break, when he'd come to make sure she was all right, she felt a horrible, welling emotion inside her. 'Oh God, I can't believe this is happening,' she cried angrily. 'How could I have been such a bloody fool?'

'It's not happening,' Avril assured her. 'There's going to be some perfectly rational explanation, and I'm going to find out what it is.'

'No, for God's sake, don't go talking to Rosa,' Carla cried.

'Why would I waste my time? It's John I'm going to talk to.'

'No! He's shooting, and the last thing I want is this turning into an issue . . .'

'It's already an issue,' Avril said firmly. 'Now you lie down, or do whatever it takes to get your blood flowing again, and I'll be back as soon as I've had a chance to speak to him.'

'Avril, no! I absolutely forbid it!' Carla cried, but Avril was already on her way out, and overcome by another pressing need for the bathroom there was nothing Carla could do to stop her.

It was the end of the afternoon before Rosa, doubling as the Horme – the Sultan's chief wife – was dismissed from the set, by which time Avril had spoken with John, so was now fully aware of who Karen was. Since John had insisted on speaking to Carla himself, Avril had been happy to wait for Rosa to come free, and now wandered over to meet her as, still masked in a silk barakoa, and richly bound in a brocaded girdle and white tulle pants, she wound a path through the camera mounts and standby lights, to go and get changed.

'Rosa.' She spoke softly, as John was addressing the remaining cast.

Loosening her mask, Rosa turned round, and Avril didn't miss the quick look of unease that flashed through her eyes.

'I'd like a word,' Avril said. 'Phoebe's still on the set, so we shouldn't be interrupted in your suite.'

'Actually, I'm on my way to costume,' Rosa responded grandly.

'No you're not,' Avril informed her. 'You're coming with me.'

Rosa's face twitched, but clearly realizing that she'd be the loser if she fought this out, she marched across the foyer, and headed down the path to the suites.

Avril followed at her own pace, and was surprised to find that Rosa had left the door open when she got there.

'If this is about Karen . . .' Rosa said, as Avril walked into the room.

'No, it's not about Karen,' Avril replied. 'John's going to deal with that. What I'm going to deal with is this.'

Rosa looked at the small sheaf of paper Avril was holding up, but when she reached out to take it, Avril snatched it away.

'Before I tell you what this is,' she said, 'I want you to know that whatever mitigating circumstances there might be for your actions, like you were dropped on your head as a baby, or rejected by a Jehovah's Witness, I'm not interested, OK? As far as I'm concerned you're a sad, vindictive bitch, and that's how I'm going to treat you.'

Rosa's eyes were blazing. 'You've got some nerve coming in here speaking to me like that!' she spat. 'You're nothing but a cheap little tart . . .'

'Stop right there,' Avril said calmly. 'Just stop, or you're going to find yourself with a lawsuit on your hands that'll ruin you even more surely than what I've got here.'

Rosa's nostrils flared, but Avril could see she was nervous. For a moment she only looked at her, then, tearing her eyes away, she glanced down at the printed notes she was holding, and said, 'This is the article Gus is sending to the industry papers, like *Stage*, and *Broadcast*, and *Variety* . . . I expect you subscribe to them, don't you? I know most people in the business do, especially directors, and casting agents, and producers . . . You know, the types you rely on to give you work.' She smiled, and watched Rosa's face grow paler. 'I expect a lot of your friends and colleagues subscribe to those papers too, don't they?'

'I don't know what any of this is supposed to be about,' Rosa snarled, 'but if you think you're scaring me . . .'

'I'm succeeding,' Avril butted in. 'I know. And you're right to be scared, because I know I certainly would be, if I were in your shoes. So now, I won't keep you in suspense any longer, because I expect you're dying to know what Gus has written. I'll read it aloud, it'll have more impact that way. Oh, you can sit down if you like.'

Rosa remained where she was, standing behind a large basket-weave chair, hands clenched on the back of it, face taut with uneasy anger.

'OK,' Avril said cheerily. 'It's quite a long article, so I'll just read the bits that are relevant. Ready?'

Rosa glared at her.

'I guess that means yes,' Avril responded. 'OK, here we go. ". . . and it was alleged by Rosa Gingell, one of the support cast, that several members of the crew were taking drugs. However, after this journalist made enquiries, it transpired that two drivers, who roll their own cigarettes, were the most likely victims of this allegation, though when I put it to Miss Gingell that she could have been mistaken, she emphatically denied it and accused me of being part of a cover-up. Fortunately, no harm has been done as a result of Miss Gingell's suspicions, though it certainly could have been, which is why *There and Beyond*'s executive producer, Carla Craig, has vowed never to have Miss Gingell near the programme again. As to Miss Gingell's suggestions that Carla Craig and Unit Production Manager Frazer Jackson have been bribing local officials to turn a blind eye to the drugs, again there is no evidence to support Miss Gingell's claim, though Miss Craig readily pointed out that fees were frequently being paid for permissions to film, or the hire of facilities. Anyone thinking that Miss Gingell's fanciful imagination had exhausted itself by now would be mistaken, for she has been quoted by several members of cast and crew, in her remarks concerning unit publicist Avril Hayden . . ."'

At this Avril glanced up and grinned at Rosa's sunken expression. 'Never thought anyone would repeat it, did you?' she said.

Rosa stayed silent, so Avril continued,

'"... I would strongly recommend that any director or producer seeking to cast Miss Gingell in the future would do well to heed my advice and steer clear of this remarkably disruptive actress, whose appetite for rumour and gossip could be extremely damaging if allowed to go unchecked."'

'You wouldn't dare,' Rosa hissed, suddenly finding her voice. 'No way in the world would you go to print with that.'

Avril laughed. 'Do you want to try me?' she said.

'And who the hell's going to be interested in what goes on around some tinpot production like this?'

'I already told you, the trade papers,' Avril responded. 'So now, I'll leave you to mull this over, and prepare yourself for the follow-up publicity which should come sometime around the end of next week.'

Avril was already at the door when Rosa, in a voice that was shredded with anger and tears, said, 'You're doing this because I told Carla John was married, aren't you?'

'Rosa, you made your bed long before you blurted out that little nugget,' Avril replied.

'Well he should have told her himself,' Rosa cried. 'He shouldn't go round . . .'

'A word of advice,' Avril cut in, 'before you appoint yourself moral guardian to the world at large: take a look at your own troubled little soul. I think you'll find it'll keep you busy enough to stop worrying about what other people are doing . . .'

'No matter what you say about me,' Rosa shouted after her, 'it still doesn't change the fact that John Rossmore is married!'

Carla was lying on the bed, staring up at the fan, and feeling so wretched she just wanted to die. Though her stomach was calmer now, it was still too delicate to risk leaving the suite, and the anger she felt at herself, for how she'd allowed herself to get into this position when she'd known all along how disastrous it could be, was only making her worse. Dear God, how could she have done it? Just what kind of an idiot was she? How many times did she need to be betrayed before it got home to her that no-one, just no-one, was to be trusted?

She shifted restlessly, as though kicking away the memory of these past few days, for it hurt too much to think of it, and even if there were a rational explanation for Karen, which she couldn't possibly begin to imagine, wasn't the state she was in now proof enough of how a relationship between her and John just couldn't work? They were supposed to be making a programme, for God's sake, not conducting some kind of pretend romance that was only going to seem real while they were here. What on earth had got into her when she, of all people, knew how easily these exotic islands could persuade someone they were in love, when all they were really in was a dream? How many cast and crew had she seen fall for it in the past, and now here she was, in it up to her neck. Her only excuse was the mind-altering power of her sexual urges, which had been ignored for so long that his attention, their attraction, had caused her to lose sight of what was really happening. But she could see it now, and how pathetic, how insane, she was, throwing herself into an affair that had never been destined to go anywhere but right where it was. And like hell was she going to think about how tender and loving and genuine he had seemed, how beautiful and right it had all felt, because, God knew, she'd been there before, and look where it had got her then . . .

Swinging her legs to the floor, she went to her computer and connected it to the mobile phone. Why not get it all over and done with in one go? Richard's email still needed to be read, but whatever it said, it was over with him too. She'd had enough. She wasn't going to be anyone's fool any more. Let them lie and cheat and destroy somebody else!

Minutes later she was staring at the screen in total disbelief, while her body trembled with shock and her mind struggled to grasp the reality of what she'd just read. Though his message had started by saying that he wished he was there with her now, what it had gone on to say, was that hearing her voice had made things clear to him, and he knew now that he must call a halt to their emails and say a final goodbye.

'I've been fooling myself into thinking that we could find happiness again,' he'd written, 'but I know now that I love Chrissie and our daughter too much to cause them the kind of pain I know it would cause if I left. They love me, and depend on me, and maybe it was hearing your voice that woke me up to the truth of how very much they mean to me too. You're stronger than they are, Carla. You don't need me the way they do. I know you'll find love with someone else, someone who's more deserving of you than I could ever be. In my heart I will always love you, and I wish you nothing but happiness in your life. *Adieu, ma chérie*, and truly blessed is the man who will win your heart.'

Her fingers were shaking so hard as she typed out an answer that it took much longer than it might have, but it wasn't until after she'd clicked on 'send' that she allowed herself to think about what she'd said, and then bitterly regretted her panicked reaction. But why shouldn't she insist on seeing him? If nothing else he owed her an explanation for the way he had behaved eighteen months ago, when he hadn't spoken a single damned word to her, not even to say he was sorry her mother had died. And what about all these emails, and the questions he had consistently avoided? And Zanzibar? Why was he lying about Zanzibar? She wanted some answers, goddamnit, and this time she was going to bloody well get them, no matter how hard they might be to hear, and maybe then she'd be able to move on without any fear of making the same mistake as she'd just made with John.

Thinking of John caused a horrible, deep ache at the centre of her heart, but she pushed it away. She wasn't going to cry over this. She wasn't even going to lose any sleep. She was just going to work out a way of getting him out of her life too.

'Actually, yes I do mind you moving in here,' Avril retorted, as Carla dumped her bags in the dressing room and looked round for somewhere to put her computer.

'I'm sorry, but there isn't anywhere else,' Carla replied.

'You could at least have given him the chance to explain before you walked out. For God's sake, they're due to break any minute . . .'

'I don't want to discuss it. If you don't want to tell me anything, that's fine, but I'm not sharing a room with a married man! Now, if it's OK with you, I'll put my computer on the edge of this table.'

'No, it's not OK with me. You've got your own suite.'

Carla returned to the dressing room, took out a toiletry bag and disappeared into the bathroom. Ten minutes later she came out again, face freshly scrubbed, hair wet, and eyes glittering with false brightness. The sound of voices outside told her the unit had wrapped, which must mean, hopefully, that the schedule was complete.

'Is this right for the party?' she said, looking down at the berry-coloured dress she was wearing.

'Carla, I can't believe you're doing this,' Avril cried.

Ignoring her, Carla said, 'Did Frazer call to say if they got everything in?'

'Yes, and they did. The night-shoot boys are just having something to eat, then they're off again. That includes John. He called too . . .'

'Is Frazer back in the production office? I'd better go over . . .'

Her heart somersaulted as someone knocked on the door, and her eyes shot to Avril.

'That'll be John,' Avril said, starting across the room.

'No, don't, I need to think,' Carla cried, in panic. 'Tell him . . . Tell him I'm not feeling well again . . .'

'You look OK to me,' Avril responded. 'And there's no point putting this off. You need to hear what he has to say and . . .' She broke off as she spotted him vaulting over the garden wall and striding up onto the veranda.

Carla gasped as his shadow fell over the room, and, taking a step back, she said, 'John! Frazer said you'd finished . . .'

'How much have you told her?' he asked Avril, though his eyes were fixed angrily on Carla.

'Nothing,' Avril answered.

'Then if you'll excuse us.'

'No! Stay!' Carla protested.

He waited for the door to close behind Avril, then took a step towards her.

Immediately she stepped back. 'This is not a good idea,' she said coldly. 'We're here to make a programme, and allowing ourselves . . .'

'I'm not married!' he seethed, cutting across her. 'And that you would think I'd deceive you like that makes me so damned angry . . .'

'Then why did Rosa say you were?' she shot back.

'Because I was. Karen and I are divorced.'

'But she's still obviously a very big part of your life.'

'Yes. She is. And probably always will be.'

'That's OK. It's none of my business. What you and your ex-wife . . .'

'It is your damned business, now for Christ's sake let's calm this down so that I can explain without having to gag you to make you listen.'

Carla's eyes flashed. 'I don't want an explanation. I just want you to understand that this . . . *affair*, has to end . . .'

'I've warned you once,' he said, taking another step towards her.

'Not because you're married, or even not married,' she shouted, darting round the bed to put it between them, 'but because it has to!'

Stopping, he glared at her with an expression of pure frustration. 'You'd do that, without even listening to what I have to say?' he demanded.

'Yes. Because whatever the situation is between you and your wife . . .'

'Ex-wife!'

'. . . has no bearing on this, except to say that it woke me up to how impossible it is for us to go on . . .'

'What the hell are you talking about? What's impossible?'

'*Us!* As a relationship! It's not based on reality. It's something that happened, the way these things do on film sets, and now we're going home . . .'

'I'm not going to let you do this!' he raged. 'I don't know what's going on in your head, but you know very well that what's happening between us . . .'

'Nothing's happening! Not any more. And not because of your ex-wife, but because I *don't want* it.'

His face was so taut and bloodless it was hard to read, but she knew she had hurt him and instantly regretted it. However, her mind was made up, she had to break this off before it got any more out of hand than it already was. 'I don't want it,' she repeated quietly.

He was shaking his head. 'I don't know if that's true,' he said, 'but if it is, then I've got to tell you, you put on a mighty convincing show . . .'

'It's not a show,' she broke in. 'I do find you attractive, I readily admit that, it's just . . . Well, it's . . .' She dashed a hand through her hair, as her resolve started to fracture. 'Look, I don't want to get into my past,' she said, determined not to back down, 'but I will tell you that it's still having a bearing on the way I think, and on what I do, which is why we can't go any further. I slept with you because I hadn't had sex for a long time, and because there really was some chemistry between us. But to try fooling ourselves into thinking it can go . . .'

'Fooling ourselves! Jesus Christ, I've read you wrong if that's how you see our relationship.'

'And it seems I read you wrong too,' she snapped back. 'Why didn't you admit you'd been married? Why let me find out from someone like Rosa? She was at your wedding, so you had to know she knew about Karen.'

'To be frank, it was a long time ago and I'd forgotten she was there,' he answered. 'She's a friend of Karen's, not mine, and hardly that . . .'

'Do you still live with Karen?'

'For God's sake!' he cried. 'Of course I don't live with her. I told you, we're divorced.'

'But you still speak every day, and she still matters more to you than being truthful with me. Well, that's OK. I know what it's like to be in love with . . .'

'I'm not in love with her,' he cut in. 'But I can see now that that has no bearing on this, does it, because what we're really coming down to is that you're still in love with Richard.'

She'd already taken breath to deny it, when she realized that maybe it would serve her better not to.

'Am I right?' he demanded.

Still she didn't answer.

He was staring at her hard, a new anger darkening all other emotion in his eyes. 'You accuse me of not being truthful with you,' he said harshly, 'but how about you being truthful with me?' Before she could speak he said, 'It's OK, I don't need to hear it. Your past is your own. I just want you to know that I never intended to hide anything from you, but our relationship is only three days old, for God's sake, and Karen . . .' He raised a hand, then dropped it, and, managing a calmer tone, he said, 'I came here to tell you about Karen, so that's what I'm going to do. God knows I wouldn't have chosen to do it this way, but I'm not prepared to have you thinking for one more minute that I set out to deceive you.'

She watched him as once again he struggled with his temper. 'I thought there was a chance you already knew this,' he began, 'the papers got hold of it a while ago . . .' He waited to see if anything registered, but it was evident she had no idea what he was leading up to.

'Karen and I have a son,' he said abruptly. 'His name's Lucas. We speak most days because of him, and I try to be there every night when he goes to bed.'

The lingering hostility in her eyes told him that she really didn't know what was coming, and were he not so angry he'd have felt sorry that she was having to hear it like this. 'Lucas has been severely handicapped from birth,' he said. 'He's ten now, and we don't know how much longer he's going to live.'

Shock registered instantly on her face, but before she could speak he said, 'I didn't want the divorce, Karen did. She couldn't cope with marriage and a handicapped child and Lucas needed her more. She wanted to devote her life to him, and having me around made it too difficult . . . She runs a school now, in Islington, for children with Lucas's condition. It's become her great passion in life, and when Lucas finally goes it'll give her some of the comfort she'll need to carry on helping those who are like him. Or so she tells me.'

Though most of the room was in shadow, she could see the pain deep in his eyes, and knew that at that moment it would be wrong for her to speak.

'I suppose the press'll be back on her doorstep when that

happens,' he went on, 'but until then I've got an arrangement with them: my scandal for their silence. All the rubbish Lionel makes up sells more papers than a handicapped child, so they're happy to run it, and on the whole Karen's not bothered by anyone looking for a new angle on the John Rossmore story. She doesn't want Lucas exploited that way, and nor do I.'

There was a tense, almost unbearable moment, as Carla tried to imagine how terrible this tragedy had been for him, but how could she when it was beyond anything she'd ever known?

'Karen and I broke up almost seven years ago,' he continued, 'and though I've never stopped loving her, I can now finally say, hand on heart, that I'm no longer in love with her. It's taken a long time to get there, and frankly, there've been times along the way when I thought I'd never stop wanting her and our marriage back. That's not to say everything was perfect between us, because it wasn't. The strain of having a child like Lucas takes its toll on a marriage, and there was a lot of blame and resentment and guilt to be dealt with before I finally agreed to go. She's never cut me out of his life though, and he knows very well that I'm his father. He can even say the word, though you wouldn't recognize it unless you were used to hearing him speak. Karen called today because he was upset that he hadn't seen me, and she thought it might help him to hear my voice. I think it worked. It usually does, but believe me, I live in constant fear that something will happen while I'm away and he'll die thinking I've left him.'

He took a breath, and his face looked almost haggard as he glanced at his watch. 'So there you have the truth about Karen and Lucas,' he said. 'We're surviving the best we can, and compared to some we've a lot to be thankful for. But it hasn't been easy, which is why I'm not going to get on your case about Richard, because I know how everyone needs their own time to come to terms with pain and disappointment, and if you still love him I'm not going to try to force you into a relationship with me. We just need to be adult about this, and find a way of working together if we can, or dissolving my contract if we can't. It's your call. Let me know what you decide, but I want you to consider this when you're thinking it over: first, you're the only woman I've felt this strongly about since Karen and I broke up. That in itself's a pressure, I know, but I think there's a chance we could be good together, though frankly I don't even want to try while you're still in love with another man. And second, for as long as he's alive Lucas will always come first.'

Seconds later the door closed behind him, leaving Carla reeling from all the emotions he'd just put her through. Worst of all was the shame she felt for allowing her insecurity and foolishness to hurt him the way she had, when he was such a good man, with real kindness and integrity, and just didn't deserve any more pain. She should never have let him leave here without telling him how sorry she was for doubting him, nor should another minute go by with him believing she still loved Richard. But though she desperately wanted to go after him, now wasn't the time. She'd have to wait, talk to him later, when he returned from the shoot.

Slumping down in the chair behind her, she sat in the small orange glow of a lamp, and thought of the way she'd panicked earlier when Richard had tried to say goodbye. How trivial her experience with Richard now seemed, in the light of John's with Karen and Lucas, but at least it had made her see that it wasn't love that had made her send a message back to Richard, it was the wretched perversity of considering him a safe haven when she'd thought she'd needed somewhere to hide from the pain of more treachery and deceit. Just to think of John in that vein appalled her now, but she hadn't known about Lucas then, so was still fearing all men were like Richard. Which only made trying to run back to him so much more pathetic, because it was like a victim turning to their abuser for comfort. God, how desperately she needed to get a grip on what was happening between them, for the man she'd reached out to was the man she'd known before he'd betrayed her with Chrissie – a man who might very well never even have existed. With mounting dismay she thought about what he was now doing to Chrissie, for the emails he was sending were every bit as duplicitous as the relationships he was supposed to be having with the women Rosa had mentioned. It was odd, and infuriating, how that could still hurt, but she understood that if Rosa was being truthful, then, in its way, it meant he was betraying her all over again. So how many times was she going to allow it to happen? Just when was she going to strip him of his power to affect her? It had to be now. She couldn't allow it to go on any longer, but as she started to open her computer to send him an email Avril came back into the room.

'OK?' she said, going to perch on the edge of the bed.

'He told me about Lucas,' Carla answered, turning to look at her.

Avril nodded. 'I was just talking to Gus about it,' she said. 'He knew. Says everyone does, but they can be pretty sensitive when it comes to kids like Lucas, it seems. So, how have you left it?'

As Carla told her she reached for paper and pen and started to write.

'What are you doing?' Avril asked.

'Leaving a note for him to find when he gets back.'

'Saying what?'

'That my feelings are every bit as strong as his, and that I totally understand Lucas will always come first.'

Avril frowned.

'What? You think I should just take my things back over there?'

'No, what I think is that you shouldn't rush into anything. It's not that I'm doubting your feelings, here and now, because I know you two have found something special, but for both your sakes you need to get Richard right out of your life, because John just doesn't need to find out later that you made a mistake. Nor do you need to find out that you can't handle playing second fiddle to Lucas. You've both been through enough, and this has all happened so fast between you, so why not wait just a couple of days, get back to London, let some normality return to the field, then see how you feel?'

Carla inhaled deeply, and gazed out at the moonlit ocean. Avril was right. If she wanted to be fair to John, and to herself, she needed to get some perspective on things before making any kind of commitment, no matter how clear it had all seemed a few moments ago.

'I was about to email Richard when you came in,' she said.
'To say what?'

Carla gave a dry laugh. 'The last part of his email, that we didn't read the other day, was ending it all between us,' she said. 'Can you believe that? So, in a panic, I sent a message back virtually begging him to see me. Needless to say, I've changed my mind now.' She paused, then said, 'I really don't want to see him, but at the same time I can't help wondering if I'll ever truly be able to move on if I don't get at least some of the answers he owes me . . . It'll always be there, in the back of my mind. Why did he let Chrissie tell me about them? Why didn't he get in touch when Mum died? What made him send that email asking me to be godmother to his daughter? Was he ever here, in Zanzibar? Which reminds me, Paola says she didn't see anyone with Chrissie either. And I asked Jaffah again, he's absolutely positive Chrissie was alone.'

Avril was shaking her head. 'So why would he say he was here if he wasn't?'

'And why would he end our relationship now?'

'I wish I could say it's mere coincidence,' Avril answered, 'but somehow I don't think it is.'

Carla sat with that for a moment, then said, 'You're right, I owe it to John to make sure this is all completely behind me before I make any kind of commitment to him.'

Picking the phone up as it rang, Avril said, 'Hello?' She listened to the voice at the other end, then started to laugh. 'She had it coming, but I'm sorry if you got it in the neck. I'll buy you a drink to make up for it.' Ringing off, she said, 'Gus. Rosa's just given him an ear-bashing about the article he wrote, and is threatening to sue him.'

'She won't get very far with that,' Carla remarked, closing down her computer.

'How can she, when he's not going to print it? It was just a lesson she needed to learn in what a lying, malicious, disruptive old boot she is.'

'She didn't tell any lies today though.'

'She did by omission, because she obviously knows John and Karen are divorced, but failed to tack the ex on the front of wife when she was merrily informing you he had one. Makes you wonder what she gets out of pissing people off, doesn't it? Anyway, I promised Gus I'd try talking you and John into giving him an exclusive on your budding romance, and before you go flying off the handle, I know the timing's not right at the moment, but it's worth you remembering that everything John does is of interest to the public, especially his affairs. We know now that it's part of the pact he has with the press to keep them away from Lucas, so maybe that's something you should consider when you're deciding how you want to proceed, because you know how particular you are about your privacy, and it's pretty well guaranteed you can kiss it goodbye if you get involved with John Rossmore.'

'Oh God, why can't life be easier?' Carla groaned.

Avril shrugged. 'I don't have much of a problem myself,' she answered, pulling her T-shirt over her head. 'Now I'm going to take a shower while . . . You get it,' she said, as the phone rang again.

Half an hour later they were strolling through the lamplit gardens up to the hotel, watching big coral-coloured crabs scuttling over the path, and fireflies winking from the darkness of the trees. As usual the night was a-twitter with the buzz and squeal of nocturnal life, and the air was thick with the beautiful orangey scent of frangipani flowers. Carla was thinking of John, and trying to envisage the scene when she told him that everything was sorted out with Richard now, and that there was no doubt in her mind, no matter how famous he was, or committed to his son, it was definitely him she wanted. Smiling as she imagined his response, she gazed up at the starry night, and the glistening white palace walls with their onion-domed windows and red, purple and green stained glass, and said, 'This place is such a paradise, it makes you wish you could stay here for ever, doesn't it?'

Since neither of them had any way of foreseeing the terrible chaos that was waiting for them back in England, the wish, though heartfelt, was purely idle, and Carla couldn't help laughing when Avril wryly responded, 'Mmm, except by then I'd have learned the language.'

Chapter 21

Sonya couldn't remember ever being in such a terrible position. Keeping secrets never had been her strong point, and a secret like this was just too much for one person to handle, no matter who they were. It was keeping her awake at night, and making her feel very strange and frightened whenever she thought of it in the day. Normally she never kept anything from Mark, but there was just no way she could show him the letter she'd found, not when it was casting Valerie's death into a whole new light that was so unbelievably ominous it made Sonya dizzy just to think of it. She'd never known anything like this to happen for real. It was the kind of story you read about in the paper with morbid, even gleeful, fascination, poring over the shocking and grisly details as though they'd been plucked from some fantastic field of fiction, rather than the devastating facts of a real person's life. The people these things happened to were strangers, belonging to another kind of world, and though it was possible to feel horrified, and even traumatized, by their experiences, you then put down the paper, or turned off the telly, and got on with your life. To Sonya it was totally bewildering to know that this time she couldn't.

The letter had surfaced just over a week ago, in the pocket of an old coat that had belonged to Valerie. All this time the coat had been squashed up behind a bundle of anoraks, fleeces and macs, at the back of a cupboard in Sonya's hall. It was the coat Valerie often used to wear when taking Eddie for a walk, and Sonya had brought it here when Carla had been unable to bear seeing it around the cottage, because of how terribly she missed her mother. Even after all this time

Valerie's scent was still on the coat, and had caused Sonya to shed a few tears when she'd put it on to take Eddie out herself. He'd been staying with them while Carla was away, and though Mark and the kids normally trotted him round the block, on that day Sonya had felt like some air, so had rummaged around for something warm, but not too smart, to put on, and had discovered the long-forgotten coat.

There was a very good chance that the single page Carla had come across in Valerie's thesis was part of the same letter, but so far Sonya had been unable to find that page. She'd spent a whole day searching the cottage, so was pretty certain now that it was no longer there. Of course Carla might have taken it to London, though Sonya couldn't think why, and she could hardly ask her when Carla would inevitably be curious, and Sonya wouldn't know what to tell her. Certainly she couldn't reveal the truth, presuming the conclusions she had drawn were the right ones. But what other explanation was there? Everything was written down, in Valerie's own hand, and now Valerie was dead!

More fear and horror rose up in Sonya as she sat at her kitchen table, dreading what was going to happen next, and feeling intimidated by the letter's very presence in the house. It was in the coat pocket again now, at the back of the cupboard. She hadn't looked at it lately because she'd given up hope of it showing itself in a more innocuous light, one that would end up making her laugh at her mistake. There just wasn't any other way to read it. The facts were there, lurid and chilling, and refusing to reveal anything but their grimmest meaning. It was written to Richard, though it was unlikely he'd ever seen it, or Sonya wouldn't have spent the past week in the kind of state she was in now. If only Avril had come down for the weekend with Carla. She'd know what to do. But for some reason she'd stayed in London, and with Mark and the kids in bed with flu, Sonya could hardly go gallivanting off to town on what would appear to be a whim. Of course there was always the phone, but it just didn't seem right to try dealing with something this big on the phone. Maybe she should find out if Avril was definitely coming next weekend. If she was, then Sonya might feel a bit better about her inaction, knowing it was going to end soon.

And so much time had already gone by since the letter was written that a few more days surely couldn't make much difference, even with Carla back at the cottage and intending to stay until Tuesday.

After three rings Avril's machine at the *ménage* picked up the call. Sonya waited for the greeting to finish, then said, 'Hi, it's me, I was wondering if you're . . .'

'I'm here,' Avril's voice came down the line. 'You just caught me. I'm on my way to the airport to pick up some clients. So, how are you?'

'OK. But I have to see you. It's important. Is there any chance you can come down here?'

'What, this weekend? Believe me, I'd love to, but I've got a producer and his wife flying in from LA.'

'How long are they staying?'

'All week. If they weren't such important clients I'd leave them to fend for themselves, but they like being looked after, and yours truly is nothing if not good at showing the folks a good time. Anyway, what's so important?'

'I don't want to tell you over the phone.'

Avril laughed. 'Why ever not?' Then, 'Oh God, you're having an affair.'

'*No!* It's nothing like that.'

'All right, keep your wig on. What about talking to Carla?'

'She's the last person I can talk to.'

'Well, you're being very mysterious,' Avril told her, 'and though I'd love to stay and play guessing games, I need to be there when that plane gets in.'

Sonya hesitated, trying to decide how much she could reveal on the phone. She was just about to say she'd found a letter, when the door opened and she spun round to find Mark, hair on end, pyjamas rumpled, padding dolefully in. She hadn't even heard him on the stairs, so had no idea how long he might have been outside. But it was OK, she hadn't said anything to alert him, at least she didn't think she had. 'You made me jump,' she laughed nervously. 'I was just chatting to Avril.'

He didn't seem very interested, and gave only a nasal grunt as, going to the kettle, he set about making himself some Lemsip.

'Sorry,' she said to Avril. 'Where were we?'

'I'm not sure,' Avril answered dryly. 'But I'm presuming you can't carry on now.'

'No,' Sonya responded. 'So when are you coming down?'

'Hopefully next weekend, unless I have to fly back to LA.'

As sweetly as she could Sonya said, 'Don't you dare go back to the States without coming to see us first. I mean it. Don't you dare.'

Laughing, Avril said, 'OK, I'll try not to. Now, I have to go or I'll be late.'

'Just one last thing,' Sonya cried. 'How did it go between Carla and John in Zanzibar? Did they end up getting it together, or . . .?'

'Oh, they did,' Avril confirmed. 'But they've got a few things to straighten out before they go any further. Namely Richard.'

Sonya's heart turned over. 'Is she going to see him?' she asked.

'She's supposed to be, but don't ask me when. Now, I really do have to go. Give my love to everyone, and I'll do my best to come next Friday.'

After she'd rung off Sonya sat Mark down in a chair and carried on brewing his Lemsip. She wasn't sure what to make of Carla seeing Richard, though what was concerning her more at that moment were those letters of Richard's that had gone missing. She wondered if they had any bearing on what she'd found out, and decided that there was a very good chance they did, though exactly how was beyond her limited powers of deduction. That was why she needed Avril to take charge. Avril always knew what to do in a crisis, and whichever way Sonya looked at it, all she could see was them standing right in the middle of a colossal crisis with only her being aware of it.

Having Eddie's cute little face and fluffy body trotting along after her wherever she went was definitely one of the best parts of being home. She'd missed him even more than she'd realized, and the slobbery, tail-thumping welcome he'd given her had amply demonstrated how much he'd missed her too. He'd never been one of those sulky dogs who liked to punish their owners for going away. He was just ecstatic to discover she hadn't left him for good, then content to return to their normal routine, which for the first couple of days had involved a lot of long walks, cuddles by the fire and drinks at the pub with Graham and the rest of their neighbours.

Now it was time to go back to London and Eddie was standing in Carla's bedroom doorway, his food bowl in his mouth, which he'd very helpfully brought up the stairs for her to pack along with everything else. Since he had another bowl in London, this was pure theatrics, guaranteed to get him an extra hug and maybe even a biscuit, and after receiving both he settled down in a watchful bundle, making sure she didn't move anywhere without him.

Tomorrow would be the first time she'd been into the office since returning from Zanzibar, as she'd come straight down to Somerset from the airport, while the rest of the unit had taken a long weekend break too. Now she was extremely eager to get the next programme under way. They were due to fly to Athens in the middle of February, and though the script was more or less ready they had yet to cast it, and firm up all the complicated scheduling and travel arrangements that their trips entailed. At this moment she was working on the assumption that John would be directing. However, all the discussions they'd had about this programme had taken place before Zanzibar, and though he'd said it was her call on whether they could continue working together, she had a horrible feeling he was going to tell her he'd decided to opt out anyway. If he did, it would be a disaster in every way, which was why she couldn't really imagine him doing it, but since there were no guarantees she intended to let him know as soon as possible that she wanted them to carry on working together, at least for the rest of the series.

Regarding their personal relationship, though she was still certain she wanted it, now she was back she was even more determined to put some closure, as Avril termed it, on her relationship with Richard. During a few moments together on the plane she'd told John that was what she intended to do, and his response, though guarded, had suggested he thought it a good idea. Which was more than she could say for Graham, who'd seemed delighted to hear about her and John, despite 'this little hiccup', but hadn't understood at all why she needed to see Richard just to confirm it was over.

'I'm probably being old-fashioned,' he grunted, 'but people in my day never really went in for all the angst-airing you go in for now, and sometimes I think you all get a bit too involved with the why, when the what next can be so much more therapeutic, not to mention enjoyable.'

Carla had laughed at that. 'You've probably got a very good point,' she told him, 'but this is something I feel I have to do, not just for my sake, but for John's too, because he needs to be as sure as I am that I don't have any lingering feelings for Richard.'

'And you really don't think you have?'

'Well, I don't suppose they're all completely dead, and I'll always wish it hadn't ended the way it did, but there's nothing I can do to change that, it just might help to understand it.'

'What's to understand?'

'Well, for one thing, why he'd never discuss it. Not once did he ever agree to see me to explain what happened . . .'

'But Carla, my dear, you know what happened. He had an affair with Chrissie, got her pregnant and left. How on earth's he going to explain that when his actions have already said it all, and when no-one's ever been able to explain love anyway? Which throws up how hurtful some of what he says might be to hear.'

'But much less so now than it would have been at the time,' she responded. 'So maybe it's a good thing he wouldn't speak to me earlier. Anyway, I'd quite like to talk to him about the way things have been since, you know, all the emails and what they were really about. Was it both of us being unable to let go? Or is there really something holding us together?'

'You still think there might be?'

She shook her head. 'Not really. Though it certainly felt like it at the time.' She sighed. 'There's so much I'd like to find out.'

And she supposed she would once she got Richard to agree to see her. So far though he was proving extremely reticent, saying it would only hurt them both, and make the parting so much more difficult than it already was. In many ways she was tempted just to accept what he was saying and forget it, but in others she just couldn't let him get away without answering at least some of the questions he'd left dangling these last few months.

Right now though, as she prepared to go back to London in the morning, she was more concerned about John, and how it was going to be when she got there. Since he was about to start editing at a facility house in Soho she knew she wasn't going to see much of him, and when she did everyone else would be around, which was why she'd started toying with the idea of inviting him to dinner one night, at the *ménage*. OK, it would be jumping the gun a bit, if she didn't manage to persuade Richard to see her, but did that really matter, when she was already so convinced that her feelings for John were much stronger than any she might still have for Richard?

'I don't know, Eddie,' she sighed, looking down at him. 'It's all very confusing, when really it should be easy. Let Richard go, move on with John. There. That's all I have to do . . .'

Turning abruptly at the sound of a sharp noise outside, she felt her heart begin to pound as Eddie's back arched and he started to growl.

'What is it?' she whispered, looking across the room at the dusk-filled window. 'Is someone out there?'

Eddie continued to growl, then, running to the window, he hiked his front paws up on the sill and stared out. He was still growling, but his tail was wagging, so Carla edged closer and silently prayed that nothing horrible was out there.

'What? What is it?' she said, as he started to bark. Then, to her relief, he cranked it up to the high-pitched tone he always used when he spotted someone he knew. Even so her heart was banging against her ribs as she moved in behind him and peered cautiously down into the garden.

Everything was exactly as it should be. Shed over to the left, two spades and a fork propped up against it. Washing line empty, twirling gently in the wind. Trees, tall and looming, branches stirring, their shadows merging into night. Back gate closed to the lane, ivy growing over it. There didn't seem to be anyone there, and Eddie had stopped barking, so whoever it was must just have been walking past.

Eddie looked up at her, eyes bright, tail still wagging.

'Was it Dumbbell?' she said, stroking his head. 'Is that who you saw?'

Jumping down, he bounced across the room, picked up his bowl and swung it from side to side.

Carla laughed. 'Yes, I think it was Dumbbell,' she said, going to fuss him. 'You old romantic, you.' Looking back at the window she felt herself shudder, then chuckle, as she thought of the story Fleur and Perry had brought back from their trip to the States. 'Well,' she said to Eddie, 'whoever it was out there, I think we can rule out the CIA, come to knock off Fleur and Perry for having contact with aliens.'

Eddie's expression was curious.

'That's what they said,' Carla assured him. 'But there aren't any aliens around here, are there? No matter what Fleur and Perry say. Or ghosts. Or strange women. Because everything's got a logical explanation in the end, you just have to find it – or, in Richard's case, force it.'

Chrissie was staring down at an open drawer, full of its usual bits and bobs, though for some reason it didn't seem to contain the rope Richard liked to use when they made love. It was always here. In the chest next to the bed. It was an obvious, and handy place to keep it, though it was true they hadn't used it in a while. However, she was certain it had been there the last time she looked, and the only reason she could come up with for its disappearance now was one she didn't want to get into. If she did, it could mess up all the good results she'd been achieving with her therapeutic medicines and counselling.

Closing the drawer she perched on the edge of the bed, tensing herself, as though waiting for the panic to come. Instead, she felt only the calm, logical urge to search the other drawers to see if it had fallen down the back, which she did, but it wasn't there either, and now she was starting to perspire.

She'd been hoping, with the help of a little wine, and some naughty magazines, to surprise Richard tonight with the kind of treat he must surely be dying for. But if she was reading this correctly he'd taken the rope somewhere else, which could only mean to someone else, the way he used to take it to her place from Carla's, right back at the beginning. Later, he'd kept a supply at her flat too, but when he'd first started cheating on Carla . . .

She was panting. Fast, short, sharp breaths, then long, steadying cool ones. It was OK. There'd be another explanation, and she was a fool to start listening to suspicions that she knew very well were a Trojan Horse for paranoia. Just because the rope wasn't here in their room didn't mean he'd been using it in another room with Elinor, the nanny, or in any other place with any other person. All those visits he made to the library, the BBC, NBC, and countless other TV and radio networks, were for research. She knew that. They had nothing to do with sex, nor was he really going to hotels, or other women's apartments, or even secluded spots in the park. He was doing exactly as he said. Checking details, trawling memories and catching up with old friends. They'd even entertained a few lately, because she'd been well enough to cope, and he'd been pleased to invite them. So thinking he was involved in illicit affairs was only her imagination, because he'd assured her time and time again that he was willing to wait until she was ready. OK, for a highly sexual man that would be hard, but she believed totally in his love, and though he had a history of disloyalty, she had only to look at the way he'd stood by her during this very difficult time, always remaining patient, never being anything but tender and understanding, even crying at times when he saw her confusion and despaired of ever being able to help her, to make her know how much she meant to him. So he'd never put her sanity in jeopardy again by betraying her. He'd fought too long and hard to pull her out of the depths to risk putting her back there now.

But the rope wasn't there, and even if she managed to fight off the paranoia, she had to be careful of denial, because no matter how easy it might be to pretend she didn't know it was missing, it was. So, she owed it to herself, and all the hard work she had done, to confront him with the question of where he had put it.

'What do you mean, it isn't there?' he said later, distracted until then by the mail he was opening.

'It isn't there,' she repeated, looking at him with strong, crystalline blue eyes, though inside her heart was pounding her resolve to pulp.

'Then I don't know where it is,' he told her.

'Well, if I didn't move it and you didn't move it, who did?' she demanded.

He blinked in surprise. It was unlike her to be this firm, though he didn't appear put out, more curious, and even impressed. Then slowly he started to smile. 'I have to ask,' he said, softly, 'why were you looking for it?'

She felt her cheeks grow hot, as, unable to stop herself smiling too, she said, 'I just was.'

He looked at her with such a knowing expression, and with such obvious pleasure at what this might mean, that they both started to laugh. 'I'll tell you what,' he said, dropping his mail on the table, 'Ryan and I'll go and take a look, won't we, sweetheart?' and, sweeping the baby out of her playpen, he carried her up the stairs.

Chrissie listened, tense with dread that she might hear his footsteps go somewhere else before they went into their room, somewhere like Elinor's room, where he would find the rope and quickly transport it to its usual place. But they didn't pause until they were right overhead, when she even heard the drawer open, while he chatted to Ryan. Then Ryan screeched and he laughed, and before she knew it he was back in the sitting room, holding the rope in one hand and their daughter in the other.

'It was caught up at the back,' he said.

Raising her eyes from the rope to his face, she felt such relief sweep over her that for a moment all she could do was smile. Then she started to laugh, and, throwing her arms round him and Ryan, she kissed them both, and told herself firmly not to be so absurd, of course it hadn't been in his pocket. It had been exactly where he'd said it was, tangled up at the back of the drawer, because that sort of thing happened to rope, and besides, if he wanted to use it elsewhere all he had to do was buy more, so what an idiot she was to think that their little supply was being shared with anyone else.

Chapter 22

It had never crossed Avril's mind, when she'd decided to start looking deeper into Richard Mere and what he might be about, that she'd find herself having to deal with the kind of shock she was dealing with now. Her mind was still reeling from it, and though part of her was ready to panic, she was holding herself tightly in check for fear of doing, or saying, the wrong thing, because if she was right about any of this then she didn't even want to think of what it was going to mean for Carla.

Sighing heavily, she shook her head and clasped her hands over her face. Nothing, but nothing, had prepared her for these horrendous suspicions, which was why she'd set this time aside today, free of clients, free of phones, to try working it all through again, to see if she ended up with the same horrifically disturbing conclusions.

First she wanted to go back to exactly when, and why, she'd begun to feel uneasy about this cyber-seduction, which was hard, when she'd never really approved, but she finally settled on that peculiar visit Richard had made to the cottage one Sunday, when Graham's wife had spotted him coming out. Of course they still didn't know for sure whether or not it was him, but hadn't it been around that time that Carla had first begun her fruitless search for his letters? It was also, Avril was certain, some time around then that she'd found Valerie's thesis in a mess in the wardrobe – the very same thesis that Carla had found the page of a letter in, a letter they all presumed was to Richard.

The question of why he'd want that page, or his own letters, was one she'd address later, though it would help to know if Carla had ever told him about the page and where she'd found it. Since Avril wasn't prepared to ask, at least not at this stage, she'd have to go with the assumption, for now, that Richard knew about both.

Next, she was recalling the conversation Sonya had had with the storage people, the day they'd moved into the *ménage*. There had been a suggestion then of someone rummaging about in Carla's container prior to everything being shipped out. And wasn't it after taking everything out of storage that Carla had finally given up her search for Richard's letters? So had Richard found them in the container? Or had he found them earlier at the cottage, and was looking for something else altogether amongst the items in storage? Of course, once again she was presuming it was him, but the further into this she went, the likelier it was becoming.

Next, she recalled the day Carla was supposed to meet him at the Bluebird Café. Though they knew for a fact Carla had been there, whether Richard had actually shown up, only he knew. The significance of that particular mystery, and whether or not it was relevant, was maddeningly elusive, though Avril was convinced it mattered. Just like it mattered to know the truth about whether or not he'd ever been to Zanzibar, because the most curious part of that was that he'd tried to end his contact with Carla at the very same time as the contradiction arose. So did that mean he knew Paola and Jaffah were saying he'd never been there? Obviously Avril didn't have an answer to that, and she had to admit that were it not for the stealing back of his own letters, and the presumed significance of the page in the thesis, then she might think he was backing off now because of John, whom he probably knew about through Rosa, who had more grapes on her vine than Bacchus. But even if John were the reason, it wasn't answering the question of whether or not Richard had been in Zanzibar, when he was supposed to be in Kosovo.

Why on earth he'd lie about it was totally beyond Avril, but the fact that the mystery existed was horribly, even grotesquely significant, if she really was reading this correctly. She hoped to God she wasn't, but if he *hadn't* been in Zanzibar, then the next question was, where the hell had he been? Obviously not with Chrissie, as she *had* been in Zanzibar, and though there was a chance he'd been telling the truth about Kosovo, checking to find out if he had would be nigh on impossible, when, as a freelancer for international news, he could have been on assignment for any of a thousand different sources. He might even have gone on spec. In fact, as far as Avril remembered, he'd gone to help a family out of some trouble, rather than to report on the war. Mighty convenient that, having his whereabouts so difficult to trace!

So, running with the assumption that he *hadn't* been in Kosovo either, Avril was left looking at the most stupefying picture of all, which had him unaccounted for at the time of Carla's mother's death. Even thinking that made her head spin. And OK, as leaps of imagination went, this one was Olympian, but the springboard of getting there was the page of a letter Carla had found, that he had so far avoided explaining. As the letter seemed to suggest that Valerie knew about his affair with Chrissie, had he gone down there to persuade her not to tell Carla? Had Valerie refused? Had they argued? Had the unthinkable then happened? Valerie had died by falling and hitting her head on a rock, but couldn't the blow just as easily have been struck by a hand, holding the rock? OK, this was a bit of a Hollywood scenario, and she knew she was prone to them, so she was more than ready to ask why on earth he would go as far as killing Valerie in order to shut her up when Chrissie would already have been pregnant, meaning he had to have been planning to leave Carla anyway. Well, one answer was that people did the strangest things, and for the weirdest motives, which, though true, got her precisely nowhere.

It seemed more likely that there was a missing piece to this puzzle that might just be contained in the letter Valerie had written. So what Avril was wondering was, if Carla, when asking Richard about the page she'd found, had unwittingly tipped him off that a letter existed, so that now he was searching for the rest of it. It would be one way of accounting for his little trip to the cottage, and could also explain the mystery chap who'd cropped up at the storage company. It didn't explain the woman the kids and Maudie had seen, but

391

that would no doubt come clear once the entire picture was complete. So going back to the letter, presumably he hadn't found it in either place, because it was only now, several months later, that he was trying to sever contact. So did that mean he'd actually found the letter now, or was some new, and even more convoluted ruse of discovery about to make itself known?

So many questions, with only surmises and suspicions for answers. And then there were the anomalies, like why take his own letters? And why initiate contact with Carla in the first place, if he hadn't known about Valerie's letter until Carla alerted him? As for the bizarre invitation to become godmother, Avril wasn't even going to try to understand that. In fact, there was so much about all this that was inexplicable and alarming, to the point of actually being frightening, that she knew she had to discuss it with someone, if only to give it some kind of perspective.

For the moment at least, mentioning anything to Carla was absolutely not an option, because if Valerie's death did turn out to be an accident, as it said on the records, it would be unforgivable to put Carla through the doubt when there was no need. So maybe she should speak to Graham when she went down at the weekend. Not only was he exceptionally level-headed, he also had a mind that was possibly even superior to Richard's, and a sort of credential as a detective. So he was obviously the one to go to, though getting him alone, without making Carla at the very least curious, wasn't going to be easy.

Sighing, Avril looked at the squiggles and squares she'd been doodling on a notepad, and wondered if she should go and speak to Richard himself. Considering what she was accusing him of, she was probably unbalanced even to think it, but if she could somehow persuade John to come with her . . . It would mean having to tell him everything that had been going on between Carla and Richard since they'd split up, and Carla definitely wouldn't like that, but who else could Avril ask to go with her that she could trust to have Carla's best interests at heart?

Less than an hour later her dilemma was over, because when Carla called to tell her that Richard had just agreed to meet her, on Friday, the wait till the weekend to see Graham was no longer an option. Something significant must have happened to change Richard's mind, and apart from a sudden willingness to give Carla the closure she needed, the only other scenario Avril could come up with was the unthinkable one of him trying to force the letter out of Carla, when Carla actually had no idea where it was. Of course she could be wrong about everything here, but one thing was for certain, she was no longer hesitant about picking up the phone to call John. Carla was seeing Richard on Friday evening, it was now Wednesday, so there was still plenty of time. This was presuming John was willing to accompany her on her visit to Richard. If he wasn't, Avril had no idea what she would do, but her instincts were telling her that she had to see Richard before Carla did, so if John wouldn't come, well, she guessed she'd just have to go alone.

John was silent for a long, long time after Avril finished outlining her own reading of the subtext to the Carla and Richard story. His lean, handsome face was hard to read, but the fact that he hadn't asked any questions hopefully meant that she'd succeeded in conveying the potential danger of allowing Carla to be alone with Richard. She wondered when he'd last spoken to Carla, and exactly where their relationship stood right now; in fact she was annoyed with herself for not finding out first. But whatever difficulties they were still facing, they surely wouldn't have a bearing on John's decision to become involved, not if he really thought there was a chance Carla could be harmed.

'I understand everything you're telling me,' he said eventually, 'and I can see why you've reached the conclusions you have, but you don't really have much to back them up, and to go crashing into a man's house accusing him of something as serious as murder . . .'

Avril's spirits sank. He was right, of course, she was acting almost purely on instinct, and the rest didn't really amount to much more than fanciful misgivings and prejudice against a man who'd hurt someone she cared for.

'However,' John said, 'now you've told me all this, I can't help being concerned too, and if anything were to happen to her as a result of seeing Richard . . .'

Avril looked at him eagerly, certain he'd come up with the answer, though short of going round there and confronting Richard she couldn't see what else to do. Nor, apparently, could he, though he clearly wasn't advocating anything as heavy-handed as Avril had in mind.

'Calling to make an appointment probably isn't a good idea,' he said, agreeing with her first observation. 'We need to catch him off guard, but first we need to find out where he lives.'

'Done,' Avril told him. 'I'm still holding Gus's article over Rosa's head, so she's willing to dance to just about any tune I play right now, to keep it from going to print.'

'OK. Then we need to decide exactly how we're going to approach him. As the other man, it's going to look extremely odd if I start trying to delve into his motives for keeping in touch with her . . .'

'So let me do it. Really, I'm asking you to come for protection, just in case I'm right, so there's no need for you to go making a fool of yourself, if that's the way it turns out. In fact, if I thought the police would listen to me for more than a minute I'd go to them, but . . .'

He was shaking his head. 'They'd want a lot more to go on before they got involved,' he assured her, picking up his mobile as it started to ring. 'John Rossmore,' he said into the mouthpiece.

Avril watched as he turned slightly away, but since they were in an edit suite with all monitors and machines switched off, she didn't have much choice but to listen.

'Saturday's fine,' he said softly. 'OK, at the cottage. I know. I miss you too.' He smiled as he listened again, then ended the call with, 'See you then.' After putting the phone away he turned back to Avril. 'That was Carla,' he said.

Avril smiled. 'I guessed. So do I take it you're going down there at the weekend?'

'I've just been invited,' he confirmed.

'So she's that sure she won't have a change of heart about Richard,' Avril commented, with relief.

'It would seem so.'

Her eyes were suffused with a teasing light as she said, 'You really have fallen for her, haven't you?'

394

'It would seem so,' he repeated. 'But that's for me to tell her, not you.'

Avril drew a zip across her lips. 'Sealed,' she promised. 'But now, back to Richard. Let's work out A, when we're going to go, and B, how we're going to handle it.'

'And C, who's going to tell Carla if you're right?'

Avril's eyes filled with dread. 'Oh God, I hadn't thought that far ahead,' she muttered.

'It's OK, I'll tell her,' he said, 'but considering it's her mother we're talking about, and an ex-lover . . .'

'I'll be on hand too,' Avril promised. 'So will Graham, I'm sure. If it comes to it.'

Carla was in the *ménage*'s kitchen preparing Eddie's breakfast, when, hearing the front door open and close, she popped out to see who'd come in to the office so early. When she saw who it was her heart immediately responded, and because of the lopsided smile he was giving her, she smiled too.

'I didn't know you were coming in today,' she said, then gasped and staggered as Eddie bounded past and threw himself bodily at John.

'Actually, I was just passing,' he said, stooping to fuss Eddie. 'I'm due in the edit suite at eight.'

Her eyes were dancing. 'And you were passing, en route from Hampstead to Soho?'

His expression matched hers, as, closing the distance between them, he said, 'OK, the truth is, I couldn't wait until tomorrow. I've got time for one kiss, and then I have to go.'

'Do you honestly believe we can stop at one kiss?' she teased.

'Ordinarily no, but as I just saw Hugo parking up outside, we don't have much choice,' and, pulling her to him, he pressed his mouth hungrily to hers.

It felt so good to be back in his arms that it was almost impossible to let go, but when Hugo came in, a few minutes later, they were both at their desks. Mumbling a gruff good morning, Hugo went straight into the kitchen for coffee.

'OK, I'll have to go,' John said, 'I just want you to know that when you see Richard later, whatever the outcome, you can count on me to finish the series.'

His irony wasn't lost on her, as, smiling, she said, 'I'm hoping I can count on you for a lot more than that. Starting tomorrow night.'

'I'll be there,' he promised. 'And you've got my mobile number, should you need to call?'

'You know I have,' she laughed.

After he'd gone she returned to the kitchen, trying to shrug off the feeling that there was something he wasn't telling her. In the end, unable to dispel it, she went upstairs to her studio and, calling his mobile, said, 'Are you as worried about me seeing Richard as I think you are?'

'Of course I am,' he answered. 'I don't want him changing your mind about me.'

'That's not going to happen.'

'Good. Then I won't worry. What days are we casting next week?'

'Monday and Tuesday.'

'OK.' There was a pause, then he said, 'Listen, if you're seeing Richard just to prove something to me . . .'

'I hope I've already done that,' she said. 'And I'll go on doing it. But there are things I want to straighten out with Richard, questions I want answered . . .'

There was another brief moment before he said, 'If things don't go the way you're expecting, if there's anything . . . Believe me, I don't want to interfere, but I care about you and I don't want you to be hurt. Will you remember that, if this . . . Well, will you just remember it?'

'Of course,' she said softly. 'And I care about you too. So let's just get this out of the way, then maybe, when you and Karen are ready, Eddie and I can meet Lucas.'

She could almost see the softening of his eyes, as he said, 'He'll like that. So will I.'

Not until the middle of the afternoon did she try calling him again, but by then the edit session was over and his mobile was turned off, so accepting she'd have to wait until tomorrow to speak to him again, she finished up at the office and went upstairs to find Avril so that they could talk about her meeting with Richard tonight. But it seemed Avril had slipped out when she wasn't looking, and as neither Felicia, nor Jeffrey, knew where she was, Carla had no choice but to resign herself to a lone session of psyching up for what might once have been a momentous, and thoroughly nerve-racking event. As it stood, she just wanted it over with, though she had to admit she was curious, and even a little excited to see him again. She knew Avril would probably disapprove of this, though grudgingly understand it, if her mobile weren't flaming well switched off too!

As John brought his Range Rover to a stop both he and Avril looked across the garden square to the house where Richard and Chrissie lived. It was much like the others in the terrace, three storeys of Regency splendour, with tall casement windows, a white frontage, black railings and a blue front door. A few wisps of smoke rose from the chimney, becoming quickly invisible in the grey mass of sky.

'Let's hope he's in,' Avril commented, looking at the light in a downstairs window.

John didn't answer. He'd spent a lot of time these past twenty-four hours going over everything Avril had told him, and now, though he was convinced they were doing the right thing in coming here, after looking at the situation from several other angles than the one Avril had taken, he wasn't necessarily expecting the same kind of outcome as she was. However, for the time being he'd decided to keep his own counsel, but if he was right in his suspicions then Carla really did need protecting, though not necessarily in the way Avril thought.

Avril turned to look at him. 'I don't feel quite so sure of myself now I'm here,' she confessed.

He switched off the engine, and removed the keys from the ignition. 'Come on, let's get it over with,' he said.

It was a bitterly cold day, with damp dripping from the barren trees, and a thick brown sludge cluttering the gutters. There was no-one around, the only sound coming from the distant traffic of Knightsbridge, then the gate hinge creaking as John pushed it open for Avril to go in ahead of him. At the top of the steps she lifted the heavy brass knocker and rapped three times.

'I wonder if Chrissie's at home?' she said softly.

Evidently someone was, as almost straight away they heard footsteps coming down the hall, then the door was opening and Chrissie was looking at them in growing surprise and confusion.

'Hello, Chrissie,' Avril said, her breath clouding the air as she punched her gloved hands together. 'Do you remember me? Avril Hayden.'

'Of course I remember you,' Chrissie responded, her natural politeness struggling with a noticeable build-up of caution. 'How are you?'

'Fine,' Avril replied. 'Uh, this is John Rossmore.'

Chrissie's blue eyes looked anxiously into his. 'Yes, I recognize you,' she said.

'Who is it, darling?' Richard's voice called from within.

Chrissie spun round, and watched him with big, bewildered eyes, as he came down the hall. 'It's Avril, Carla's friend,' she said. 'And John Rossmore.'

Richard frowned, though his manner was perfectly hospitable as he said, 'It's freezing out there, won't you come in?' and, slipping a protective arm around Chrissie, he opened the door wide.

Once they were all in the warmth of the hall that smelt of babies, and something delicious cooking in the kitchen, he offered a hand to John. 'Pleased to meet you,' he said, his eyes looking directly into John's.

'Likewise,' John responded.

Seeing them standing there together, the fleeting observation that Carla really knew how to pick her men passed through Avril's mind, for, in their own individual ways, they were both exceptionally attractive. Then Richard was turning his shrewd grey eyes to her and saying, 'How are you, Avril? It's been a long time.'

She smiled, and tried not to be daunted by the extremely unwelcome understanding of just how difficult this was going to be, with him being so friendly, and Chrissie appearing so nervous. 'I'm fine, thank you,' she replied.

'Would you like to take off your coats?' he offered.

Avril glanced at John, then her eyes flew to Chrissie as she suddenly gasped, 'Oh my God! Something's happened to Carla, hasn't it? That's why you're here. Something . . .'

'Carla's fine,' John assured her, putting a steadying hand on her arm.

Her eyes came uncertainly to his, and he smiled in a way that seemed to relax her.

Watching Richard clocking the moment, Avril shrugged off her coat and handed it over. She didn't miss the appreciative sweep of Richard's eyes as they glided over the front of her sweater, though she could hardly put him down as a flirt or a lecher when her breasts were hard to miss. Nor, right at this moment, was she finding it very easy to think of him as a killer.

'Shall we go through to the sitting room?' he suggested, indicating the way.

A fire was crackling in the hearth, and an assortment of baby toys was scattered around the floor, though there was no sign of the baby. Probably sleeping, Avril thought, perching on the edge of a large leather armchair, and reaching her hands out to the warming flames.

John went to the opposite chair, while Richard and Chrissie sat together on the sofa, and though Richard appeared quite relaxed, the arm he rested along the back of the cushions behind Chrissie seemed almost protective. Avril felt glad Carla couldn't see it, for taken at face value they appeared extremely close, and no matter how over it Carla might be, this would inevitably be hard to swallow.

'Would you like some coffee?' Chrissie suggested.

Avril looked at John. 'No, thanks,' he answered.

More seconds ticked by, then Richard said, 'Well, I'm glad you felt free to drop in.'

It was a joke, not intended to embarrass, simply to lighten the mood and help them get to the point of their visit. Avril wondered if he had any idea what was coming. If he did, then he was the coolest customer she'd ever come across, because his expression was so benign he could be waiting for them to sell him a carpet. She looked at Chrissie, who appeared to be haunted by all kinds of conflicting emotions, but most of all she seemed so eager to be friendly that for the first time in her life Avril found herself smack in the middle of a situation she didn't know how to handle. She hadn't thought about how much this was going to hurt Chrissie, in fact she hadn't considered Chrissie at all until now.

Her eyes went to John. They'd agreed that she would start

the ball rolling, but whatever lines she'd rehearsed had just been erased from her memory by that pathetically disarming look on Chrissie's face. Just no way could she sit here, building up to accusing the woman's husband of murder, when she seemed about an inch away from a breakdown already.

Chrissie and Richard were looking at John too, and Avril's admiration of the man scaled new heights as, apparently recognizing her untimely loss of bottle, he went right off script and said to Richard, 'We want to ask you about your trip to Zanzibar.'

Avril blinked. So did Richard. Then, frowning, he looked at Chrissie, who was looking at him in equal confusion. 'I've never been to Zanzibar,' he said, turning back to John. 'But Chrissie has. Maybe she can help.'

Avril's heart was thumping. He'd never been to Zanzibar! So why tell Carla he had?

John glanced at Chrissie, then, with more courage than Avril knew she could muster, he said to Richard, 'While Chrissie was in Zanzibar, where were you?'

Richard's eyebrows shot up, though he didn't appear to take offence as he said, 'I believe Kosovo. Why? Is it important?'

'It could be,' John replied. 'Can you prove you were in Kosovo?'

This time Richard gave a laugh of amazement. 'Do I need to?' he asked.

To Avril's confusion John appeared slightly amused too. 'It would probably be helpful if you could,' he responded.

Richard took in a breath, then blew out his cheeks. 'Well,' he said, 'I'm sure I can prove it, but first, I'd like to know why I'm being asked to.'

John looked briefly at Avril, then to Richard he said, 'This might seem an odd question, but did you tell Carla you'd been to Zanzibar?'

Richard was completely taken aback. 'I'm sorry,' he said. 'I'm not sure I understand.'

'You've been filming there recently, haven't you?' Chrissie suddenly jumped in.

John nodded. 'And your research and set-up were invaluable.'

She seemed pleased by that, but then turned to Richard as

though wanting him to take over again now.

'I'm curious,' Richard said, 'to know why you think I told Carla I'd been to Zanzibar.'

Again avoiding a direct answer, John said, 'When was the last time either of you were in touch with Carla?'

Chrissie and Richard looked at each other again, and Richard said, 'Not since Carla and I broke up. Why?'

'Have you had any contact by email?' John asked.

Avril's eyes were fixed on Richard, watching for the slightest sign of discomfort. To her astonishment, there was nothing more than a continued bewilderment. 'No, no contact by email,' he answered. Then, with a laugh that was trying to be polite, he said, 'I'm starting to wonder if we might need a lawyer?'

'I'm sorry,' John said smiling. 'We're in a difficult position, but we do need to ask the questions.' He looked at Chrissie. 'Have you had any contact with Carla?' he asked. 'I mean, via the email?'

She shook her head. 'For a long time I was afraid to get in touch with her at all,' she said, 'and now . . .' Her eyes flicked up to Richard. 'She probably wouldn't welcome it.'

Richard sat forward, resting his elbows on his knees, and clutching one of Chrissie's hands between both of his, he said, 'I'm afraid all this intrigue is going to be difficult for us to deal with when you've gone, so if you wouldn't mind telling us exactly what it's about . . .'

Avril was about to speak when John put up a hand to stop her and said to Chrissie, 'I'm sorry if this is going to cause you some pain, but I have to ask you, Richard, if you have an arrangement to meet Carla this evening?'

Chrissie's head spun to Richard, as her cheeks paled, but before he could answer she said, 'He can't have, his publisher's coming for dinner.'

Richard looked at John.

Avril's tone was challenging as she said, 'So were you intending to stand Carla up again?'

Richard couldn't have appeared more astonished. 'Again?' he repeated.

Chrissie's fist was pressed to her mouth as she said, 'I knew it! Oh God, I knew it!'

'No!' Richard cried, pulling her into his arms. 'It's not true. I don't know what's happening here, but I'll have to ask you to leave if you're going to carry on like this.'

'What were all the emails really about?' Avril demanded. 'Were you just playing with her mind, or was there a purpose to them that . . .'

'Stop!' Richard barked. 'I don't know what emails you're talking about, nor do I know why you think I went to Zanzibar, or why I had an arrangement to see Carla this evening. Carla and I broke up a long time ago, as you well know. There's been no contact between us since, other than some unpleasant threats in the early days, all from her. I'd hoped she was getting on with her life by now, in fact I even called her at Christmas just to see how she was.' His arms tightened around Chrissie, as, looking down at her, he said, 'I didn't tell you, because nothing came of it, and I knew from her response that she wasn't ready to see you.'

Chrissie swallowed hard. 'What makes you think I want to see her?' she whispered.

Smiling into her eyes, he said, 'You miss her dreadfully, I know that. And I hoped, if we could repair some of the damage, that it might help you to get strong again.' He kissed her forehead, then turned to Avril, who was caught between feeling like an intruder, and trying to get to grips with the admission of a phone call at Christmas.

John's next words showed that he was either well ahead of her, or out of his mind. 'Someone's been sending Carla emails,' he said, 'using details and references that would only mean something to you two. Can you explain that?'

Still not rattled, though again surprised, Richard said, 'Maybe if you told me what kind of details or references.'

'Passages from French classics,' John replied. 'Mentions of operas you'd been to together, places you've visited . . .' Before Richard could answer, he continued with, 'Do you have any idea where the letters are that you wrote Carla?'

Avril blinked, as she tried to keep up.

Perplexed, Richard said, 'I imagine with Carla.'

'Actually, they're missing,' John told him. And before the significance of that had any time to register, he added, 'Did you ever receive a letter from Carla's mother, just before she

402

died? Perhaps suggesting that she knew about your affair with Chrissie?'

Stunned, Avril watched Richard's own astonishment give way to a considered response. 'I don't recall ever receiving a letter from Valerie,' he finally answered. 'Either just before she died, or at any other time.'

'Or an email from Carla? Since you broke up?'

'No.'

John looked at Chrissie. 'Then who's been sending them?' he asked.

Chrissie's eyes boggled. 'I never send emails,' she told him. 'I never use the computer.'

'I'm sorry,' John said. 'That wasn't meant to be an accusation.' His eyes returned to Richard. 'Do you have any suggestions?' he asked.

Avril watched, dumbfounded, as something seemed to happen between the two men that finally came out in words presumably only they understood. 'He's always been very protective of her,' Richard said.

'And knew you extremely well,' John added. 'Presumably well enough to pass himself off as you on the email, particularly if he had your letters . . .'

'What are you talking about?' Chrissie demanded.

'Graham,' Avril said, finally catching up. 'You're talking about Graham.'

'Are you saying that Graham's been pretending he's Richard on the email?' Chrissie cried.

Richard said, 'How long has it been going on?'

'Six months, or more,' Avril answered, still so astounded by the idea of Graham sending the messages that she couldn't even begin to connect with where it would take them.

'But why?' Chrissie cried. 'Why would he do that?'

John was getting to his feet. 'I guess we need to ask him.'

A horrible thought suddenly burst into Avril's head, and, turning to Richard, she said, 'Just a minute, if you're not seeing Carla tonight . . .'

'Precisely,' John said, cutting her off. 'Do you know where they're meeting?'

'No,' Avril answered, her face draining of colour. 'I didn't ask. But surely he'll just stand her up again, because he can

403

hardly pretend he's Richard in person, can he?'

John and Richard looked at each other. 'True,' John said, 'but I'd be happier if I knew where the meeting was supposed to take place.'

'I don't know why you're all so alarmed,' Chrissie said. 'He'd never hurt her. He's much too fond of her.'

Richard turned back to John, waiting for his answer.

'I don't really want to get into it,' John said, 'but Graham could have another agenda that's much less benign than impersonating someone on the email, even if that is benign.'

Avril swung round. Was he saying now that he thought Graham might have had something to do with Valerie's death?

'You mean he could intend Carla some harm?' Richard said.

'Until we speak to him, I wouldn't want to venture what he intends,' John replied, glancing at his watch. 'But I do think you should call Carla and tell her you can't meet her tonight. At least if she knows the arrangement's off, she won't go to wherever he's suggested.'

'Where can I get her?' Richard asked, reaching for the phone.

Avril gave him the office number, but when he got through it was to be told that Carla wasn't there. Avril grabbed the phone. 'Marjie? It's Avril. Do you know where Carla is? We need to get hold of her urgently.'

'She went to get her hair cut,' Marjie answered. 'You can probably get her on her mobile.'

Avril hung up, and dialled Carla's mobile. Though it rang, no-one answered, presumably because her bag was stuffed in a locker. Then a recorded voice came on the line inviting the caller to leave a message. 'Carla!' Avril barked. 'Call me *immediately* you get this message. I'll be on my mobile.' Ending the call she looked at John. There really shouldn't be any urgency about this, but Carla being out of contact made it feel like there was.

'Did Marjie say if she was returning to the office?' John asked.

Avril instantly redialled. The answer was no, Carla wasn't expected back before five, when Marjie was leaving. Then

Marjie added, 'Was it you who just called Carla's mobile? I heard it ringing, upstairs in the studio. She must have forgotten to take it.'

'Oh Christ,' Avril groaned. She looked at her watch. It was a quarter to five. The supposed meeting with Richard wasn't until seven, so they still had a couple of hours, and Carla was highly likely to turn up at the *ménage* sometime after five, in order to get ready.

'Call Graham,' John said. 'Ask him if he's expecting her.'

'You think she's going down to Somerset?' Avril said, confused. 'Wouldn't she think it a bit odd for Richard to arrange to meet her there, when they're both in London?'

'I don't know,' John answered, 'but there's enough time for her to get there between now and seven. Or Graham could be on his way up to London. Do you know his number?'

Avril stared at him blankly. 'Being who he is, he's bound to be ex-directory,' she said, turning to Richard. 'I don't suppose you have it?'

He shook his head, and was about to speak when she suddenly started dialling again. 'Sonya'll have it,' she declared. A few beats later she made the connection.

'Avril!' Sonya cried. 'Are you coming down? I really need to see you.'

'Yeah, I'll be there,' Avril told her. 'But first, do you have Graham's number? I need to call him.'

'Why?' Sonya demanded, her voice sounding shrill.

'It's a long story, just give me the number.'

'There are things about Graham I need to tell you,' Sonya said.

Avril's eyes opened wider. 'What about him?' she responded, turning to look at John.

'Mark'll be back any minute,' Sonya replied, 'so I probably won't have time to tell you much, but I found a letter, in the pocket of . . .'

'What letter?' Avril broke in.

'I think it's the rest of the one Carla found in the thesis.' Sonya took a breath. 'Avril, it's terrible,' she said. 'Graham's wife, she's not his wife, and the detective . . . It's all in Valerie's letter. Avril, they've killed someone, and I'm just really afraid that they . . . They might have killed Valerie too.'

405

'Jesus Christ,' Avril cried. Then, pulling herself sharply together, said, 'Just give me that number. Now!'

As she dialled Graham's house, she relayed what Sonya had said, watching the same shock register on all their faces. 'Damn!' she muttered, when Graham's machine picked up.

Slamming down the phone she turned to John. 'I wish she'd bloody well call,' she growled.

Taking the phone, he dialled the office again and said to Marjie, 'It's John. Tell me, does Carla have Eddie with her?'

'Yes,' Marjie answered.

'OK,' he said, and rang off. 'If she's got Eddie then there's a very good chance she's on her way to Cannock,' he told the others.

'Or to somewhere between here and Cannock,' Avril added, unhelpfully.

'Call Sonya again,' John said, the tautness of his face belying the calmness of his tone. 'Find out if Carla told her where she was meeting Richard.'

Having made the connection, Avril asked the question, then turned hopeful eyes on the others as Sonya said, 'I didn't know she was meeting Richard, but she did say she was coming down to Cannock tonight.'

'What time?' she said.

'I presume straight from work.'

'Are you meeting her train?'

'She didn't ask me to.'

'Well, you'd better get to the station and make sure it's you who takes her to the cottage and nobody else. Better still, take her to your house.'

'Avril, you're scaring me. What's going on?'

'I'll explain everything when I see you, just please go to the station . . .'

'Which one? I've got no idea which train she's getting, or where she's going to come in.'

Frustration almost got the better of Avril, but with supreme effort she stopped herself screaming and said, 'Go to Bath. That's the most likely. She thinks she's meeting Richard at seven, so if she is heading to Cannock she should be there around six to six thirty.'

Banging down the phone she went after John, who was

already in the hall, putting on his coat. 'I hope to God she is going to Cannock and nowhere else,' he said, handing her hers. 'Even so, we're going to be heading straight into the rush-hour traffic now . . .'

'I think I should come with you,' Richard said.

Chrissie looked at him anxiously. 'Why?' she demanded.

'I just think I should,' he answered. 'Elinor's here, and I'll be back before you know it.'

Then to John, 'I'll take my own car, and follow you.'

As they ran outside Avril's heart did an almighty flip when Richard stopped at a silver BMW and started to get in. She'd forgotten all about the car, but wasn't it a silver BMW that had been spotted outside Carla's? Turning to grab John's arm she was about to tell him, when she remembered it was Graham's apparently bogus wife who'd claimed she'd seen the car. Shaking her head, she ran on to John's Range Rover.

'So what I want to know is how come you and Richard seemed to hit on Graham at the same time?' she said, as they sped off towards Knightsbridge.

John glanced at her, then hit the brakes hard, as they approached a red light. 'There was no coincidence in the timing,' he answered. 'I had my suspicions before we went in, and it didn't take me long to realize that Richard was speaking the truth.'

'So how did Graham get into your frame?'

'When there's a woman who matters, you're always aware of the other men in her life, no matter who they are, or what role they might play, and in Graham's case, the role was never quite clear. At least not to me. It would seem not to Richard either.'

'Mmm,' Avril grunted. 'Well, despite your bit of male bonding back there I just want to warn you that Richard Mere's a damn sight cleverer than most, and though you might have let him off your hook, he's definitely still on mine. So just you keep making sure he's behind us, and not whizzing off along some back roads trying to get there first.'

Chapter 23

The light from the computer screen was casting a soft blue-grey glow over Betty's face, making her skin seem coldly waxen and her eyes unnaturally bright. The room around her was in darkness, the curtains pulled, the door closed. She steered the cursor carefully to its positions, opening each of the email addresses that was set up with a literary title, checking to see if there were any last-minute messages from Carla, either cancelling her date with Richard, changing the venue, or saying something to confuse the plans.

Finally, satisfied that everything was going ahead, she shut down the computer, then, closing the study door behind her, she walked along the hall to the kitchen. Outside the wind was howling, making the old house creak and rumble, though no rain spattered the windows yet, and the moon was still a clear round ball in the night-black sky.

Placing a fresh sheet of paper on the table, she went to a drawer for a pen, then glanced at the clock. Six thirty. Pulling up a chair she sat down to write, her aging features registering no emotion as she penned the few necessary words before folding the sheet neatly into quarters, then going into the laundry-cum-cloakroom for her coat, boots and headscarf.

With no-one else at home to call goodbye to, she let herself quietly out the back door, and trudged in her small zip-top boots past the rows of onions and potatoes, carrots and parsnips, beneath the bamboo frame laden with fat runner beans, and on along the path to the gate. Once in the lane, she belted her coat more tightly around her, and knotted the scarf under her chin. It was so bitterly cold it was unlikely she'd pass any neighbours, but even if she did, no-one would expect her to stop, or even to speak. Unless something extraordinary happened she'd be there in a couple of minutes, earlier than planned, but she knew Carla was home, because she'd seen her and the dog arrive a short while ago.

Carla was still wearing her coat and gloves as she touched a match to a firelighter, piled some sticks and lumps of coal around it, then, after making sure it was catching, she went back to the kitchen to carry on unloading the groceries she'd brought in. Hiring a car and driving down from London had shown her just how much she missed the convenience of being able to stop off at the supermarket, or chemist, or outrageously expensive lingerie shop where she'd picked out something very special for tomorrow night, without having to put someone else to the trouble of taking her.

'Yes, we definitely need to get a car of our own,' she told Eddie, slotting a pack of chicken breasts into the freezer, then closing the door quickly before she frosted up along with everything inside. 'We're not rich enough to go for anything fancy, at least not yet, but we should be able to stretch ourselves to something that'll get us up and down the M4. You'd like that, wouldn't you?' she said, peeling off her gloves and passing him a salt and vinegar crisp.

Wolfing it down, he sat waiting for another, which he got when a wave of nerves stole Carla's appetite and made her look at the clock. All day she'd been trying to imagine what it was going to be like seeing Richard again, especially here, where he'd once been as at home as she was. It was disconcerting to think of how relaxed he had been with her mother, and Eddie, and the neighbours, when she now knew that, at the end at least, it had all been a sham. It annoyed and dismayed her to know that his betrayal still hurt, though fortunately much less than it once had. Nevertheless, she regretted not putting her foot down about meeting some-where more public, for she was unsettled by the prospect of him returning to the intimacy of her home, even though he'd said they could go out when he got there. Apparently he was staying with some friends at Bradford-on-Avon, who must be new, because she didn't remember him knowing anyone there before.

409

Going into the sitting room to check that the fire was still flickering, she shovelled on more coal, gave it some help with the bellows, then banged her hands together as she thought of all the planning, and perfection, she'd be pouring into tomorrow night. By then it would hopefully be much warmer in here, and romantically cosy with lots of candles, wine and soft music. She gave a quirky sort of smile at the strangeness, yet joy, of knowing the effort was going to be for another man, and how startling, yet wonderful it was to know that the other man was John. However, Richard was yet to be dealt with, and though she might be reserving all the real effort for tomorrow night, she had intended at least to shower and change before he arrived. But with it being so cold upstairs there was just no way she could bring herself to peel off even one layer of clothing, never mind the lot. Besides, time was running out, so giving up on the idea of looking so fantastic he'd torment himself for years for ever letting her go, she was about to get out a hairbrush and some lipstick when Eddie suddenly started to bark, and her heart leapt to her throat.

'Damn you, Richard,' she muttered, not only because he was early, but because now he was here she no longer wanted to see him. What was the point of putting herself through it, when all she really wanted was to forget and move on?

'Eddie, stop!' she shouted, as his excitement seemed to grow more frenzied. 'Stop!' she repeated as he bounded into the hall, then back into the kitchen. She hadn't heard anyone knock yet, so he must have heard the car, though it was unlike him to get this worked up over someone driving up and getting out.

'Eddie! What is it?' she cried, as he bounced up and down, and kept running over to the back door. 'No, you're not going out there. It's dark and it's too cold.' As she finished speaking she was looking curiously at the slip of paper Eddie was pouncing on, as though trying to attract her attention towards it.

'What is it?' she said, going towards him.

Tail wagging furiously, he stared fixedly down at the note, waiting for her to pick it up, then followed her movements as she unfolded it and started to read. 'Dear Carla, I'm sorry to approach you like this, but it's very important that I speak to

410

you. I'm outside in the back garden, and can't come to the door because I'm afraid of the dog. Yours, Betty Foster.'

Carla's heartbeat gave a skip of surprise. Frowning, she looked at the door and imagined Betty out there in the cold, a lone figure in the darkness, watching the cottage, and sending a shiver down Carla's spine with the very strangeness of her actions. Looking at Eddie's crooked little ears and eager face, she said, 'How can she be afraid of you?'

His head tilted to one side, then began scratching at the door.

'No.' She pulled him back, then, realizing Betty was asking for him to be shut away before she came in, she found herself feeling slightly uneasy. This was such peculiar behaviour from a woman who never spoke to anyone, much less asked to be let in through the back door on a cold wintry night, that she couldn't think what to do. And in a complete turnabout from a few moments ago she found herself willing Richard to turn up right now. Then she started as Betty's voice called out softly, 'Carla, please don't be afraid. I only . . .'

Eddie's barking drowned whatever else she said, so taking him into the office and closing the door, Carla returned to the kitchen, and said, 'Betty, can you hear me?'

'Yes, dear.'

'Betty, I don't understand why you're doing this. What's the matter with coming to the front door?'

'I don't want anyone to see me come in,' Betty answered.

Carla stared at the back door in amazement. Had she heard that correctly?

'I understand that I'm probably alarming you,' Betty said, 'but I really do have to talk to you.'

'Where's Graham?' Carla asked.

'Giving a talk at a library in Bath.'

Carla fell silent and stared hard at the door as she tried to decide what to do. On the one hand, it seemed absurd to be unnerved, not to mention mean to keep an old lady out in the cold. However, some instinct, or maybe it was paranoia, seemed to be buzzing an alarm in her head, making her wonder if Betty was some kind of crazy woman that Graham kept under control with drugs, and under lock and key when he wasn't around? Far-fetched maybe, but what about all

411

those trips she made to her sister's? Maybe they were just a cover for spells she spent in a psychiatric clinic. Maybe she'd escaped and her medication was wearing off . . .

Realizing she was spooking herself to the point of needing her own psychiatric help, Carla forced her mind into the more rational reminder that she was not only a lot taller than Betty, but a lot younger, and presumably stronger too. So, unless Betty was armed with an intent to kill, which she seriously doubted, where was the harm in letting her in?

Carefully sliding the bolt back, she turned the key in the lock, then moved swiftly over to the knife drawer, just in case, and called out, 'OK, you can come in.'

The handle made a slow half-turn, then the door swung gently open, and Betty's meek, wind-mottled face appeared from the darkness.

'Thank you,' she said, though her eyes were darting anxiously around the kitchen.

Realizing she was looking for Eddie, Carla said, 'It's OK, he wouldn't hurt you.'

'I just . . . I'm afraid I have a bit of a phobia about dogs,' Betty admitted, her close-set eyes peering out of the oval frame of her headscarf, and making her look no more ominous than an old lady who'd come in the front way collecting for the Salvation Army. Also, the slight hint of a Northern accent was welcome, for it added some credibility to sojourns with a sister rather than weeks in a straitjacket.

'It's cold,' Carla said, nodding towards the door.

Betty quickly closed it, then, making to untie her scarf, asked if Carla minded.

Carla waved her on, watching her fussy little movements that ended with the scarf being tucked into a coat pocket, and betrayed no signs of a manically deranged inner person.

'You're very like your mother,' Betty commented, surprising her.

Carla merely looked at her. Then, seeing the unsettling effect her scrutiny was having, she heard herself saying, 'Would you like to come in by the fire?'

Betty nodded. 'That would be nice, thank you.'

As Carla led the way through Eddie started barking again, and Betty instantly drew back. 'It's OK, he's in the office,'

Carla assured her, the strangeness of the situation making her feel slightly out of kilter with herself. Then chattily she added, 'I'm expecting someone shortly, so I'm afraid I don't have much time.'

Betty turned as she reached an armchair. 'Is it all right if I sit here?' she asked.

'Of course,' Carla answered. 'I'd offer to take your coat, but the fire hasn't really got going yet.'

They both looked down at it, watching the flames flying up the chimney, too new to give off much heat, but managing to add a sprightly animation to the small, chilly room. Then, perching on the edge of the chair, Betty said, 'I've been trying to talk to you for a while, but with the dog always here . . . It was me on the phone on Christmas Day, when you were at the pub. Graham knows it was me, but he wouldn't tell you that.'

Carla was too taken aback to make any kind of immediate response, but after sitting down on the sofa, while watching Betty's curious distraction, she said, 'Why didn't you just call me here?'

Seeming not, hear the question, Betty said, 'I've come a few times, but I'm always so nervous of the dog . . . I kept hoping you'd look out and see me.'

When she stopped Carla gave a quick glance at the clock. Richard should be arriving any minute.

Interpreting the glance, Betty said, 'I'm afraid Richard's not coming.'

Disbelief widened Carla's eyes, but before she could fully register that, Betty said, 'The emails, they've all been from Graham.'

Carla stared at her, so unnerved by this astounding statement that she was back to thinking the woman insane, and that she had somehow to get her out of here.

Betty said, 'Actually, the last email, the one asking you to come here tonight, that was from me. I'm sorry I tricked you, but I was afraid if I told you I wanted to see you, and asked you to keep it secret from Graham, that you'd tell him anyway.'

At last Carla found her voice. 'I'm sorry, Betty,' she said, 'but I'm not following any of this. In fact, I'm . . .' She jumped as the phone suddenly rang. 'Totally confused,' she added weakly, then was about to get up, when Betty's words stopped her.

'Please don't answer it,' she said.

Carla blinked.

'In case it's Graham,' Betty explained. 'Or anyone else. I really need to tell you what's been going on, because I can't sit by and allow all these lies to continue.'

Hearing the answerphone pick up in the study, Carla sat back and waited for Betty to go on.

'Perhaps I should begin by telling you that I'm not Graham's wife,' Betty said, glancing down at her joined hands. 'I'm really just a housekeeper, and, I suppose, a friend.'

Though mildly stunned by this revelation Carla quickly realized that, as a truth, it had some merit, considering the almost separate lives the two of them led. 'So why say you're his wife?' she asked.

Betty blinked a couple of times, then said, 'It was decided, some time ago, that it would be easier that way.'

'What would?' Carla said, trying to think of a scenario that would suit this description, but what she came up with was so bizarre, she decided just to let Betty continue.

'Barry Fellowes,' Betty said, 'who you all think of as a detective, is my real husband. We met Graham fifteen years ago when Barry answered an advertisement Graham had put in the local paper. We were all living up north then, and Barry hadn't worked in a while, so he was keen to get the job Graham was offering. It was just a handyman's position, with a bit of gardening, and the occasional driving, but it provided a little cottage in the grounds of Graham's house that was a lot better than the council flat we were in at the time. So he went for the interview, and when he told Graham about me, Graham took me on too, as his cook-housekeeper. He wasn't all that well known as a writer then, but he comes from a moneyed family, and Barry and me, well, we'd never even set foot in a house like Graham's before, so we thought ourselves very fortunate to have this chance. And right from the start it all worked out very well. We got along nicely, all of us, and Graham was the best employer we'd ever had. Still is, I

414

suppose, but everything's very different now to what it was back then . . .'

She paused, blinking rapidly for a moment, then, after glancing anxiously at Carla, she continued. 'We'd been with him about a year when he offered Barry a kind of bonus in return for helping him research one of his books. The two of them often used to sit up late into the night talking through plots and motives, and all that sort of thing, still do in fact, but Graham had never offered to pay Barry before, and definitely not the kind of money he was talking about now . . . At the time I didn't know anything about it, Barry didn't tell me because he knew I'd never have let him take the money, never mind get involved. The first I knew about anything was when the police came to tell Graham that someone had been found dead in the woods at the back of his property. Of course, I didn't have any idea how the poor chap had come to be there, or even who he was, so when the police questioned me it was easy to be ignorant, because at that point I was. They questioned Graham and Barry too, and for a long time I thought they were as baffled as me. But then Barry told me what had really happened.'

She took a breath, and Carla noticed the way her mouth was trembling as she tried to go on. After a few halted attempts, she said, 'Graham was writing about this character who was a bit of a simple bloke, ordinary like, who gets offered more money than he could ever earn in his life to kill someone. That was the basis of the book, and the bloke being offered the money was the point where the story started, which meant that straight away Graham wanted Barry to tell him how he felt about the offer, you know, all the conflicting emotions, like doubt, greed, fear, excitement, so Graham could write them all down. Then they spent months recording everything Barry was experiencing as they went through the motions of picking out their victim, and hatching out a plot on how to go about it without getting caught. Barry says it all took on a momentum of its own, that it wasn't really serious when they first got started, but I don't know. All I know is that when the time came Graham was there, in the woods, when Barry brought the old drunk over from Barnsley, and bashed in his head with a stone. Then he got Barry to tell him everything he'd been feeling,

415

from the time he'd picked the man up to the point when he knew the man was actually dead . . . The two of them discussed it for months, along with all the details of the investigation. That was an important part of it too, because Graham was now having some first-hand experience of being interrogated by the police, and the chance of being found out, the fear and all the other things he felt, all went into the book. Well, I expect you've read it. *Tragic Endeavours*. It was his first big bestseller.'

Dimly aware of how slowly she was breathing, Carla thought about the book, and how it was lending an awful truth to Betty's words. Then there was that extraordinary moment in the pub, the night *There and Beyond* was first transmitted, when he'd confessed to seeing someone murdered. But such lack of respect for human life, and outrageous exploitation of a humble man's morals, didn't fit at all with the Graham she knew, until she realized, with a cold, sinking dread, that it would fit with the man who'd been sending emails she'd believed were from Richard. Recoiling from that, she looked at Betty, whose right cheek was glowing red from the fire. Seeming to decide that Carla was now ready to hear more, Betty continued.

'It was about the time the book came out that Graham decided we should all move south,' she said. 'Well, we say it was Graham's idea, but really it was Barry's, because he had a fancy for living in a big house of his own, now he could afford it, and if he bought himself somewhere near where we were people would wonder where he'd got the money. So we all came south and that was when Barry and Graham said that it would be better if we told everyone I was Graham's wife. That way no-one would wonder why he wasn't married, being so eligible like, and it would prevent him from having another woman move in, which Barry didn't want, because he was afraid of anyone finding out our secret. Of course, we don't ever call it blackmail, what goes on between the three of us, but really, that's what it is, because we've all got this hold over each other now, and though the characters in Graham's book *Quiet Chaos* are two women and a man, he's based it on the way we all live, and the harm we could do each other, if we wanted.'

The phone was ringing again, but this time Carla didn't

even attempt to get up, nor did she hear the rain that had started drumming against the windows.

'Of course, me and Graham, we've never lived together as man and wife,' Betty said. 'At least not, you know, in the biblical sense. We have separate rooms, and I expect you've noticed how often I go away ... Barry's got us a big house, just outside Taunton, which needs a lot of looking after, but it's private, and no-one round about really knows who we are, or thinks of Barry as a detective, the way they do here. It was a cover Graham came up with, because no-one would be suspicious of a detective making regular visits to someone who writes the kind of books he does.' She took a quick breath, but didn't continue until a distant rumble of thunder had subsided into the wind and rain. 'We've had some really bad periods over the years,' she said, her eyes reflecting the troubled state of her mind. 'Times when things have turned so ugly ... All the blame, and the threats ... Of course it's pressure as well as guilt that gets us all riled up ... We all want to get out of the situation, but there's no way we can now, so we have to get over it, and I suppose, in its way, it makes us a bit like any other family, except with us we're really stuck together. But I have to keep reminding myself that it could be a lot worse, because underneath it all Graham's a lovely man, and does everything he can to help us through the bad times. Well, you know what he's like, and I can tell you, he thinks the world of you. You're the daughter he never had, and no-one's ever mattered more to him than you, except your mother, of course, when she was alive.'

Carla tensed at the mention of her mother, but said nothing as Betty's pale eyes seemed to drift into some other kind of thoughts that even a new crescendo of thunder didn't appear to disrupt.

'Lovely woman, Valerie,' she said. 'I'd like to have known her, but Graham and Barry thought it would be safer if I never got on terms with anyone, then there wouldn't be any danger of me and Graham contradicting one another, you know, about our pasts or what-have-you, that would make people suspicious.' She stopped and stared forlornly down at her lap, apparently contemplating the hopelessness of her existence.

Watching her, Carla couldn't help wondering why she was telling her all this now, and was about to ask when a loud rap on the front door set her heart pounding and Eddie barking. Her first thought was of Richard, then, remembering, her eyes returned to Betty, who appeared suddenly very tense and anxious, and on the point of springing to her feet.

'Are you expecting someone?' she whispered.

Carla shook her head, and they continued to look at each other as Eddie stopped barking leaving only the storm breaking the silence. Seconds ticked by, then the sound of a key going into the lock set Eddie off again and turned Carla rigid. Telling herself that it had to be Avril, or Sonya, she stared out into the hall, so on edge that she didn't even call out for Eddie to stop.

The sound of the front door closing brought her to her feet. Her heart was pounding and the fire was burning her legs as Eddie's bark turned to a whine, the way it often did when greeting someone he knew. She knew it must be Graham, and fear slid through her to realize he was in the study with Eddie! But he wouldn't hurt Eddie. There was no need. He just wanted to reassure him, and settle him down.

Her eyes remained fixed on the doorway as she strained her ears for a voice, then her heart jolted at the sound of the office door being quietly closed. There was a brief silence, then the floorboards creaked. A moment later Graham's large frame filled up the doorway, seeming to trap them in the room. Then his eyes found Carla's and it was as though the air was suddenly thickened by the strain of his pent-up emotions, while rain from the grooves of his hair ran down his face like tears.

For several long, disorienting seconds they merely looked at each other, as she tried to reconcile the familiarity of his face and warmth of his aura with the cold-blooded actions Betty had described. In a way it was like looking in a mirror and seeing the wrong reflection, for no evil showed in his persona – in fact nothing, except her perception, had changed since the last time she'd seen him. Yet the very fact that he'd let himself in, and that he was now standing there, unwelcomed and attempting to gauge her thoughts, removed them from the norm in a way that was frighteningly strange.

Finally he turned to Betty and began slowly to shake his head. 'You're not experienced enough with the computer to cover your tracks,' he informed her.

Carla looked at her too, and saw an uneasy defiance in her eyes. 'I had to come,' she told him. 'You know that.'

'No, Betty, you didn't,' he responded. Then, looking at Carla, he said, 'How much has she told you?'

Unwilling to mention the murder, Carla said, 'I know she's not your wife.'

For a moment Graham pulled thoughtfully at his beard, then, indicating the other fireside chair, said, 'May I?' Without waiting for an answer, he unbuttoned his coat and came further into the room. When he was seated, he addressed Betty again. 'Does Carla know that you've tried speaking to her before?' he asked. 'Have you told her that the woman her niece and nephew saw was you, trying to pluck up courage to get past the dog? And the female intruder Maudie spotted? Have you admitted it was you, and explained what you were doing? And the phone call to the pub on Christmas Day? Of course, your incompetence on all occasions denotes an underlying willingness to be caught, we all understand that, it's just unfortunate that this time you've managed to get much further. Now, what I need to know is how much further?'

'She knows about the emails,' Betty said quickly.

Graham's brows went up, and after slowly nodding his head he looked up at Carla. 'Won't you sit down?' he said.

For a long time she only looked at him, waiting for him, even willing him, to deny Betty's words. But he didn't, and as the horrendous, unthinkable truth of what he'd done washed over her, her sense of violation could hardly have been any worse. She looked at his hands, and his face, the crook of his legs inside his trousers, and the swell of his chest beneath his shirt. Then she thought of all the things he might have done to himself in response to the intensely intimate instructions she had given, she thought, to Richard. Masturbation was only the beginning; she couldn't bear to go any further, for never, in her worst nightmares, had she ever imagined it was Graham, the man she'd almost considered a father, who was receiving those emails, and doing God only knew what as a

419

result of them. Nor could she bear to think of the brazen acts she had carried out on herself, using her fingers, and mirrors and ropes and candles, all the time thinking it was Richard asking her to do those things, sitting somewhere in his own quiet space at the hour they arranged, knowing everything from the moment she disrobed to the moment she reached self-imposed fulfilment. And it had only ever been Graham sitting in that quiet space, thinking, seeing, controlling . . . Dear God, how many times had he looked at her, knowing she wore no underwear, because *he*, not Richard, had told her not to? And all the frankly obscene words she had used to describe her lust, intending to turn Richard on – what had they done to the man who was really receiving them? *Oh God! Oh God!* Her stomach churned and her head reeled at the sheer revulsion of it all. It was so perverted and disgusting and outrageously invasive that just to look at him now was making her skin crawl, for it was as though he had touched the most intimate parts of her with the most intimate parts of himself, and she *just couldn't stand it*!

'Has Betty told you the reason for the emails?' he asked her.

'No,' she responded, her voice breaking through a wall of repulsion.

He took a moment to digest this, apparently summoning an excuse for the inexcusable. Suddenly she wanted to yell at him, scream and rant, bang her fists in his face, but all she did was stare down at him in unrestrained disgust. He knew what he'd done, so he knew how she must be feeling, and she didn't want him to make any mistake.

When finally he spoke his words almost took her breath away. 'I did it for your own good,' he said.

Her mouth opened, then, pressing a hand to her head, she sank down on the sofa. 'You've lost your mind,' she told him.

He was nodding. 'I know you think that's an extremely odd, and even unkind thing to say,' he responded, 'but it's true. I did it for your own good, and I think Betty would bear me out on that.'

Carla looked at Betty, but it appeared she had lost her tongue, for she merely continued to stare down at her tightly bunched hands.

'You were in a great deal of pain,' Graham said, recalling

her attention, 'which was hardly surprising considering the level of betrayal and rejection you'd suffered at the same time as the death of your mother . . . Even the strongest individual would have been incapacitated by such a series of blows, and if you have any idea how much you mean to me . . .' He stopped as Carla flinched, then continued with, 'It was very difficult seeing you struggling so hard to overcome it all. Months went by and the hurt just never seemed to leave you. Or maybe it did by degrees, but it carried on holding you back, making you afraid. I knew you were trying, but with your mother no longer here to help you, and your father heaven only knows where . . . You needed someone to coax you out of the despair, and I believed if I could eliminate at least one part of your grief, by making it appear as though it had no actual substance, then there was a very good chance of you making a swifter and more thorough return to the life you should have been leading. Of course your mother's death was irreversible. Nor could I undo Chrissie's or Richard's betrayal. But rejection lends itself rather more readily to perspective, and since perspective is much easier to change, I realized that was what I must do. So I devised a way of making you see the rejection as a deeply regretted mistake, which wasn't difficult when none of us ever wants to believe we're wrong about someone we love, nor do we ever find it easy to let them go. It therefore stood to reason that you'd accept that love again in whatever shape or form, and as the email was the perfect tool, I used it to help you rediscover your confidence and strength through the continuance of a connection you had trusted so completely, and needed so desperately, that it was unlikely you'd question it too closely. Although you did question it, but only ever in a way that would give you the answers you needed. And as angry as you might be now, I don't think you can say that the desired results weren't achieved.'

As appalled that he could think she'd approve of his actions, as she was at the actions themselves, she felt so much outrage gathering inside her that it was hard to keep her voice steady as she said, 'You're surely not trying to tell me that you believe betrayal can cancel out rejection, because that's what this amounts to, and you know it. You've betrayed me now more insidiously than Richard or Chrissie ever did, because this kind of exploitation and manipulation, no matter how worthy or altruistic you try to make the motive, is monstrous and totally unforgivable. Jesus Christ, I bared my soul in those emails, thinking I was talking to Richard, and all the time . . .' She put her hands over her face, as the near incestuousness of the sex once again swamped her. 'My God, it makes me feel ill just to think of it. What a fool I must be . . .'

'No, never a fool,' he argued. 'Only someone who was wise enough to see this as an easier and quicker path back to the life they'd abandoned.'

Her head snapped up in furious amazement. 'How can you say that,' she cried, 'when I had no idea you were behind it, pulling all the strings, experimenting with my psyche, as though you were some kind of god with a new creation. I truly believed those emails were from Richard, and now, just to think of the way you exploited all my confidences and played games with my mind, not to mention . . . God, I can still hardly believe you did it,' she gasped. 'You're a sick and cruel man, you must know that.'

His eyes went down, and she saw that a small tic was jerking one lid. 'Yes,' he said, 'I was always afraid you'd think that, but it was a risk I was prepared to take, just to see you whole again.'

Unable to look at him any longer, she shielded her eyes with her hand. It was all just too awful and humiliating and outrageous to take on board in its entirety.

'Tell her about the letters,' Betty suddenly said.

Carla glanced up at her, then returned her gaze to Graham, who was still looking down, watching his thumbs circling each other and seeming almost diminished by her aversion to his atrocious methods of therapy.

'Yes, the letters,' he said, finally looking up. 'Of course, they were very helpful. Mimicking Richard's style, and knowing the complete depth and tenor of your relationship, would have been almost impossible without them.'

Carla was aghast. '*You* have my letters from Richard?' she exploded.

He nodded.

'But how on earth did you get them? Sonya would never

have . . .' Dashing a hand through her hair, she said, 'This is so much worse than I realized. So much worse . . .'

'Yes,' he agreed. 'It is.'

Her eyes were scathing as she turned them back to him. 'You've trespassed on something that was so precious and private to me that you've got to know I can never forgive you. In fact, if I could I'd . . .'

'Tell her why it's worse than she realizes,' Betty interrupted.

Graham's face was bleak as he looked at Betty.

'Tell her about the book,' Betty insisted. 'Tell her how you've been harvesting . . . That's what he calls it,' she said to Carla, 'harvesting. He's been harvesting your responses, and using them for the central character in the book he's writing now. So there's not quite as much altruism in his motives as he's willing for you to think.'

'It began because I care about her so much,' Graham angrily responded. 'You know that, so don't try to paint it any other way. The using of her responses came much later, and only because she had such a fascinating ability to make anything I threw at her work . . .'

'Stop discussing me as though I weren't here,' Carla seethed.

Graham was immediately contrite. 'I'm sorry,' he said quietly. Then, after a pause to collect himself, he said, 'What Betty is referring to is your remarkable capacity for giving every quotation or innuendo I cited a merit or a meaning I had not foreseen. In other words, you were so willing to believe that it was Richard who was sending you those messages that no matter how obscure they were, you always managed to turn them into a message that was not only uplifting for your spirits, but nourishing for your heart. Of course, I tried always to stay with the works he'd mentioned in his letters, but even if I ventured outside them, you invariably gathered them into the realms of understanding that only a woman in love, and so in need of reassurance, can possess.'

Carla's eyes were blazing. 'You mean you were challenging my pathetic powers of self-delusion to see if there was anything I couldn't turn into a nice soothing balm for my belittled ego. Well, I'm sure I wasn't a disappointment, because we all know that the human capacity for self-deception is almost limitless when it's time to face the rejection and let go of love. The problem is, when we're in the thick of it, we never seem to realize we're doing it – unless you've got a friend like Avril who keeps trying to make you face it. But I wouldn't, so I can see what a gift of a study I was for you. Why make it up, when you've got me to do it for you? Give her a few quotes from Rousseau, or a maxim from La Rochefoucauld, then sit back and see how her poor deluded mind turns them into proofs of love, and reasons to hope. Very convenient for a man who doesn't think like a woman, but needs to write like one. Ingenious, in fact. What I want to know is what the hell you were planning to do if Richard *had* come back into my life?'

Graham sat in the aftermath of her outburst, as though allowing the air to settle and some calm to return, before he spoke again. 'We thought,' he said finally, 'when he called you at Christmas, that that eventuality had in fact arisen. But it seems we were wrong.'

Carla's eyes closed as she grasped the one single occasion that had been true. It surprised her to find that it gave her a steadying kind of warmth, until more anger erupted with the realization of Graham's remarkable good fortune that nothing had been said in that call to blow his despicable scheme wide apart. Then she was glaring at him again as she said, 'Of course, it's why there was the confusion over Richard's visit to Zanzibar, isn't it? You didn't know that he'd never been. You just assumed he had, because I assumed he had.'

He didn't deny it, nor did he offer any excuse or apology.

'Oh God,' she groaned with a laugh of disbelief and disgust. 'It's sick. So unbelievably sick.' A second or two passed, then her rage mounted again as she cried, 'Just what would you have done if I'd agreed to be godmother?'

He was shaking his head. 'I knew there was no risk of that,' he told her.

Inflamed even further by his arrogance, she shouted, 'Of course you did. After all, wasn't it you who suggested that he'd probably only used the question to get me to respond?

424

Of course it was you, because it's always been you, avoiding giving answers that I was too afraid to press for, in case I learned something that would hurt me all over again. So there was another little exercise for you, the denial and cowardice a person goes into as a means of self-protection. Did you get that? Yes, of course you did. It wouldn't be like you to miss it. And what about standing me up? How convenient it was for you that I was so fearful of it happening that I didn't wait more than fifteen minutes, then sent an email immediately I got back to say what I'd done. Once again, I played right into your hands. How lucky you've been with me. And how very contemptible and dangerous you are.'

'No, please don't say that,' he protested. 'You're whole and happy again now. You're riding many exciting waves in your career, you're on the brink of a new relationship with a very special man, and we have always rejoiced in the many rewards of our friendship. This doesn't need to come between us. It can be put down to what it was, a rather misguided but extremely well-intentioned attempt to help you through an exceptionally bad spell in your life.'

Carla's outrage could find no words, so she merely turned to Betty as Betty said harshly, 'I didn't only tell her about the emails.'

Carla eyes shot back to Graham, and she saw a man she had once known seeming to shrink inside his skin rather than face the cruel light of yet more exposure.

'I had always hoped,' he said gruffly to Carla, 'that you'd never need to know even half as much as you already do, but it would appear that Betty has done her worst, so in order to give the situation any understanding, or forgiveness, I can see that I must tell you certain other facts that are going to be perhaps even more shocking and painful to hear than those you already have.'

Unable to imagine anything that could even come close to being worse, she merely stared at him with flatly hostile eyes.

'The page that you found in your mother's thesis,' he began, startling her with such an unexpected change of subject, 'was part of a letter she wrote, I believe to Richard. I needed to find the entire letter, which I knew had never reached Richard, or we certainly wouldn't be sitting here

425

now. I also needed to find it without alerting you to its contents, or even indeed that it had any particular significance. Our means of doing so have been both enterprising and costly, and I'm afraid rather intrusive, since we not only had to perform several searches of this house without being detected, we also had to equip your telephones, and indeed the house itself, with certain electronic devices that would allow us to listen to, or record, your conversations, so that if you ever found the letter we'd know straight away.'

Stupefied beyond speech, Carla could only watch as he got up to put more coal on the fire. His actions seemed to lend yet another bizarre dimension to the already staggering complexity of his role in her life.

'It was during one of our early searches for that letter,' he said, as he sat down again, 'that we came across Richard's letters to you. I still have them, of course, and you are welcome to them back at any time.'

Carla made no response, only allowed her repugnance and anger to show as she continued to glare at him.

His eyes dropped for a moment, then, after a brief look at Betty, he said, 'Getting back to our methods of tracing the letter your mother wrote ... You might recall an occasion, one Sunday afternoon, when you and Sonya were talking on the phone about Richard's letters, and it was mentioned that they could be under the stairs. Thanks to our electronic devices we were able to hear your conversation, so I immediately called to invite you and Avril to come and help celebrate my birthday. Which you did, and while you were with me Barry Fellowes, whose correct identity I imagine you're now acquainted with, came here to the cottage to look under the stairs. Unfortunately he didn't find the letter, so we had no choice but to go on listening and looking, and since a good deal of our devices have been installed through the walls of the house next door, our main problem has been Maudie and her almost constant vigilance.'

Carla thought of Maudie's sharp little features peering out through the cloud of her white net curtains, always knowing something was going on next door, but never understanding what. And to think, in her concern, she'd asked Barry

426

Fellowes himself to check over old Gilbert's house to find out what was going on. Were it not so pitiable, it could almost be laughable.

'Fortunately for us,' Graham continued, 'Maudie never appears actually to have seen anyone, though Sonya certainly did, the day she arrived unexpectedly and caught me coming out of the house. I believe I'd come in that time to replace a file we'd taken that contained details of the storage company you were using in London. Though there was an itemized list for each of the containers, we weren't expecting the letter to be mentioned, but it helped us to know what was in each box, so that Barry could keep his search to a minimum when he went to see if the letter had somehow found its way into storage. Prior to that, as I recall, we claimed Betty had seen someone who looked like Richard outside the cottage while you and Avril were in Monte Carlo. We did this for two reasons, one, because Betty and I were still inside the cottage, looking through your mother's thesis, when Barry called to tell us that Sonya was on her way to the village and was likely to arrive at any moment. We left the thesis in rather a mess, I'm afraid, so we thought it better to suggest that Richard had been around that day, rather than any other kind of intruder. This was working on the assumption that if you thought there was a chance it was Richard, you'd be unlikely to call the police.'

Carla didn't mention that she'd never found the thesis in a mess, though Avril might have, as she was using that room at the time. However, it did account for how the mail had got to her desk that weekend, since Sonya was certain she hadn't picked it up. What a silly mistake for such a clever man, though it had hardly caused him a problem.

'The second reason we suggested Richard was there,' Graham said, 'was to make you think he was serious about a reunion. By then we knew what model of car he drove, because we'd hired a private detective to watch his house, as a kind of precaution.'

Carla's eyes were now painfully wide. 'A precaution against what?' she said, too bemused now to be angry.

'Well, we needed to know where he was at any given time in case he turned up on the TV somewhere in Afghanistan, or Africa, when we were saying he was in

427

London. We also needed to get an idea of his relationship with Chrissie . . .'

'Why did you need to know that?' she cried, hating this more than ever.

'In case it was breaking up and he showed any signs of returning to you. I'd need to know that, wouldn't I, considering I was pretending to be him.'

Feeling a wave of revulsion shudder through her again, she said, 'This is all so warped and horrible that I'm not sure I want you to go on.'

His eyes were gentle as he looked at her, waiting for her to make up her mind.

'Just what the hell do you think's in this letter?' she finally asked.

'Oh, we know what's in it,' he answered, glancing at Betty, 'because just like she came to you tonight, Betty paid your mother a visit too, and apprised her of our little secret. Didn't you, Betty?'

It took only a moment for Carla's mind to soar through the entire extent of his meaning, then explode in utter horror as she realized that if her mother had known about the murder, if she'd threatened to go to the police . . . 'No,' she whispered, a thick, pounding heat burning in her chest. 'Tell me it's not true. Oh, please God, no, no, no.'

'It's not true,' Graham said firmly. 'It's not what you think, but it's because of what you think that we had to find that letter before you or anyone else did.'

Carla was on her feet. 'You killed her,' she cried breathlessly. 'Oh my God! The blow to her head. You killed her. You killed her.'

Both Graham and Betty rose, but before either of them could reach her, she was gone, out through the kitchen, into the garden, away from their shouting and pleading for her to come back and listen, to give them a chance to explain. But no explanation was needed. Her mother had known about the murder they'd committed, and now her mother was dead, killed in the exact same way. Was that what they were intending for her now? To bash in her brains, rather than risk letting her live another day with their hideous secret? Oh God, why, oh why had Betty told her?

428

Throwing open the gate she staggered against the wind into the lane, and began heading through the driving rain to Maudie's. Jagged forks of lightning flashed down from the sky, lighting the way for a brief, dazzling moment, then suddenly she became aware of a figure looming out of the darkness ahead. Terror struck her heart as she realized it was Barry Fellowes, and, spinning into a forceful gust, she pushed her way back into the garden, and made for the shed. She tripped on a flagstone, then lost her footing in the mud, but finally she managed to tear open the door and with violently shaking fingers pulled the key from the lock, before closing and locking the door behind her.

By now her heart was thudding so hard she could barely even hear the rain above it, nor, in her agitated state, could she dare to hide behind the old bicycles and boxes, for fear of knocking something over. So standing as still as she was able, rain dripping from her hair on to her face, limbs juddering like crazy, she strained her ears to hear anything beyond the pounding might of the storm. Then her heart twisted with terror as she heard the clatter and squeal of the gate opening and closing, followed by the noise of someone squelching through the mud towards the shed. There was a moment of nothing but the wind and rain, then she almost screamed, as the door suddenly rattled.

'It's not going to do you any good hiding in there,' Fellowes called out. 'So open the door, or I'll have to force it.'

Carla stayed where she was, hardly daring to breathe, as tears streamed down her face. *Dear God, please help me, please help me,* she prayed fervently and silently, for this was the man who'd beaten an innocent drunk to death, and who had very probably wielded the rock that had killed her mother. So what was he going to do to her now? The same? Or did they have something else planned for her? Oh God, why had Betty told her? And how in hell, trapped here in this shed, was she ever going to escape them?

Chapter 24

'Oh, for God's sake!' Avril cried, as they sped round a bend in the motorway to be confronted by a twisting chain of red tail lights that snaked as far as the eye could see. 'What is it? Roadworks, or an accident?'

'Roadworks,' John answered. 'They've been here for weeks. Damn!' he muttered, thumping the wheel. 'I should have remembered.'

'Is Richard still with us?' she said, turning to look back.

'Is it him? I can't tell,' John responded, glancing in the rear-view mirror, only to be blinded by the headlights behind.

'I think so. Oh God! What are we going to do?' she seethed, as they came to a stop. 'We can't even turn round. And why doesn't she answer the damn phone?' she added, shaking her mobile in frustration.

'Try again,' John said, looking at the time. 'Jesus, it's after half past seven. If they were meeting at the cottage she'd be there by now.'

'Unless they weren't actually meeting there,' Avril responded, still dialling.

A moment later Richard came up to John's side window. 'The next exit's only about half a mile,' he shouted, over the wind and rain. 'Do you want to take the hard shoulder?'

'Yes,' John shouted back. 'Do you know the way from there?'

'More or less. Shall I lead?'

John gave him the thumbs up, then closed the window as Richard ran back to his car.

'Still the machine,' Avril said angrily. Then, as Richard

430

passed in the BMW, and John pulled on to the hard shoulder behind him, she said, 'Have you got a map?'

'On the back seat.'

'I still don't trust him,' she stated, leaning over to get it. 'He might try to lose us, so we'll need to know where we are.'

'Your attitude's not helping,' John told her sharply. 'He's stayed with us this far, now let's just concentrate on getting there, shall we?'

Suitably chastened Avril fumbled around for the map-light, then attempted to locate where they were. She'd never heard John use that tone before, so he was obviously even more uptight than she'd realized, and knowing there was a good chance they were on a wild goose chase anyway, since Carla wasn't answering either of her phones, wasn't helping to calm anyone's nerves.

'Try Sonya again,' he suddenly barked, as they followed Richard onto a roundabout at a dangerously high speed.

Avril did, but there was no response from her either.

'Where the hell is everyone?' she shouted, then almost screamed, as a car suddenly pulled out of a side road right in front of them. John yanked hard on the wheel, swerving the Range Rover across the road, bumping the offside wheels up on to the opposite bank, narrowly missing a tree, then braking hard as they hit the road again, taking them into a short, semicircular skid.

'Are you OK?' he asked, obviously shaken himself, as he righted the car, and started to drive on.

'Yeah,' she gasped, still holding the dash. 'Are you?'

'I'd feel a hell of a lot better,' he answered, 'if we didn't appear to have lost Richard.'

Carla was staring wide-eyed at the shed door. She hadn't heard anything except her own heartbeat and the storm for several minutes, though she still didn't dare to move. The cold and damp were seeping deep into her bones, as was the fear. Seconds ago something had scurried across her foot, making her gasp, and now the dank, earthen stench of wet wood and rusting metal seemed to be stealing the air. There had been no sound of Fellowes moving away, nor of anything else beyond the rain drumming the pitch roof like nails, and the thunder rumbling darkly through the sky like an omen. It was a nightmare, please God, it had to be, because if it wasn't then the reason she was here, freezing and shivering in terror, had to be real, and if it was real she didn't know what the hell to do.

Feeling more tears scalding her cheeks, she carefully lifted a hand and pushed them away. If her suspicions were correct, if they really had killed her mother . . . She almost choked on the horror, for it was so painful to think of her mother dying that way . . . Dread seared through her chest, and she was about to take a breath to steady herself when her whole body stiffened at the sound of someone calling her name.

'Carla!'

Instinctively she drew back into the shadows. Over her shoulder was a small, rectangular window, but through it she saw only silvery spikes of rain, rushing through the moonlit darkness.

'Carla, hiding like this isn't going to help.' It was Graham, and he was right outside the door.

Despite the thudding fear in her heart, she tried to breathe more slowly, but her chest was so tight the air could barely get through.

'Carla. Don't make them hurt Eddie,' Graham pleaded.

Carla's eyes widened, as terror punched a hole in her fear. Eddie! How could she have forgotten her precious Eddie?

'I know how much he means to you,' Graham called.

Carla's eyes were wild as her head spun with confusion. How was this happening? How had he turned into this monster?

'Please,' Graham coaxed. 'We both know you don't want anything to happen to Eddie.'

Panic flared in her head. They were threatening Eddie! Dear God, they were going to hurt her dog. How could she let them do that? Poor, defenceless Eddie, who thought he was with people who loved him. An image of his little face flashed in her mind, his big brown eyes clouded with confusion, as someone started bashing in his head . . .

Suddenly her hand was on the key, turning it, and the wind swung the door wide.

'If you dare to hurt Eddie, I swear *I'll kill you*,' she seethed into Graham's face.

'Please, come inside,' he said, trying to take her arm.

Snatching it away, she ran over to the back door. 'Eddie!' she called. 'Eddie! Come here!'

She heard him whine, then saw him in the hall, being held on his lead by Barry Fellowes.

'Let him go!' she screamed. 'Let him go *now*!'

'It's OK,' Graham said, coming up behind her. 'No-one's going to hurt him. It was the only way to make you come inside and listen.'

'Then let him come to me *now*,' she raged, rain streaming down her face with the tears. If she could get hold of him, and somehow bypass Graham . . .

'He'll stay right where you can see him,' Graham assured her, 'but for the moment, we'll let Barry hold him. Now please, let's go inside.'

Feeling sure she shouldn't do it, she stepped in through the door, and beckoned to Eddie again. Though he tried to come, he couldn't, and as Graham closed the door she rounded on him in fury. 'Let him go!' she snarled. 'If you want me to listen then you have to let him go.'

Graham's eyes flickered over to Fellowes, then, with a sorrowful shake of his head, he said, 'I promise, no-one's going to hurt him, but if you're afraid, which you obviously are, we don't want him attacking us. Now, come along into the warm. Betty's gone. It's just us . . .'

'Why's Betty gone?' she cried.

'Because of the dog,' he reminded her.

She was shaking her head. 'I'm staying here,' she said, edging back towards the door. 'I'm not going into the sitting room, and I'm not listening to a word you say until you *let my dog go*.'

Again Graham looked at Fellowes, then, sighing, he turned back to Carla. 'No-one killed your mother,' he said. 'She died, just as you've always believed, by falling and hitting her head on a rock. The fact that it happened so soon after Betty told her our secret, combined with the fact that it bore such a similarity to the way we had disposed of the drunk, was nothing more than an unfortunate, though of course tragic, coincidence. That was why we had to do everything we could to find the letter, because it stood to reason that anyone who read it would think exactly as you're thinking now, and though an investigation would probably have cleared us of suspicion in the case of her death, we certainly can't be cleared in the other case.'

Carla's eyes were staring at him hard, hair plastered to her face, water dripping from her clothes, but though her heart was still racing, and her body trembling, she felt slightly less panicked now as she struggled with whether or not to believe him.

'So you see, we don't mean you any harm,' Graham said. 'We only want the letter.'

Carla glanced at Fellowes, then took another step back towards the door. 'I don't know where it is,' she told them. 'I've never seen it, except for that one page.'

Graham's head went down. 'It has to be somewhere,' he said, stroking his beard.

'But even if I had it,' she shouted rashly, 'you can't expect me to be a part of the cover-up, any more than my mother could. So it seems that you don't have any choice but to kill me too.'

Graham lifted his head, but before he could speak Eddie began such a frenzy of barking that it was impossible to hear anything else. Graham turned to look at him, while Fellowes struggled to hold him. Graham shouted something. Fellowes grabbed Eddie's throat. Carla screamed for him to stop. Then suddenly the door burst open and Betty stepped into the room, a gun clenched tightly in her hand.

John's Range Rover was speeding through the country lanes, keeping hard on Richard's tail, now they'd finally caught up with him. The rain was still pounding the windscreen, making visibility dangerously poor, and occasionally the wind slammed so hard into the side of them that the vehicle rocked on its chassis. They were little more than three miles from the village now, but with no answer yet on the phone they still had no way of knowing if their urgency was called for, or futile – or even if Carla was there. However, the fact that her phones had gone unanswered for so long was alarming them greatly, since none of them could come up with any logical explanation.

Avril had stopped calling Richard on his mobile now. The lanes were too dark and winding for him to do anything but keep the car on the road. She'd tried Sonya several times more, but there was still no answer there, so Avril had started hoping that Sonya and Carla were somewhere together, and preferably somewhere safe. But that hope was dashed when her mobile suddenly rang and Sonya's voice exploded down the line.

'Avril! Thank God! I went to the station, but she wasn't there. Then Courtenay fell down the . . .' The line suddenly broke up, swallowing the next few words, until she said, '. . . take him to hospital. I haven't had a chance to call till now.'

'So you don't know where Carla is?'

'No. She's not answering her phone.'

'I know that.'

'Nor's Graham. Oh God, do you think I should call the pub and get someone to go over there?'

Avril's eyes rounded. 'Yes!' she cried. 'Do it now!' Then, clicking off, she said to John, 'Why didn't we think of that? To call the pub.'

His eyes remained concentrated on the road ahead.

It was debatable who heard the sirens first, him or Richard, for they seemed to slow in unison, and as the blue flashing lights came speeding up behind them they both pulled in to the side of the road.

'Shit!' John muttered, 'this is just what we need.' Then his eyes widened as first one, then another police car went roaring past, heading straight for the village.

'Oh my God,' he murmured.

'It might not mean anything,' Avril declared.

In front of them Richard's car was stuck in a ditch, wheels spinning, mud flying. Immediately John pulled the Range Rover alongside him. 'Get in!' he shouted.

Richard glanced over, then gave his car one last rev, which was all it needed to get it back on the road, and seconds later they were all once again speeding towards the village.

Betty's eyes moved from Graham to Fellowes and back again. The gun trembled in her grasp, her face was bloodless and scared. Outside the wind continued to howl. Rain splashed in through the open door.

435

Long seconds ticked by. Carla stood rigidly where she was, too terrified to move. The gun was no longer pointing at her, but there was still no knowing what Betty intended to do.

'Betty,' Fellowes said.

Betty glanced at him, but kept the gun trained on Graham. Carla could see how hard she was breathing.

'It's got to stop,' Betty said harshly. 'Do you hear me? It has to stop. One person dead is enough.'

Graham's face was strained, though his voice was steady as he said, 'But Betty, you're the one holding the gun.'

'It's wrong,' she snapped. 'What you do. What you made Barry do. The way you try to control people's lives.'

'Betty, just put the gun down,' Fellowes said.

Betty was still looking at Graham. 'All this time, what you've been doing to Carla . . . The way you've listened to her through the walls of this house, the things you got her to do . . . You're a wicked man, Graham.'

A horrible heat passed through Carla's head. She didn't want Betty to go on. She didn't want it confirmed that sexual gratification had been a part of Graham's plan. It was better not to know.

'I care deeply for Carla,' Graham said gruffly. 'You know that, Betty. I was trying to help her . . .'

'I know what you were doing,' Betty interrupted, 'and it's obscene . . .'

'Stop!' Carla cried. 'Please, just stop!'

Betty glanced at her.

Carla suddenly saw red. 'Put the gun down,' she shouted. 'Just stop this and put the gun down.'

Graham started to move forward.

Betty swung round and Eddie growled. In an attempt to avoid Graham, Betty stepped back hard into Carla. Carla gasped. Then suddenly Eddie was rushing forward.

'Stop him!' Betty yelled.

'Eddie!' Carla shouted. 'No! Stay!'

Eddie stopped. The gun was pointing straight at his head. Without thinking Carla grabbed it, and shoved Betty hard into the Aga. 'Eddie stay!' she shouted again, then the breath left her body as Fellowes grabbed her, trying to wrest the gun from her grasp.

Immediately Eddie pounced, clamping his jaws round Fellowes's arm.

Fellowes kicked him hard in the gut. Eddie yelped. Then Fellowes grunted in pain as Carla kneed his groin with all her might.

She was still holding the gun. Her eyes were wild, her breath short and erratic. She'd never held a gun before. She didn't know what to do. *For God's sake, what was she going to do?* 'Eddie! Go outside!' she shouted.

Graham looked at her beseechingly. 'Carla, no-one's going to hurt you, or Eddie,' he said, edging towards her.

'Stay back!' she cried. 'Just stay back.'

Graham spread his arms, as though to show he meant no harm.

Carla looked at the open door, then back to Graham. Eddie was still at her side, but if she left he'd leave too. She just had to get past Betty. But Betty didn't mean to harm her . . . Except Betty was screaming . . .

Then another voice spoke from the darkness outside.

'Carla! Carla! Are you all right in there?'

Carla swung round as Maudie's anxious face peered in through the door. The old woman turned instantly white when she saw Carla with a gun. 'I saw the door open,' she said feebly, then gasped as Fellowes lunged for the gun, and in one deft movement grabbed Carla round the neck and jammed the weapon into the side of her head.

'Get out!' Fellowes snarled at Maudie. 'Just get the hell out and take that damned dog with you.'

'Eddie no!' Carla cried, as Eddie pounced on Fellowes's ankle. 'Maudie, please, get him out of here,' she implored.

But Maudie could only gape in horror at the way Eddie was tearing at Fellowes's trouser leg.

Furious, Fellowes lowered the gun, ready to shoot.

Carla jerked back with all her strength, screaming, 'Eddie! Stop!'

'I called the police!' Maudie suddenly shouted. '*I called the police!*'

Fellowes turned the gun towards her.

'No!' Betty screamed, and slammed a pan into his outstretched arm.

He howled with pain, and, breaking free, Carla dived for the gun as it hit the floor. Somewhere, amongst all the madness, she registered the sound of police sirens. Snatching up the gun, she backed around the table and pressed up against the sink. She was looking at Graham with wide, panicked eyes and a reeling brain. Then she looked at Fellowes, who was nursing his shattered arm, and Betty, who seemed as agitated as Maudie. 'Get out!' she shouted. 'All of you. Just get out.'

No-one moved.

Then Graham stepped forward. 'Carla,' he began.

'*Get out!*' she screamed.

'It's the police, they're here,' Maudie blurted, as someone banged violently on the front door. And seconds later, with no warning whatsoever, two policemen forced their way in past Maudie through the back door.

Minutes later the kitchen was so full of people that Carla could hardly move. The gun had been taken from her, and four policemen, all in uniforms and luminous jackets, were attempting to take charge. Maudie was still there, and so, for some reason, were Fleur and Perry Linus. No-one seemed to have any real idea of who to speak to first. Two policewomen came in, walkie-talkies squawking, as one headed towards Betty and the other to Maudie. The trauma was still so recent that it was hard for Carla to register what was happening. Then she saw Graham, watching it all, absorbing every detail of the participants' behaviour. His manner sickened her, and made her angry, but she was too numb to speak. She looked at Betty, who was sitting at the table, her face buried in her hands, while Fellowes attempted to explain what they were doing there. For a long time it seemed as though everyone was talking at once, until in the end one of the officers shouted for silence, then announced that he was taking everyone to the station.

As they all began moving out Carla stood up against the dresser, Eddie pressed in close to her side. The mayhem seemed to go on and on, looming in and out of focus, as she struggled to fight back the nausea. Then suddenly a new shock rendered her almost senseless.

'Richard?' she whispered, as he shoved his way past a policewoman and came into the kitchen.

438

'Are you OK?' he asked, moving swiftly towards her, his face taut with concern.

She looked at him, too stunned to answer, and did nothing as he gathered her into his arms and held her tight, the way he always used to. For a moment she wondered if the past two years had all been a dream. Maybe she was going to wake up any minute and find that none of this had happened. There were no police in her kitchen, Graham hadn't become a monster, Richard had never betrayed her, and her mother was still alive. Then a policeman shouted to the crowd outside to go home, and, coming to her senses, she pulled away.

'It's all right,' she gasped. 'I'm OK.' But she wasn't, for the shock of him turning up like this, on tonight of all nights, when she was still so confused about what was truth and what was lies, and shaken by the fact that she'd held a gun in her hands, not to mention that she'd been terrorized and stalked by a man she'd almost considered a father, and still didn't know whether her mother had been murdered, or had died in an accident . . . Her eyes closed as the staggering weight of too many emotions threatened to engulf her. Then Avril was beside her, hugging her hard. 'What the heck has been going on?' Avril demanded.

'Don't ask,' Carla answered, too dazed to feel any more surprise. Lifting her head she saw John standing in the doorway, watching her. She moved towards him, her heart suddenly so full that tears were welling in her eyes as he drew her into his arms.

He was still holding her when, moments later, a police officer said, 'You need to come with us too, Miss.' He looked down at Eddie and wearily shook his head. 'And there was us thinking the worst we had to deal with tonight was a couple of trees down over on the Trowbridge road.'

Eddie sat to attention, and gave a few nervous wags with the tip of his tail. Overcome by a wave of love, Carla stooped to put her arms around him and kissed him on the head. Then to John she said, 'I can't leave him here on his own, not after all he's just been through. Will you stay with him?'

John smiled. 'I'm coming with you,' he told her. 'But we'll take him with us.'

'If there's someone who can take care of him,' the policeman said, 'it'll be better not to bring him along.'

Knowing there would be any number of volunteers outside, Carla dug Eddie out a few biscuits, then Avril took over, while she ran upstairs to change into dry clothes. Only then did she really start to wonder how on earth Richard, John and Avril had happened to arrive when they did – and apparently together. But that particular mystery would have to wait, because she was just too bemused and exhausted to go into it now, and besides she was going to need every ounce of what little energy she had left to get through the next few hours of police interrogation.

It was nearing midnight by the time Carla and Avril finally came out of the police station, to find the storm only marginally less belligerent, and the moon still smothered in cloud. John and Richard were behind them, though Maudie, Fleur and Perry had left a while ago. It seemed that Fleur and Perry, with their alien search technology, had managed to tune in to the equipment Graham had installed in Gilbert's cottage, and having heard what was going on at Carla's had called the police only minutes before Maudie had spotted the back door open, and made a call herself. Apparently it was common practice for Fleur and Perry to make recordings of all their contacts, so most of what had occurred at Carla's was on a tape that was now in police hands. If any privacy laws had been violated, then it seemed the Avon and Somerset Constabulary was turning a blind eye, since they had the far more serious matter of a fifteen-year-old murder to deal with. A murder, as it turned out, that they were already aware of, for they'd long ago been contacted by the Yorkshire police, informing them of their suspicions regarding Graham Foster and the two members of his household staff. It was thanks to this warning that Valerie Craig's untimely, and similar death had been investigated much more thoroughly when it had happened than her family knew. So the coroner's verdict of accidental death had been reached with all the forensic, medical and circumstantial evidence necessary to clear it of murder.

'I can't tell you what a relief that is,' Carla said to Avril, as they stopped at John's car. 'To think of her being murdered ... I don't think I could bear it, and then having to go through the investigation ...' She shivered, and turned to John and Richard as they joined them. Still stunned by the fact that Richard was there, and not yet having had a chance to ask why, she slipped her hand into John's and took him to one side.

'Do you mind if I ride back with Richard?' she said. 'I'm not sure we really need to talk that much, but as he's here ...'

Tilting her chin up, he kissed her gently on the mouth, and said, 'I don't mind. But for God's sake, don't overdo it. You've been through a lot already tonight ...'

'I know.' Her eyes went off to one side, as the wind tore between them. 'I still can't get to grips with the fact it was Graham,' she said. 'All those emails ...' She laughed dryly. 'Boy do I feel a fool. I don't think even the police know if there's a crime in there somewhere, it's all so new and uncharted. Perhaps if he'd been impersonating Richard in order to extort money, or to conspire in a recognized crime ...'

The police hadn't questioned her about the sex, and she wasn't going to tell John about it either. It was simply too humiliating, and she just hoped to God that it wasn't more research for Graham's book, because if it ever got published ...

'Come on,' John said, giving her a quick hug. 'It's freezing out here, and I for one could do with a drink.'

A few minutes later Carla was sitting beside Richard in his BMW, watching John's tail lights through the rhythmic sweep of the wipers as they cleared the rain from the windscreen. Though Richard was explaining how he'd come to be there, she was only half-listening, for her thoughts kept wandering off in so many different directions, recalling disjointed scenarios from the past few months, as well as this evening, some that burned with a newfound clarity, and others that had no real significance at all. For a while her thoughts settled on the evening when she'd first told Graham about the single page she'd found in the thesis. She couldn't recall him showing even a moment's unease, or urgency, though he'd obviously known right away what it was. Probably she'd been too absorbed in herself to notice even if he had been alarmed, but then it was forgotten as she began wondering what had run over her foot in the shed tonight. Then she was thinking about Fleur and Perry's transit van buzzing around the countryside in search of spaceships, which soon yielded to the strangeness of Graham putting more coal on the fire tonight. Then she was thinking of Eddie on his lead being held by Barry Fellowes; the phone going unanswered; Rousseau's *Philosophical Dictionary*; the fact that Richard hadn't turned down her mother's request to be there when she disclosed his betrayal to Carla, because the letter, which she now knew Sonya had the rest of, hadn't been about that. Then she was reliving the questions the police had asked tonight, which led her back to times she'd spent with Graham, discussing possible meanings for the emails.

Richard was still talking, so she tried again to listen, but soon she was noticing the familiar comfort of his car, with its smell of leather and smoothness of speed. It was virtually indistinguishable from all the other BMWs he'd owned, except for the baby-seat strapped into the back. She wondered if she should ask about the baby, or Chrissie, but she didn't want to, so she only looked at him as he stopped speaking, and found herself thinking that perhaps, in his perverse and exploitative way, Graham really had done her a favour, for she felt peculiarly removed from Richard now, as though Graham's deception, and her own self-delusion, had become entangled with the memories that were real, making them feel strangely false too.

'So you really thought all those emails were from me?' Richard said, sounding both amused and surprised.

She turned to look out of the window.

'I'm sorry they weren't,' he said, in a conciliatory tone.

'Don't be.' She stared out at the passing darkness, focusing neither on her own ghostly reflection, nor on the anger she could feel building inside. Instead she thought of the many times she'd shared her feelings with Graham, telling him everything he already knew. There were so many instances, all rushing to be remembered, but galling as they were, none were as hard to face as her belief in the connection of her and Richard's souls that had enabled them to understand and read each other in a way that was existentially profound, and karmically bestowed. How grand and privileged she'd felt in the might of that love and fated power of its journey. How pompously and completely she had considered them to be special and tragic and above mere worldly affairs. And all the time she'd been thinking that way he'd been loving someone else, knowing and feeling nothing of the allure or attachment she had believed in so utterly, and had clung to so desperately.

'Why?' she suddenly said. 'Why are you sorry the emails weren't from you?'

He glanced over at her. 'Because it seems to matter to you that they were,' he answered.

She turned away again. 'Once maybe,' she muttered. 'Not now.'

She heard him take a breath to respond, but there was a moment before he said, 'Good. I'm glad it doesn't matter now.'

More anger welled up inside her, but she was too tired to vent it with any more than the childish retort of, 'It doesn't.' She was going to thank God to her dying day that he'd never seen those emails – and she had to take steps now to make sure no-one ever did.

'So there's no confusion about your mother?' he said.

'Not about the way she died, no,' she replied. 'But I'm still wondering why you never got in touch when it happened. You'd known her all that time, she'd made you a part of our family . . . She really cared about you, and you didn't even bother to send a card to say you were sorry, or a flower to put on her grave.'

'I didn't think you'd welcome it,' he answered. 'But believe me, I felt her death very deeply.'

She waited for him to add, so did Chrissie, but he didn't, and maybe because of that small sensitivity her anger deflated. It was funny, she was thinking, she'd had so many questions to ask him, but now it was hard trying to remember which were relevant. Actually, not so hard, because really, in the end, everything boiled down to why. Why had he started an affair with Chrissie in the first place? Why hadn't he told her himself it was over? Why did he refuse to speak to her afterwards, when she'd so desperately needed the answers?

'I thought we were so close,' she told him. 'I never dreamt you were hiding so much.'

'If you're asking me to explain,' he responded, 'then I can only tell you this: I loved you then, and I love you now, but not in the same way I love Chrissie. When it happened between me and her, I knew right away we were different – special, I suppose – but we both cared so deeply about you that we could never find a way to tell you.'

She said nothing as she remembered how he'd once felt it was different for them, that they were special, and meant to be. It seemed he'd forgotten that now, though she suspected, if she reminded him, he'd insist it was true, but had just been on another level to the bond he shared with Chrissie. Then she recalled John's belief that it was possible to have more than one soulmate. Maybe he was right. She thought of Avril and inwardly smiled. It could be that John was one too. It certainly felt that way, though it was still so early in their relationship she guessed only time would tell.

She said, 'So you thought Chrissie getting pregnant would be a way to tell me?'

There was only a slight awkwardness to his tone as he said, 'Whether she got pregnant on purpose, or by mistake, I don't think even she knows for certain, but I would have married her anyway, just as soon as we'd found a way of breaking it to you.' He glanced over at her. 'Do you think you could have stood to hear me say any of this back then? God knows, it can't be pleasant now.'

He was right, and wrong, for it was a lot worse than simply unpleasant – and to have heard it back then would have just about killed her. 'How long were you seeing her, before she got pregnant?' she asked.

'Almost a year.'

Her heart folded around the words, for it was still hard to think of the betrayal without recalling the times she'd spent with them both, totally believing in Richard's love, and never dreaming that all he wanted was to be with Chrissie. Then suddenly, out of nowhere, came a terrible yearning for none of it ever to have happened, for them to be driving along now, as they had so often in the past, totally relaxed in the strength of their love, complete in their sense of togetherness. But the feeling passed, and though she knew he still had the ability to hurt her deeply, she understood that it was mainly the unwillingness of old habits to die that was keeping her connected to him now.

'I don't expect you to care,' he said, 'but it's been a very difficult time for Chrissie. She hated hurting you so much that when she found out your mother was dead she begged me to go back to you.'

Carla didn't comment.

'The guilt has been hard on her too,' he continued. 'And since Ryan was born . . . She's come very close to breaking down altogether. She's still a long way from being over the worst of it.' He laughed, dryly. 'One of her greatest wishes is for us all to be friends, but in her heart she knows it can't happen. Apart from anything else, she doesn't trust me. I betrayed you, so I could betray her too. She doesn't understand that she's different.'

Carla thought of the three women Rosa had mentioned, but only asked about one. 'Does she know about the air stewardess?'

The lengthy pause before he answered told her it was true, though she thought he was going to lie, until he said, 'No. She doesn't. Kate's married too. We have an arrangement that in no way interferes with the rest of our lives.'

'I wonder if Chrissie would see it like that?' Carla responded.

'Of course she wouldn't. But it doesn't change for a moment the way I feel about her. I love her in a way I've never loved another woman.'

Carla was silent then, as she waited for the ache inside her to die away. She thought of John and Avril, and what they might be talking about now. Nothing so difficult, she imagined. Then looking up ahead she saw they were approaching the pub where Eddie was waiting, no doubt with all her neighbours, who must be agog with all that had happened. Before they got out of the car she said, 'I'm sorry it's been so hard for Chrissie, but I wouldn't have been a few weeks ago. And as for us ever being friends . . . Does she know you're here now?'

'Yes.'

445

'Then tell her, if it can happen, and I really don't think it can, then it'll be because of her, never because of you.'

Very soon they were perched on stools in front of the bar, listening to Fleur and Perry as they continued filling everyone in on their part in the drama. Carla, with Eddie at her feet, was tense with the fear that they'd reveal the sexual part of it all, but no mention was made, and she could only thank God for their discretion – or better still, their ignorance, for there was a strong chance that nothing had actually been put into words. After a while she tried to eat the shepherd's pie Sylvia had prepared for their return, though, on the whole, she only managed to look around at them all in the cosy firelight, and feel very tired, but safe, and relieved to be there.

'So what's going to happen to Graham now?' Sylvia wanted to know, plonking free drinks down in front of John and Richard. Carla and Avril already had theirs, but Carla wasn't making much headway with that either.

Everyone looked at Angie and Pete, Cannock's resident lawyers. 'There's rarely ever any bail set for murder,' Pete answered.

'Murder,' Beanie repeated wonderingly, as though this was the first time she'd ever uttered the word aloud. 'It hardly bears thinking about, does it? I mean, you'd never have thought, would you, him being such a gentle-seeming soul.'

They were all silent for a moment then, as they confronted again the astonishing ingenuity of the deception that not one of them had ever even begun to suspect. To think that they'd known him, chatted with him, bought him drinks, respected him, never delving into Betty's shyness, just accepting it as one of those queer quirks some people had; never doubting the identity of Fellowes with his smart suits and detective-looking car . . . That they could all have been so taken in was, well, disconcerting to say the least.

'But he didn't do it, did he?' Joe Locke pointed out. 'It was that detective bloke what did it.'

'Yeah, but Graham put him up to it, so that makes him just as guilty, don't it, Pete?' Beanie said.

Pete nodded.

446

'What about Betty?' Gayle Locke asked. 'Did they arrest her too?'

'Oh yes,' Maudie answered, still flushed from all the excitement.

'I wonder what's going to happen to the Old Rectory?' Lloyd said.

'Be a bit spooky to live there now, wouldn't it?' Sylvia shivered. 'They've got it all cordoned off up there, did you see?'

'Why would it be spooky?' her husband demanded. 'They didn't kill anyone there, did they? It happened in Yorkshire.'

'Maybe you'll all take notice of me next time I tell you there's squatters,' Maudie said, waspishly.

'They was hardly squatters, was they?' Jack retorted. 'And you was the one who got Jekyll checking up on Hyde, so to speak, when you got that Fellowes bloke to look over old Gilbert's house, so you don't have that much to crow about.'

Sylvia dug an elbow in his ribs as Maudie bristled, and the others stifled a laugh.

'So who was it they offed then?' Lloyd wanted to know.

'We already told you,' Perry responded. 'A drunk, up in Barnsley. Don't know his name, but I expect the poor bloke's got one. Or he did have, when he was alive.'

For some reason everyone turned to Carla, as though she might know the man's name, but at that moment she was looking at John, who seemed to be looking at her rather strangely, and then she realized how close she was sitting to Richard. Was that what was bothering him? It wasn't where she wanted to be, but when she tried to get up Richard put an arm around her, and pulled her against him. Then everyone was talking again, asking questions, making comments, spouting wisdom, though all she could hear was the voice inside her head telling her to move away from Richard. She didn't understand why she couldn't. Then John got up, and seeming not to see her, began shaking everyone's hands and, bidding them goodnight. The voice inside her was still urging her to go to him, yet the strange stupor she was in wouldn't allow it. Richard's arm felt burdensome and wrong, but when she turned her head to tell him no words came out. It was as

447

though she was halfway in a faint, unable to pull herself out of it, or to plunge entirely into it.

Then she heard John say, 'Come on, let's go.'

Taking his hand, she was about to get up when Richard said, 'Are you all right?'

Turning to him, she said, 'I think so, but I'll be glad when it's all in the past.'

He smiled as he said, 'You will get over us, you know. Everything takes time, I'm just sorry you were taken in by those emails. It can't have helped, but I'd like to see them sometime.'

Carla stiffened, as John's hand tightened on hers, and Avril gestured for her to go no further. Now wasn't the time, but the look in Avril's eyes promised that it would certainly come, and Avril would make sure it was soon. For the moment, however, all Avril said was, 'Richard, darling, I'm sure Chrissie must be wondering what on earth has happened to you by now, and as I'm in need of a lift back to London . . .'

It was in the early dawn light that Carla slipped quietly out of John's arms, tugged on a tracksuit and went downstairs to stoke up the Aga. She'd slept heavily in the aftermath of all that had happened, but now she was awake she knew it wouldn't be possible to go back, so not wanting to disturb John she decided to take Eddie for a walk.

As they strolled away from the village, watching the ash grey sky starting to glow red on the horizon, she was thinking of her mother and how she'd turned to Richard for help when she'd learned the truth about Graham. Knowing how attached Carla was to Graham, and what strength she and Richard drew from each other, it seemed her mother had wanted Richard to be there when she broke the awful news. How ironic that Richard was planning to break some awful news of his own at the very same time, and Carla guessed she could only feel thankful that her mother had never known about that.

She still wasn't clear as to why Betty had told either of them the truth about Graham, though it had been such a terrible burden to carry all these years that sharing it, and then having someone else take the responsibility of revealing it, was possibly at least a part of her motive. Or maybe it was all much more sinister than that, part of some diabolical master plan that even now was being stored up in Graham's mind, making him half-delirious with the thrill of what he could and couldn't control, for the sake of his art.

Not wanting to go any further with that, she turned her thoughts to John and smiled warmly as she wondered what her mother would think of him, and his fame, and his relationship with her daughter. No doubt she'd love him, though, like many others, she might be in awe of his looks for a while. But his easy-going charm would soon have her drawing him into their family the way she had with all her children's friends and lovers. Only Greg's wife had ever resisted, which was a shame, but it hadn't been in Valerie's nature to force anyone against their will.

Carla's mind returned again to the letter her mother had written to Richard. She guessed it would always be a mystery how that one page had come to be caught up in the thesis, while the rest of it was in her coat pocket. Though there seemed to have been some kind of plan, divine or otherwise, for it was quite remarkable how everything had played its part in bringing Graham's crime to light. How appalled, and no doubt fascinated, he must have been when Valerie died such a similar death to the murder he'd paid Fellowes to commit, and what ghastly serendipity had played itself out since, from the discovery of that single page in the thesis, to Fleur and Perry's quirky search for aliens, right down to poor little Courtenay falling down the steps at Bath railway station and ending up at the hospital with six stitches in his head. If that hadn't happened then Sonya might well have got to Carla before Betty had last night, and though the letter might well have been evidence enough to condemn Graham and Fellowes, Carla might never have got to find out as much as she had, about the emails, the purpose behind them, or the warped kind of caring that, the sexual part of it aside, she couldn't fully deny had helped.

After walking for half an hour or more she returned to the cottage, gave Eddie an early breakfast, then took off her tracksuit and slipped back into bed. John was still sleeping, so she snuggled in behind him and was just wondering about Avril, and what she and Richard might have talked about on their way back to London, when, in that strange linking up of minds that sometimes happened, the phone beside the bed suddenly rang.

Reaching out for it, John lifted the receiver and brought it to his ear.

'Carla?' said the voice at the other end.

'I'll pass you over,' he answered. 'Avril,' he said to Carla.

Carla took the phone, then settled into his arms as he turned onto his back to hold her. 'Hi,' she said. 'I was just thinking about you. Are you all right? It's not even seven o'clock yet.'

'I know,' Avril answered. 'But I need your advice.'

Carla frowned. 'On what?'

'Well,' Avril said, 'remember you told me how Richard's thing was being tied to the bed?'

Carla was already starting to smile, and turning the receiver so John could hear too, she said, 'Yes.'

'You know, it's strange,' Avril said, 'but Richard and I got awfully tired on the way back to London last night, so we stopped at this hotel, and it just so happened that he was carrying some rope, and now, of all the blessed things to happen, he's still at the hotel tied to the bed, and I'm in a taxi on my way back to London. With his clothes.'

Carla and John were already laughing.

'So what I want to know,' Avril said, 'is who I should call to set him free? The hotel manager, or the *News of the World*?'

Carla's eyes were full of mischief as she looked at John and debated the issue. She could see how intrigued he was to hear her answer, but though she'd have loved to have chosen the *News of the World*, in the end she took enough pity on Chrissie to say, 'Why don't you call Gus, and let him do the honours?'

'Now why didn't I think of that?' Avril responded, clearly very impressed with the answer. 'But it wouldn't be fair to wake him up at this hour, would it?'

'Absolutely not,' Carla agreed. 'Call him around nine. And when he introduces himself to Richard I don't think he need go to the trouble of explaining that there's no film in his camera, do you?'

'No. Too much detail,' Avril replied. 'And clothes? Maybe I should bike the ones I have here round to Gus?'

'Mmm. But I think it would be a nice gesture on your part to send one of your warm dressing gowns round too. Gus can give him that first, then produce his own clothes when they get back to London, before he has to face Chrissie.'

'Yes. Yes, that works.'

'Oh! And just for that one shot,' Carla added, 'you know, in the dressing gown, do you think Gus might have a film in his camera?'

'Oh, I'm sure he would,' Avril assured her. 'Just for that one shot. It'll be a kind of keepsake?'

'Exactly.'

'OK,' Avril said. 'Love to John. Speak to you later,' and she rang off.

Though John was laughing, he was all but writhing in Richard's embarrassment as Carla dropped the receiver back in place, then rested her arms on his chest.

'So,' she said, trying not to laugh herself, 'let that be a lesson to you, John Rossmore – never get tied up with Avril.'